RADIO DREAMS

DANCING FEET
SONGS & BOOKS

A DUET MEMOIR

RADIO DREAMS

THE STORY OF AN OUTLAW DJ AND A COSMIC COWGIRL

JOE GRACEY ★ KIMMIE RHODES

Special thanks to The Buddy Holly Education Foundation for their sponsorship and to all my friends, fans, and family for your support. This labor of love would not have been possible without your help.

Published and distributed by
Dancing Feet Publishing (Gracey-Rhodes, Inc.)
PO Box 342032, Austin, Texas 78669, USA

To contact Dancing Feet Publishing or for information on related audio and video documentaries, blog posts, events and exhibits, and recorded music projects, including *Radio Dreams Audio Documentary and Retrospective*, please visit:
www.radiodreamsbook.com | www.dancingfeetpublishing.com
or e-mail: info@dancingfeetpublishing.com | radio-dreams@kimmierhodes.com

Cataloging-in-publication data is available from the Library of Congress.

ISBN 978-0-9990-6990-5 (cloth : alk. paper)
ISBN 978-0-9990-6991-2 (pbk. : alk. paper)
ISBN 978-0-9990-6992-9 (library e-book)

Consultation, Design, and Production
Lindsay Starr Communication & Book Design

Copyediting and Proofreading
R. G. Fuentes

FOR BLUE

RICH FROM THE JOURNEY

Kimmie Rhodes

We stood before the waving sea
And stared at vast infinity
And praised the life that brought us here
To take our ride upon this sphere
For when we reach the distant shore I know we'll be returning
Rich from the journey . . .
Rich from the journey . . .

You never know what's up ahead
The tempest rolls and the skies are red
But off into the world that waits
Between tomorrow and today
To seek our fortunes and our fates
Driven by this yearning
To be rich from the journey . . .
Rich from the journey . . .

And when it's time to leave the harbor of this dream
We'll have a heart that's filled with memories

So, sail away sweet soul in peace
Hoist your sails into the breeze
Beneath these stars so hard to read
God speed the winds that carry me
And tell my friends to look for me
For soon I'll be returning
Rich from the journey . . .
Rich from the journey . . .

CONTENTS

FOREWORD

THIS IS THE STORY of two great people—Kimmie Rhodes and the late Joe Gracey—told through the lens of Kimmie's memory and Gracey's writings. It is a truly inspiring account of their love and strength together, withstanding challenges that would have defeated all but the most resilient of souls. They met in 1980, soon after Gracey had lost his voice to cancer, and were together until he passed away in November 2011. It is a poignant and beautifully woven patchwork of stories and memories of their upbringing and their lives together, intertwined with the culture of Texas—the food, the radio, and the birth and history of the vibrant Austin music scene, from rock 'n' roll through outlaw country to *Austin City Limits.*

I am proud to be working with Kimmie on an audio companion to this book, for which I have been exploring the archive she has compiled over the years. It is a treasure trove of tapes, cassettes, records and notes, Joe Gracey air checks, vintage broadcasts, phone messages from Willie Nelson and Beth Nielsen Chapman, and interviews with such musicians as Joe Ely, Delbert McClinton, and Rodney Crowell. These days, Kimmie is still writing, playing, and performing as she always has done, while also pouring her passion and instinctive knowledge into major film documentaries and projects for the Country Music Hall of Fame. And she continues to be inspired by Joe Gracey's legacy. I feel blessed to know Kimmie, her son Gabe, and her daughter, Jole. They enrich our lives.

BOB HARRIS, OBE, BBC Radio 2, author of
Still Whispering After All These Years

—★—

Dear Kimmie, I would like to personally thank you for the wonderful support you provide to the Buddy Holly Educational Foundation, which I cofounded with Peter Bradley Sr., to help fulfill the "dreams and wishes" that Buddy shared with me. We truly appreciate your great artistic contributions to the very important and successful Chris Difford songwriting retreats in the UK, which TBHEF sponsors. These fantastically creative events, at which established singer-songwriters help educate and cowrite with aspiring new young talent, is very special to me, as it is exactly what Buddy would have wished for his music legacy. I am delighted to endorse your excellent book, as you are a highly respected and much-loved artist-songwriter hailing from Buddy's birthplace, Lubbock, Texas. Also, it gives me great pleasure that you have received one of our unique guitars, titled "Lonesome Tears," and have joined our close-knit family as an ambassador of TBHEF. I hope your instrument brings you much pleasure and that the spirit of Buddy's music legacy inspires you to write more wonderful songs. Good luck in all of your future music endeavors.

MARIA ELENA HOLLY, cofounder of The Buddy Holly Educational Foundation

— ★ —

Kimmie Rhodes is a favorite singer of mine. Her *West Texas Heaven* album should be handed out to every aspiring vocalist, to offer lessons in tone, taste, and phrasing. When she wasn't out there singing, she was completing *Radio Dreams*, a book that reveals an extraordinary love story, accompanied by a soundtrack filled with great Texas music.

PETER COOPER, museum editor, Country Music Hall of Fame and Museum, author of *Johnny's Cash and Charley's Pride*

— ★ —

I believe that *Radio Dreams* is really a cultural touchstone that poetically weaves together the humorous, heartfelt, and heart-wrenching stories of two "Super Roper" soul mates set against the eclectic backdrop of Austin's "cosmic" music scene. No doubt that "Willie, Waylon, and the boys" are proud of their "Outlaw Sweetheart," Kimmie Rhodes, for her courage in pouring her heart onto these pages as only a true artist can.

ERIC GEADELMANN, filmmaker, co-curator Country Music Hall of Fame and Museum *Outlaws and Armadillos* exhibit, author of *They Called Us Outlaws*

Smart and a smart-ass both, Gracey was a pillar of a burgeoning music community on the verge of being discovered nationally and internationally. He welcomed music fans to some of the most exciting and eclectic music being created as one of the voices who did radio commercials for the storied Armadillo World Headquarters. It was Ol' Blue Eyes, as he called himself, who coolly and casually opened his microphone so Willie Nelson and his friend Kris Kristofferson could perform an impromptu concert for listeners at home. Gracey not only played Ernest Tubb and his Texas Troubadours; he also took the time to explain ET's significance and line out Tubb's hip bona fides for a generation that had previously ignored their parents' and grandparents' music.

He turned on music lovers to exotic sounds in their own backyard, such as Tex-Mex conjunto music as articulated by his friends Doug Sahm, Ry Cooder, and Flaco Jimenez, and western swing, the almost-forgotten Made-in-Texas country-jazz hybrid popularized in the 1930s, kick-starting its revival by putting Asleep at the Wheel and Alvin Crow into heavy rotation. Gracey played a critical role in defining Super Roper Radio, as KOKE was known, demonstrating how the Rolling Stones and Gram Parsons were related to George Jones, Bob Wills, and the Texas Playboys. In that respect, he was as influential as Willie Nelson, Austin's musical godfather, in bringing the hippies and the rednecks together through the common love of music.

JOE NICK PATOSKI, Wittliff Collections at Texas State University, author of biographies of Stevie Ray Vaughan, Selena, Willie Nelson, and the Dallas Cowboys

Kimmie's visit and engagement with the students of my Women and Texas Music honors course has confirmed my belief that the lives and careers of individual artists are not only significant for what they tell us about their particular journey and contribution, but they also provide us with valuable insights into the broader human experience. These memoirs have much to offer us all.

DR. KEVIN MOONEY, Texas State University

—★—

Kimmie is some perfect hybrid of a songbird and poet and a hell of a lot of fun. I cherish her.

JASTON WILLIAMS, playwright, author of *Greater Tuna*

—★—

I felt a strong connection with Kimmie and Joe from the moment I first heard *West Texas Heaven*. There's a truth and a soulfulness in Kimmie's music that spoke to me from that point on and continues to speak to me today. Once our paths crossed in person, as Kimmie and Joe visited Ireland and came into my studio to talk and play; that friendship grew, leaving me with many sweet musical and personal memories that I treasure. I was honored to welcome the guys to the BBC studios on many occasions, and every time their travels took them here, I'd look forward to the music and the chat that we would share. Kimmie and Joe were a perfect musical pairing. They would lean on each other musically as they crafted their session tracks, and they always seemed cosmically intertwined. They just seemed to know what the other would do or say next. My sweetest memory came when my wife, Kerry, and I welcomed our first child into the world in 2006. Little Tara was brought into the world with the sound of Kimmie's song "Love and Happiness for You" in her ears. Thank you for the memories, the music, and love, Kimmie, and we hope to see you back in your second home of Ireland as soon as your wings can carry you.

RALPH MCLEAN, BBC Radio Ulster

—★—

Kimmie Rhodes and her husband, Gracey, were the perfect musical match. Gracey's musical, practical, and commercial mind got the very best out of Kimmie's poetic, insightful, artistic soul. They both wrote songs, but Kimmie wrote more of them. Gracey was the support, strength, and the rock that gave Kimmie the strength and security to perform, to tour, and to try new things. They traveled the world together and made a huge impression here in Europe. Ireland, one of the Celtic countries, which gifted the rudiments of country music to America, became a second home to them. Here they gained a loyal fan base that Kimmie and her son Gabriel still have. The stories they wrote in songs have many other stories behind them, and I know that's what we'll discover in this book, which became a labor of love for Kimmie after Gracey's untimely death. Their lives together and in music have been a great gift to all of us. I thank God for them daily.

BRIAN D'ARCY, CP, priest, journalist, BBC Radio Ulster, author of *A Little Bit of Healing*

An angel named Kimmie Rhodes Gracey was sent to me just when I needed one most. In 2012 I was diagnosed with a recurrence of tongue cancer and faced a dire uncertain future. Local doctors doubted my ability to speak following the recommended surgery. I quickly made plans to be treated at MD Anderson Cancer Center in Houston. Before those plans were secured, a friend sent Kimmie to me. Kimmie's husband, Joe Gracey, had been diagnosed and treated at MD Anderson starting in the late '70s for the same type of cancer that had recurred for me. The medical protocols at the time resulted in his losing his tongue and his speech. In spite of this disability, Joe went on to have a successful career, not only in music production but also in gourmet cooking, leading to his appointment as a columnist for *Saveur* magazine. His was a lively, robust life for thirty-five more years until he succumbed to a cancer in his early sixties. Kimmie, a highly talented and acclaimed singer-songwriter was sent to assure me that in spite of absent speech, I would live a full and extraordinary life, as had Joe. This disability had not slowed him at all but rather had opened opportunities for both of them to express their creativity in new directions. She was open and honest about the realities of this disease. No Pollyanna, she spoke frankly about the challenges and fears that they had faced. More importantly, she was overwhelmingly grateful for the thirty-five years that they had gained. She also acknowledged the hope they had experienced with the exceptional and skilled care they received in Houston.

This is just what I needed to hear. I was so touched by both the message and the messenger that I picked myself up and determined that I would not be cowed by this turn of events. Little did I know that this was the beginning of a friendship in which Kimmie and I were able to help the other through each of our own barriers and move full-face forward. It has been a blessing to have her friendship as I have worked my way to survivorship. Her kindness and sharing have helped me evaluate my own situation and given me the courage to move ahead. It was also gratefully the beginning of a deep relationship with MD Anderson Cancer Center. Ever thankful to them for saving my speech and my life, I was searching for ways to give back. Through the ensuing five years of care and recovery, I have been fortunate to speak for and contribute to publications for MD Anderson audiences. My particular story of fully regaining my speech has been helpful to many who look for hope in any way while facing cancer themselves or their loved ones. Many times Kimmie and I have worked together to promote early detection, securing second opinions, and broadcasting the tremendous attributes of MD Anderson. I am so thankful for her friendship; her openness and acceptance have helped me to honestly face issues presented by cancer and recovery. She has pushed me to be more public about my experience so that others in similar situations can experience the hope, gratitude, and sense of safety that are present for me now.

CORA "CORKY" HILLIARD, cancer survivor

Hittin' town in February of 1973 was a dream come true. Our first record came out when I was twenty-one years old; Austin was our first taste of success. I met this DJ on KOKE-FM named Joe Gracey. He also wrote a music column in the local paper, the *Austin American-Statesman.*

He was playin' our music so I went to meet him. He wanted to meet the young guy with the weird band name who sounded like Ernest Tubb!! He was the first radio guy who dug where we were comin' from. We became close friends. We shared a house on South 6th Street in 1976 or so. He was partying and DJing and I was on the road most of the time, so we were perfect roommates. I could go on and on. . . . Stories of crazy broadcasts from 6th Street at the Ritz and the wild-on-air shenanigans with Speedy Perez, Huey Meaux . . .

RAY BENSON, Asleep at the Wheel, recording artist, author of *Comin' Right at Ya*

—★—

Kimmie Rhodes is infectious. The story between Gracey and her is well worth the journey: a great love story at a time when music was turning toward a progressive future. Whether we were laughing, recording, or writing, joy was our experience with these two talented people. So glad Waylon and I were part of it.

JESSI COLTER, singer-songwriter, recording artist, author of *An Outlaw and a Lady*

—★—

Of all Joe's qualities—his deep knowledge of music, musicians, and of anything technical—what always stood out to me was his kindness and grace. I think often about the days I spent with him at *Austin City Limits*. His presence was always reassuring, always graceful. God certainly gave Joe Gracey the right name. In the pressure-packed environment of *Austin City Limits* tapings, Joe always made me feel like everything would be all right.

LYLE LOVETT, singer-songwriter, recording artist

—★—

What would life be without Joe Gracey and Kimmie Rhodes? A lot less artful, daring imaginative, compassionate, and fun. My treasured times with Joe in Ireland, lessons in life from his Magic Slate, and the angelic voice of Kimmie coming at you with that look in her eye that says, "I hope you know how real this song I'm singing is." And talk about good old "Hey, can I do a favor?" friendship, poured from a bottomless pitcher of love. What a precious gift they bring.

GARY NICHOLSON, singer-songwriter, recording artist

— ★ —

Kimmie makes me feel like jelly; she turns me inside out with her songs and her wit. She is inspiring to be around, and I would love nothing more than to write with her, to share in the wonderful light she shines as a writer.

CHRIS DIFFORD, singer-songwriter, recording artist

— ★ —

My experience with Kimmie from day one and throughout our lifetime of friendship has been that she is the epitome of someone who lives by the glass-half-full standard. When I was going through chemotherapy with treatment for stage two breast cancer in 2000, Kimmie came and stayed with me for several weeks. She refused to let me watch any news or any violence on television. She made me leek-and-potato soup around the clock and wonderfully overall created this Walt Disney kind of atmosphere within which I could brace myself against the hell of the treatments I was going through, making sure that I didn't have any more negativity in my life.

With all that life has dealt her, her attitude has been the gift to all of us. I have been a witness to Kimmie's incredible unfolding life following the death of Gracey, and I can't imagine the sense of responsibility she must feel to curate and direct his incredible story into the world. She was his voice for over thirty years, and now she's doing an amazing job of being the steward of his memory. In fact, you can't separate the story of Kimmie from the story of Gracey, nor would you want to, but her story continues with so much strength and resilience that is brought forward in the heart of this woman. I am proud to call her my friend. I expect amazing things to come after Kimmie has completed the placement of Gracey's legacy. I have been really lucky to be a part of both of their lives.

BETH NIELSEN CHAPMAN, singer-songwriter, recording artist

I was hooked on Kimmie sometime in 1992, I guess, the day I heard the line "cheap and square and strange," which she used to describe the place where she grew up, at least in that song. One, because it mirrored life in the little North Carolina town I grew up in, and two, because it changed—or more specifically her writing overall changed—the way I listened to songs. For an old-line '70s Nashville publisher and hillbilly song-plugger guy, I worked with a whole lot of commercially successful songwriters, and there is a pretty predictable formula to the way most of them put songs together.... It has to be if they want to get covers on major radio artists, not that there's anything wrong with that. I was privileged to work with every one of them!

Kimmie came along not knowing those rules or, like a lot of Texas songwriters, choosing to ignore them. She was just so fresh! So far from formulaic, calculated. Her writing is so much more literary. It hits me like Emmylou's work or Lucinda, Nanci Griffith, those guys. To me, her work, her music, is equal parts song, book, theater, and philosophy. Then you throw in Joe Gracey, bon vivant with a heart of gold, rapier wit, Austin radio's Galileo . . . who gave me one of the most memorable musical nights of my life in Austin, and you have an irresistible combination: Mike Nichols and Elaine May. (I know, I know, who the hell are they?!) Anyhow, Kimmie and Joe were two of the most unique humans I was ever blessed to meet. Thank you, "Baby Girl," for bringing me Austin songwriting, Joe Gracey, and your sweet spirit, gifts that will forever make me "richer" from the journey.

DAVID CONRAD, trustee, Country Music Foundation
Board of Directors

When I think of soulful and thoughtful songwriters, there is one name that always comes to mind: Kimmie Rhodes. I had the great fortune to work with Kimmie when I was the vice president of motion picture music for the publishing company that she was signed to, Rondor Music. She was quite often the first writer whom I turned to when there was an assignment to write a song that required a thoughtful lyric because I knew that whatever she would write would come straight from her heart.

I remember one particular assignment was to ask her to write an end title song for the remake of the Christmas classic, *Miracle on 34th Street*. I told her that I knew it was a tough assignment to write a Christmas song in the middle of the summer, but I knew that she would find a way to create something magical. About a week later, I received a FedEx package—a demo cassette of the song she had written called "Miracles on Christmas Day." I listened to the tape sung by an angel and immediately called her to ask how something so beautiful and so "seasonal" could come so quickly and from the heart of Texas. She told me that she rented the original film to watch it again, immediately went into her studio, and turned her air conditioner down as low as it would go. She created Christmas in August, and out flowed one of the most beautiful Christmas songs I had ever heard. Unfortunately, the song never made the final cut of the film, but the "Miracles" demo sung by my Christmas angel from Texas continues to be my go-to Christmas song every year.

DEREK ALPERT, president, Concern Foundation

—★—

This is a love story. Love of music, love of life, love of one another. In the early '50s, two of music's most unique people were created for the purpose of creating more. Joe Gracey and Kimmie Rhodes represent all that is good, crazy, and exhilarating about the world of words/tunes. The fact that they chanced upon one other is one of life's wonderful and unpredictable mysteries. Coming from absolutely different backgrounds and cultures, they melded into Austin music's most significant couple. Yet they remained individuals with their special talents overlapping in some respects, vastly diverse in others. Joe—all bustle and rock 'n' roll and soul and wild. Kimmie—so quiet and sweet and strong and focused. Yet they united within the most important realm of all—making beautiful music, channeling others' offerings, using unbridled energy to connect, and weaving humor and heart to get it all done. Both were strong-willed, thus continuing to leave a permanent mark on all that is good about the world of song. Both had an ear for a story, and both could magnify the simplest of tales into fables, mysteries, heartbreaks, romantic ballads, all the while remaining unpretentious, self-effacing, yet Texan proud.

On so many levels, they were the yin and yang of country, rock, outlaw, classical, soul, R&B, gospel, and the multiple other components that form the kaleidoscope of Texicana music. Each sang like birds, railed against injustice, fought for righteousness, and suffered fools not gladly. Yet each had a great deal of compassion in their hearts for others and all that ultimately matters in this brief adventure called life. And live they did: Joe, taking existing music and re-presenting it into a nationally recognized radio format that made the sum of the parts greater than the whole, and Kimmie taking her tumultuous childhood memories and molding them into a sound that Emmylou Harris describes as "the voice of a beautiful child coming from an old soul." Joe, writing in a prose somewhere between Ernest Hemingway and Dan Jenkins for the Austin newspaper, cooking magazines, rock 'n' roll periodicals, you name it. Kimmie, authoring hundreds of songs only partially revealed in recorded song yet adopted by musical greats such as Willie Nelson, Trisha Yearwood, Wynonna Judd, and multiple other significant collaborators.

But alas, time has its way, and time took its toll on Joe. I loved Joe like only a little brother can. He was my hero, mentor, and delight. He lived longer after he had cancer than before he contracted it. He lost the incredible tool that got him to the spotlight, his DJ and singing voice, only to seek a new and grander spotlight. Kimmie is the sister I never had but always will. She gave Joe a shelter and safe place after his traumatic and ridiculously ironic disease. She gave him strength and drew on him for more strength to become one of Austin's all-time great singers, songwriters, artists, and personalities, which she remains today. I have never seen two individuals so completely artistically intertwined yet delightfully independent.

In *Radio Dreams,* two of showbiz's most iconic characters share their unique thoughts and words. Sit back, relax, laugh, cry, and prepare to feel with all your heart. This book is magic, just as the authors will always be magic. Joe says it best in this book in response to what life gave him: "Life regained is in some ways better than life untroubled." Read the story. Enjoy the journey. Regain the life!

BROTHER BILL GRACEY, singer-songwriter, recording artist

I guess the Jackalope Brothers could lay claim to discovering Kimmie, if our friend T. J. McFarland hadn't already told us about her first, but really, Kimmie discovered herself that day she came to town. It wouldn't do to say that Kimmie kidnapped us, since no one would go the ransom anyway, but we were hers and she was ours from the day we met. And, it wasn't so very long after when Joe and I were doing a bit of day drinking one summer afternoon at the Tavern that we saw Kimmie drive by in her little yellow Volkswagen, and Gracey says to me, "Yonder comes my third wife." And so it came to pass.

That was way back then. Years fly by. Joe is gone but dang sure not forgotten. I think of Gracey every day. I miss my old Brother Jackalope. Kimmie Rhodes waltzed into my life all those years ago. I keep the windows and doors to my heart open all the time. Kimmie comes and goes as she pleases.

BOBBY EARL SMITH, singer-songwriter, recording artist

The legendary radio station KOKE-FM could never have had the cultural impact it did in Texas without Joe Gracey, or Ol' Blue Eyes, at the KOKE console. Joe was a powerful voice for Texas roots music from Bob Wills to Jimmy Reed to Flaco Jimenez to Doug Sahm to the Flatlanders. His spot-on music savvy, Lester "Roadhog" Moran impersonation, Texas vibe, and sense of humor defined KOKE-FM and the entire Austin music scene in the late '70s and for years to come. Joe's daily 10:00 a.m. to 2:00 p.m. *Super Roper* radio show was the mover and shaker of *Groover's Paradise*. It made Austin the Live Music Capital of the World that it is today. Joe's end of show sign-off, "Drink lots of water, stay off your feet, and come when you can," defined Austin as much as armadillos, Shiner beer, Soap Creek Saloon, and the hippies and rednecks who embraced KOKE's progressive country music.

KANDY KICKER, KOKE-FM

—★—

Joe Gracey was the personality of the "progressive" movement when there was a serious need for better relationships between the participants. He was also a major part of the movement's frontal lobe as well. He was the one who recognized the kinship between Willie and Dylan and could put together sets that bound music lovers together while agitators just jawed and whined. If Joe had been left alone, or put in charge, the marriage of genres would have taken on a majestic proportion instead of just clawing out a niche. Ol' Blue Eyes was cool, funny, and smarter that most all of the people involved. He was who I wanted to be: everyone's favorite guy. Whereas Arlie Duff was famous for "Y'all come," Joe was cracking us up with "Stay off yer feet, drink lots of water, and come when you can." All that, and he ended up with Kimmie, too, just deserts for a cultural leader.

EDDIE WILSON, Armadillo World Headquarters,
author of *Armadillo World Headquarters*

—★—

Kimmie Rhodes is a great storyteller, songwriter, and musician who sings like an angel. Joe Gracey was a great musicologist, record producer, and chef, with the perfect voice for a disc jockey until he lost his voice. Together they made beautiful music on and off the stage and in the studio. Their story tracks the evolution of Texas music and their love affair with Texas, music, and each other.

MIKE TOLLESON, cofounder of Armadillo World Headquarters

—★—

"I loved to see Joe Gracey laugh!"

DELBERT McCLINTON, singer-songwriter, recording artist

— ★ —

Kimmie and Gracey cooking together was an exercise in synchronicity. T. J. (McFarland), who introduced them, said, "They finish each other's sentences, like they are one mind." Hard as it may seem to believe, he finished more of hers than she did of his.

CHARLOTTE HERZELE, MEd, MPH, PhD

— ★ —

I saw Kimmie at the Cactus Café in Austin some years ago, and she had her son Gabriel and Joe Gracey playing with her. My favorite line from the show was when she introduced them, saying she "liked to use what she found lying around the house." My takeaway that night: I learned the lesson that if you want to write a beautiful song, it helps to have a beautiful voice. Kimmie's range and the incredible sweet pure quality of her voice is a wonder. She just works at her job and has for a long time, writing great and beautiful and fun songs, and I don't think she's ever gotten the acclaim and appreciation she deserves. That's the tip of the iceberg of my personal regard for Kimmie. It's been great being her friend.

MARCIA BALL, singer-songwriter, recording artist

— ★ —

Kimmie Rhodes: The soul of a poet and the voice of an angel.

RODNEY CROWELL, singer-songwriter, recording artist

— ★ —

Kimmie has the voice of a beautiful child coming from an old soul. She touches us where the better angels of our nature dwell, and I believe we need that now more than ever. If you haven't before, do yourself a favor and bring her into your listening life.

EMMYLOU HARRIS, singer-songwriter, recording artist

Everyone's got a Gracey story, and I've got a few myself. I'm thinking of a wild trip to the Mexican border in particular. Gracey, among other things, was a great producer. During the many hours we spent in the studio on other projects, notably on Kimmie's records, he taught me a lot about recording, a lot about life, and that being sick wasn't necessarily the end of the world. I miss his incredible touch on the mixing board, his cooking, his humor, and, most of all, I miss his soul.

WES McGHEE, singer-songwriter, recording artist

Joe Gracey was quite possibly the most passionate and original food writer you've never heard of. That's fair enough, because he wasn't really a food writer at all—he was a musician and music producer by trade. But he was also a guy who thought nothing of driving two hours for his favorite barbecue, he made his own sausage, and he once spent three days with his wife sampling boudin all over Cajun country, an adventure he chronicled on *Letter from Graceyland,* a blog he started in mid-2007, which he described as "musings on food, cooking, travel, music, and life its own self from Joe Gracey Jr., music producer, food and travel writer, cancer survivor, frequent contributor to *Saveur* magazine, musician, gourmand, and borderless bon vivant."

Gracey had an expressive face. I always thought he would have made a great (silent) comedian, and, in fact, one of his idols was W. C. Fields. Even more remarkably, although he had no tongue and thus no taste buds, he could somehow taste food and wine, whether through a few errant receptors scattered around his mouth (as he liked to claim) or simply through aromas. I talked to Kimmie when Gracey was in palliative care. "Do you want me to tell him anything?" she asked. I couldn't think of anything intelligent, so I just said, "Tell him I'll see him on the other side." I could almost hear her smiling sadly on the other end of the phone. "Foie gras in heaven," she said, in a wistful voice. "Foie gras in heaven," I replied, although I wonder if I shouldn't bring along some boudin or some Jésus de Morteau.

COLMAN ANDREWS, *Saveur* and *Gourmet* magazines, The Daily Meal website

★

The first time I met Kimmie Rhodes was at a typical 10:00 a.m. demo session at Almo/Irving Music Publishing in Nashville. Introductions and pleasantries all around then quickly down to business. Her songs were simple but told beautiful stories, her voice, angelic. In fact, her songs and voice moved me to tears by the end of the session. I ran on for a minute about the hurt I was feeling from some things I had experienced the past year. Kimmie said very sternly, "You need to come to Austin and let me and my husband, Joe Gracey, take care of you for a while. You need some healing." Well then, just two weeks later I was picked up at the Austin-Bergstrom International Airport and driven west for about an hour.

We walk into her house and she presses play on her answering machine, and there's Waylon singing "Happy Birthday" to their daughter, Jole. I knew immediately this was going to be a healing time for me. Joe and I became brothers in just one meal. He and Kimmie introduced me to the finest food I have ever eaten. Man, watching those two cook was like going to school. They taught me about wine and their love for France. What a life-changing experience. We have shared such happiness, and we have shared heartache. It has been a pleasure to know Kimmie's family and for her family to know mine. Our spiritual journey will continue.

JOHN GARDNER, house band drummer, Sunbird Studio

★

In 2012, Austin's global education nonprofit, the Nobelity Project, began construction of the Joe Gracey Library and Music Lab in rural Kenya. It wasn't until we officially opened the library, with the school's principal wearing a sharkskin suit and playing Elvis Presley songs on the guitar, that we knew what a great impact Joe's lab was going to have. The Gracey library prompted much more partnership work at Amboni primary and a new Simbara secondary school, which was just starting on adjacent grounds. The students at both schools love their time in the Gracey library and lab. Planting a tree in Joe's honor at the school was an emotional moment for us. We've watched that tree grow for years and watched those kids grow, too. (Anyone who wishes to make a donation to that work in Joe's honor can do so via *www.nobelity.org/donate.*)

TURK PIPKIN, The Nobelity Project

PREFACE

IT'S GOOD TO WRITE A MEMOIR. Everyone should give it a try sometime, whether you are a writer or not. It helps puts things into perspective, which for me has brought understanding and gratitude. Processing the past has helped me move forward—beyond any hard times—and it's been liberating as a songwriter to write free of rhyme and time limitations, although it was helpful to have been "pre-versed" at finding core meaning. It's comforting to peruse Joe Gracey's memoirs because, for at least a little while anyway, the void left by his absence has been filled with words that ring with his unique sense of humor and his own beautiful truth.

By the time I met him in 1979, Gracey had started writing a book that he was forever meaning to finish. He gave it the title "Radio Dreams," because of a recurring dream he had about getting into situations in which he was trapped outside a radio station, helplessly listening to the "dead air" that is every disc jockey's nightmare. Because he lost his voice to cancer in his late twenties, he was forced to communicate through writing. So, much of what he had to say on all kinds of subjects was left behind not only in his unfinished manuscript, which gives us the personal account of his childhood and early radio days—or "dreams," as it were—but also in the many letters, blogs, e-mails, essays, and articles that he wrote throughout his years, making it possible to piece together the rest of the story. Even before his loss of speech he wrote about something almost every day.

I know his friends and fans will be happy to "hear" his sweet, smart voice again and enjoy his personal account of who he was and why he so passionately tightened his embrace on an existence that shaped him into someone who owned a wisdom earned through quiet courage in the face of hardship, but which he tempered with levity and wit in a very cool way.

Throughout the years I watched him make his way through the world, realizing that even with his faults (and in spite of my own) I had been given the best man ever. I learned so much from him, and many a morning when we would wake I would tell him, "You're everything," which always made him smile. As his perennial sidekick and interpreter, I gained deep insight into his essence and eventually got good at anticipating what he would probably be going to say next. Over time I finished many sentences for him to spare him the frustration of being left behind in group conversations. This book, composed from the bottomless rubble of archives that fell to my safekeeping, also added to by the pummeling of things sent to me from friends after he left us, is my responsible attempt to return him to the conversation once more.

Because I started singing as a child and had a colorful (if not checkered) backstory, people have always encouraged me to write more than just songs on the subject. So, inspired by Gracey's narratives, I decided to make this book a dual memoir, and, in as loving and forgiving a way as possible, recount my earliest memories, including my musical influences, up to the point where I met Gracey, when our adventures together commenced and then carried on for an incredible three decades.

On the day we met, I think Gracey recognized in me what he saw in himself, someone who was trying to "begin again." Like an experienced big brother, he offered the encouragement that I was missing, so my bent toward ideas that were "too grand," inherited from my father, seemed okay. Hardly attainable goals suddenly looked promising and worth the effort. Life felt overwhelmingly karmic and right when Gracey would play guitar and I would sing his songs, which he was no longer able to sing himself. We started out as best friends, with that deep bond between us, and grew into knowing that fate's flawless timing had brought us together because we needed each other.

Early on, Gracey eagerly shared with me his relationship with Cowboy Jack Clement, so "The Cowboy" became a beloved mentor to me as well. Cowboy sang a song for me the first time I met him: "We must believe in magic. We must believe in the guiding hand. For if you believe in magic, you have the universe at your command." Maybe he admired my dumb blind faith, but most assuredly he noticed how innocent and oblivious I was to the unlikely prospects of becoming a singing star. Either way I know he appreciated how much I loved music, so I've always felt like Cowboy gave me those lyrics as a sort of talisman, just as when the Wizard of Oz gave Dorothy the ruby slippers. Gracey, having recently lost his voice to cancer, in his own silent way sang along. He had already bravely headed in a new direction, having been encouraged by Cowboy to become a record producer because of his background in radio and experience in knowing what a great record should sound like. We all basked in the fallout from the power of Gracey's courage, enthusiasm, and excitement, magnificent in those days, when he had just been handed another chance to live, howbeit with major obstacles to overcome and a challenging reinvention to realize.

Gracey's determination and generosity and "that magic we must believe in" led us down countless roads that we watched wondrously unravel into everything we believed: days and nights filled with music, love and happiness, well lived with our children, our family, and our friends. By choosing to compile selected writings and documents from a mountain of archives for inclusion in this book, I hoped not to write a musicology textbook. (Lord knows there are many who would be far better at that than I!) Rather, my aim is to present the story of two people who made a stand together among constellations of souls who have given their hearts and lives to communicating through the songs they penned and/or music they loved. And I thought it would be more real to give our writings a chance to traverse a lifetime one day at a time. I like to think of the individual memoirs as pearls and the manuscript as the years that strung them together into a wearable strand.

Please allow forgiveness for any mistakes regarding facts, dates, and names, as I was loath to change the writing too much for fear of losing the spirit in which they were written. Much gratitude to our dear friend and Jackalope Brother, Bobby Earl Smith, and wonderful "Brother Bill" Gracey for their patient fact-checking attempts at toning down Gracey's tendency to brag, and even lie (after all, he was from Fort Worth, Texas, and W. C. Fields was his hero!) concerning events that happened before I came into the picture.

Special thanks to those who supported this effort in all ways imaginable and unimaginable and especially to those who tolerated my dogged and shameless requests for a million favors and my passion for completing this book and for understanding that it was not just "widow's grief" that caused my tenacity but an undeniable desire to express my gratitude for the days of love and life I shared with Gracey by honoring his contributions to Texas music and celebrating all that he was and meant, not only to our family but also to his many friends and fans. Besides, I have never liked being expected to wear the mark that the ugly, outdated word "widow" connotes. By including my personal recollections in the mix, I honor my loved ones, whose kindness shaped my story.

And, lastly, these days it's difficult to find someone whose reality has not been touched by cancer in some way. Any painfully honest and deeply personal thoughts have been shared only with hope that those who have been affected by the disease and loss might find kinship, courage, and peace through our musings.

KIMMIE RHODES

2018

ABOUT THE AUTHORS

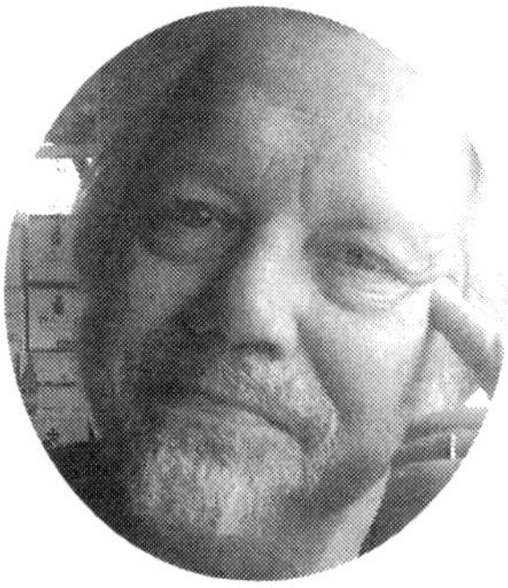

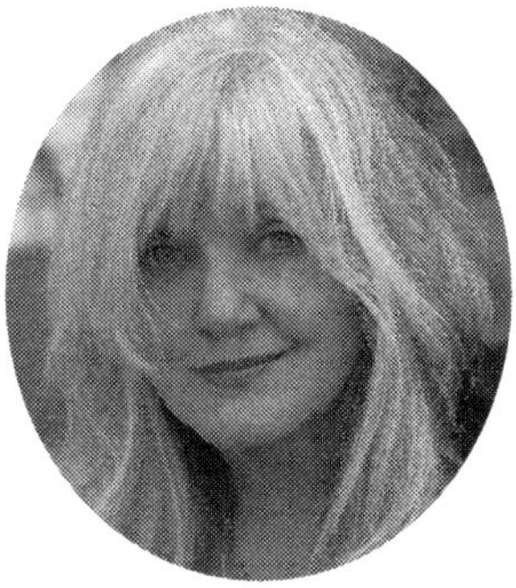

JOE GRACEY, from Fort Worth, Texas, was a natural-born communicator from an early age who became a country music disc jockey for KXOL-AM and FM while still in high school. He attended the University of Texas at Austin, earning a degree in American studies while moonlighting on Austin Top-40 station KNOW-AM and writing the *Austin American-Statesman*'s first rock music column. In 1974, he joined Austin's KOKE-FM, the world's first progressive-country radio station, and helped the station earn its *Billboard* magazine Trendsetter of the Year award. Gracey also served as talent coordinator for the first season of *Austin City Limits*, the longest-running music series on American television. Gracey left radio to establish Electric Graceyland Studios, where he produced some of the first recordings by blues legend Stevie Ray Vaughan. In 1979, Gracey lost his voice to cancer, but he continued engineering, producing, and performing as a bassist and rhythm guitarist. In 1996, he engineered Willie Nelson's groundbreaking album, *Spirit*. In 2003, he recorded *Picture in a Frame*, Nelson's duets album with Kimmie Rhodes, and the Grammy-nominated Nelson–Ray Price duet album, *Run That by Me One More Time*. A gourmet cook and wine connoisseur, Gracey contributed articles and recipes to *Saveur* magazine. Gracey's head and neck cancer returned in 2009. After a long battle with the disease, he died on November 17, 2011.

TEXAS-BORN SINGER KIMMIE RHODES is a multi-platinum-selling songwriter whose work has been recorded by Willie Nelson, Wynonna Judd, Trisha Yearwood, Amy Grant, CeCe Winans, Joe Ely, Waylon Jennings, Peter Frampton, Mark Knopfler, Emmylou Harris, Townes Van Zandt, and Babe the Pig, among others. She also has released sixteen solo albums, written and produced three musicals, and published a novella/cookbook, *The Amazing Afterlife of Zimmerman Fees.* Rhodes served as an associate producer for the documentary *They Called Us Outlaws,* dedicated to the memories of Joe Gracey and Waylon Jennings and presented by the Country Music Hall of Fame and Museum in Nashville.

RADIO DREAMS

1

RADIO DREAMS

JOE GRACEY

IT IS DAYTIME and I am out on the street, two blocks away from the radio station. There is a gray metal public-address horn on the corner of the building where I work, inexplicably broadcasting my radio show out into the parking lot. I realize that the record that I had put on is now about to run out and I am out here for some reason, much too far away to get back in time, even if I run. I listen helplessly as the sound of the needle in the end grooves begins to repeat endlessly. It is the DJ's worst nightmare. I wake up. . . .

When you work on the radio, especially in 1960s-era Top 40 radio, you learn that dead air is the cardinal sin for the operator of the control board. Everything has to move fast, fast, fast, be overlapped and slammed home and yelled loud and insistent. No gaps or pauses allowed. Dead air is anathema, not tolerated. Being a DJ in a format like this is exhilarating, a mad dash from the beginning of your show to the end, slugging coffee (or worse) and lighting cigs and talking fast and moving your hands over the controls in a constant ballet, a coordinated, practiced caressing that never stops. Records are cued up by rocking them back and forth by hand, then rolled back to a precise point before the start of the music, so that when I touch the turntable start switch, the song starts exactly when I know it will. Ads are on endless tape loops inside plastic cartridges shoved into automated tape players in correct order, cued and awaiting my finger on the start button, their last line typed on the label so I know when to jump in. Everything is within easy reach of my hands, the microphone suspended a certain exact distance from my mouth, always the same spot in relation to my face, my ashtray and coffee cup always exactly where my hand falls to them, my ad copy and promos positioned exactly eye level on a pedestal over the board, where all of the volume and start/stop controls are. It is my world for four hours every day, my reason for being, my connection to people that is much more intimate than I can ever be face-to-face. When I turn on the microphone switch, I can feel the electrons coursing through the giant power tubes in the transmitter on top of the hill, pausing just that tiny moment to listen to the sound of air before I begin to speak, my deep resonant voice causing the massive tubes to pulse purple and red in the night, the antenna tower blinking red, and the wind singing in the wires. Oh, baby, I love being on the radio. . . .

IT IS 1956 IN FORT WORTH, TEXAS, in a suburban frame house in a new part of town. In the kitchen, a five-year-old boy hears "Heartbreak Hotel" come on the radio and is swept up into it. "Mommy, why don't you like Elvis?" he asks. Mommy, whose strong opinions on everything from Communists to Christmas include frequent denunciations of Elvis, is only able to say, "Well, I like his singing, but I don't like the way he moves," which means nothing to the boy. The boy—me, Joe Ellsworth Gracey Jr.—loved the way music sounded on the radio. Everything sounded good on the radio.

I was born in a Texas town in the middle of oil fields and cattle ranches. My first memory is of the smell of burning hide as the cowboys branded the calves at roundup. My grandfather set me on the top rail of the silver-painted pipe fence to watch. The calves bawled, jumped up, and ran around. The air stank. Dust clouds filled the sky.

My second vivid memory is of standing in the front seat of our car watching the dust motes falling through the hot, still West Texas air, while listening to "How Much Is That Doggie in the Window," or one of the many terrible pop songs of the pre–rock 'n' roll era while my mother shopped for groceries. (Imagine living in a time and a place where you could leave an unattended three-year-old in public.) I memorized those songs and liked them because they were all that we had to listen to. It was a long way from that song to "Blue Suede Shoes" and "Hound Dog," songs that would change our world. My father, a conservative lawyer and WWII vet, said that *Mad* magazine and the Beatles ruined my generation. In reality, Elvis ruined it, if you think it was ruined, which I don't.

When I was three we moved to Fort Worth and I got my own little record player and some albums of Glenn Miller's band. I remember one record called "Mairzy Doats," which I played over and over, but one day I somehow got a copy of Tennessee Ernie Ford's "Sixteen Tons"; it changed my life. I sat in a little rocking chair and listened to that single a billion times. I can still see the old purple and silver Capitol Records label going round and round. The song had elements of the blues, pop (it had a clarinet), and country. It was truly cool and was a great Merle Travis song to boot. His deep voice, the dark mystery of the lyrics, the sound of the upright bass, the clarinet, the little reverb trail on the record all mesmerized me. I was hooked—hooked as a singer, hooked as a picker, and hooked as a record producer—at only five years old. I never had a chance to become anyone else. One day as a man, I shook hands with the great Merle Travis and felt a circle closing in my life.

I think back to my mother's insistent drumbeat:

> Travel is good; food is worthwhile; new experiences will make you a better person.
>
> English is a beautiful language and writing an art that is worthwhile. Reading is fun, but it is also a learned skill and one that will repay you a thousand ways. Intelligent people read newspapers and books and learn from them, and never stop. A writer is as much an artist as a painter or a violinist or a dancer.

I would simply not be who I am had she not been there to weave that into the base fabric of my being. I would not be writing now, for the same reasons. I didn't just make those things up; she taught me those things, over and over again.

Mother, Mary Ann Gracey, was a "closet liberal." We were raised to have respect for other cultures and races and languages. I learned from her to despise racial and cultural bigotry. I learned the story of the Jews and the terrible history of the African Americans. I learned to respect and tolerate other opinions as long as they were morally acceptable. There were no closed minds in my home. Everything was open to discussion and debate, and sometimes opinions changed. We somehow even managed to get through my Vietnam protest, long hair, and dropping out of the fraternity. She hummed along to my Beatles records, drove me to Dallas to get my first bass guitar at Sears, and took

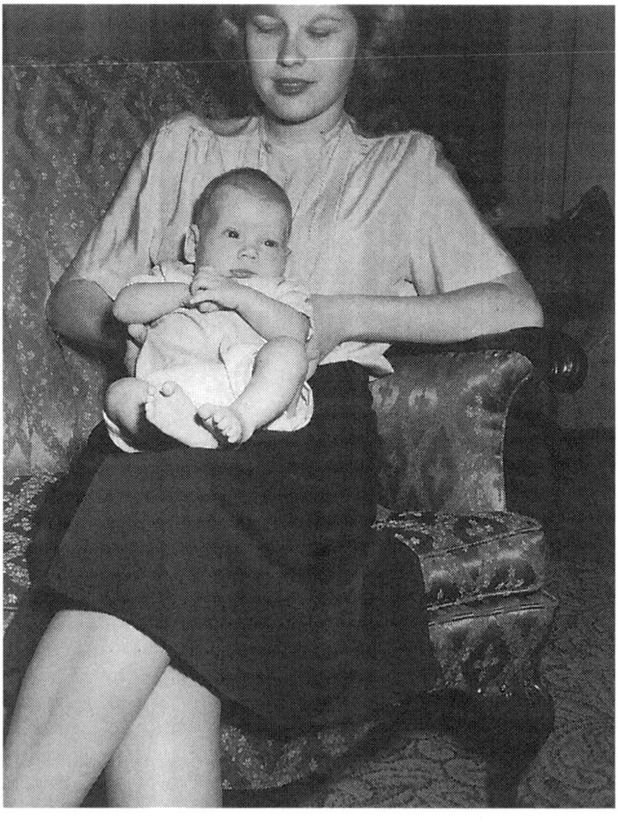

Baby Gracey with mother, Mary Ann.

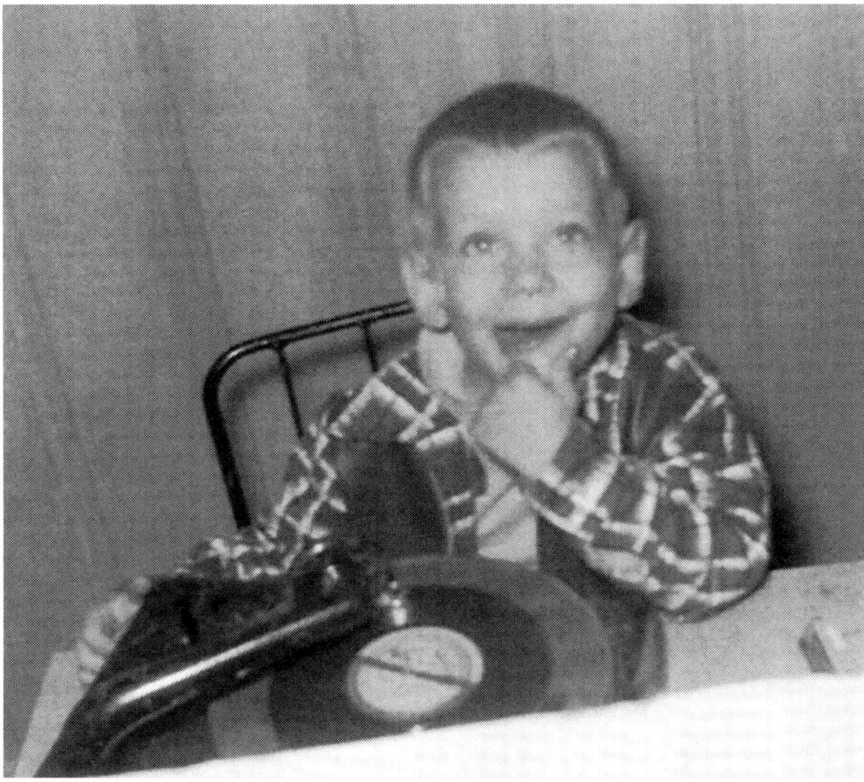

Little Gracey spins a record.

me to my first radio job. She cussed the liberal media but loved Walter Cronkite and was proud of me when I started writing for the *Austin American-Statesman,* even if it was a column about rock 'n' roll music. She thought it was funny when my father's friend Walter Caven said, "Our kids would be fine if we could just knock some of these damned principles out of 'em."

Mary Ann guided us in ways overt and subvert. She offered good advice when my brother was casting about for a successful career path. Most of the time she kept her own counsel when we would make bad choices. She tolerated my wild lifestyle, perhaps knowing that I just might grow out of it someday. She sat by my bed for months when I was twenty-seven and fighting cancer at MD Anderson and called her friend in Houston to get me a badly needed competent doctor.

She took us to the library and the bookmobile religiously, long before there was anything called a summer reading program. She bought us Glenn Miller and Broadway musical records and took us to Casa Mañana theater and the symphony and the Louvre in Paris and got us into chic restaurants in New York so we would know what really good food was and be citizens of the wider world. She gave us the tools to live amazing lives, and she did it on purpose, too. I can't take a step now without thanking her for it.

MY DAD, JOE E. GRACEY SR., was a war hero. As a kid I became very interested in war: guns, tanks, ships, planes. I read *Sergeant Rock* comics and built models of all the WWII ships and planes. I was really just "all ate up" with it. It still interests me; I even have large sections of my bookshelves filled with books on war-related topics.

I used to ask my father about the war, not being old enough to realize that it might be painful for him, but he would tell me about his experiences in a low-key manner, never exaggerating or playing the hero. He was a US Navy gunnery officer on a destroyer. When war broke out, he realized he was going to be drafted, and, not wanting to crawl through the mud with a rifle and be shot at like many of his buddies, he opted to join the Navy instead. Being a recent college grad, they made him an officer. When they found out he was an avid hunter and a great shot, they sent him to gunnery school at Notre Dame. There he learned the ranges, types, and various abilities of the guns aboard US ships and how to man the gunnery tower on a large ship, which coordinated targeting and set the ranges on the vessel's weapons.

A gun turret sat on top of the central tower above the bridge—the ship's topmost part. The gunnery officer manned the turret, which rotated 360 degrees, giving him a clear view, as he used his rangefinders. Hooked up to the turret, the antiaircraft weapons fired in unison at the same target. The officer also calculated the ranges and angles for big guns that lobbed heavy shells—some as big as a small car—into enemy targets many miles away. This made him a very important part of the ship's ability to shoot, but it also made him the target for enemy planes.

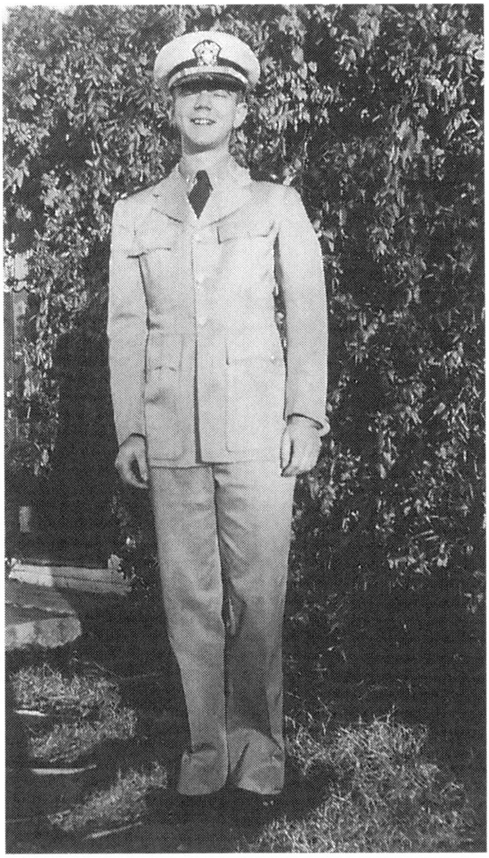

Joe Gracey Sr. in uniform.

He had shipped out of San Diego for the Pacific and was assigned to a destroyer, the USS *Helm*. He would spend the next three years fighting in every major battle from Coral Sea to Okinawa, under Admiral Chester Nimitz (a German-Texan from Fredericksburg). The destroyer, relatively small, fast, and lightly armed with only five-inch cannons and forty-millimeter antiaircraft repeaters, had several duties in the fleet. One duty was to protect the perimeter of a battle group headed by a cruiser or battleship that usually contained at least one carrier.

Enemy subs prowled around the groups, like giant, silent steel sharks, looking for a way in to sink a carrier, which was using sonar systems to constantly search for submarines. Enemies who thought that their sub had been located would generally steer downward and wait, engines off, silent, hoping the stalker would move on. The helm contained sixty-gallon oil drums filled with TNT and a depth sensor, which they would set to activate at the depth they suspected that the sub was hiding. They'd roll these drums over the side of the ship, where they would sink silently through the cold waters; when they reached the programmed depth, the dynamite would blow. He told me that they did this several times and soon after bits of flotsam floated to the surface, along with pieces of human bodies, usually lung tissue because it floated. He said it made him feel sorry for the men who died. They would pull in some bodies and bury the Japanese submariners at sea. When a man was buried at sea, they would strap the body to a five-inch gun shell for ballast and slide him over the side into the icy sea. They did this many times with American soldiers, too.

I never heard my father utter words of hatred for the men he fought and killed. Instead, he would express sadness at their deaths. I don't think he was particularly fond of the Japanese or their prewar culture, but then most Americans of that era felt the same way, for good enough reasons. He didn't go to war out of loathing but rather out of desperation to save his homeland from evil.

He said that toward the "shank end" of the war, the Japanese would send out Kamikaze planes; their dedicated suicide pilots would make of themselves a flying bomb to target the decks of US ships. Twice he managed to cripple a Kamikaze plane, and the pilot attempted one last dying crash into his tower perch, but the plane sailed mere feet away, over the deck and into the sea. He could see the look on the pilot's face as he went by, just a kid. Dad was only twenty-two himself.

He was there until the end, when they went ashore in Okinawa harbor. He brought back a Japanese officer's sword, a taste for Aussie mutton, and a disdain for shipboard cooking. He and his mates said that "chicken soup" on the menu "meant hot water that the cooks had let a chicken run through once."

I realized years later that my father suffered from depression, related no doubt to post-traumatic stress disorder, but nobody called it that in those days; he just suffered, as did we all. Nonetheless, he was a hero, a genuine, no-bullshit hero, who just had a terrible job that he had to do, which he went and did.

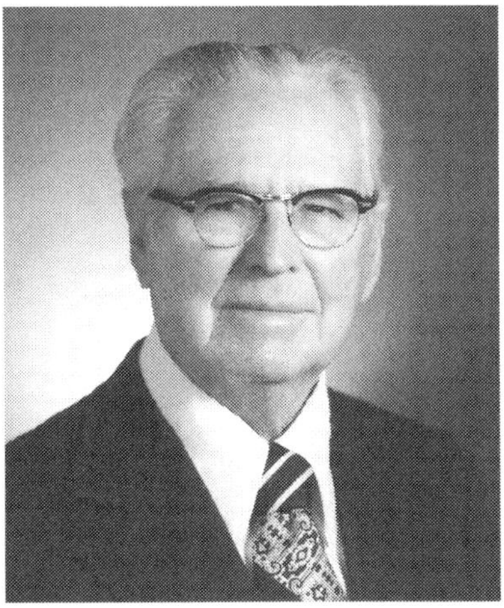

Cecil "Daddy Pop" Morgan.

He often took us bird hunting and fishing. He was an ace shot because he had such good hand-eye coordination, which I seem to have inherited.

Sometimes Dad comes to me in dreams to tell me things, and I know now how much he really loved and admired me, even though he was too frozen to ever say it to me. He was a good man and a good father, and I wish I had managed to tell him I thought so before he died. I guess this is me telling him now, wherever he is.

So, here's a toast to Lieutenant Junior Grade Joe Gracey Sr., his compadres Walter Caven and Bostelman and Crimp and all of the men who went off to fight in the most honorable war this country has known, if there is such a thing. They were just boys, but they were heroic boys who paid a terrible price that nobody else ever truly understood.

After the war, Dad became a corporate defense lawyer who represented the Rock Island and Union Pacific railroads. He was a very meticulous, careful grinder who never went to trial unless he was grossly overprepared. He always won. He expressed amazement and admiration for my lawyer grandfather, Cecil A. Morgan Sr., who he claimed could go into court totally unprepared and "pull law out of his ass" all day and still win somehow. He also claimed that Cecil "made about half of that law up out of whole cloth." I find this hard to fathom.

My great-uncle, Charles Goodnight (who, with Oliver Loving, blazed the famous Goodnight-Loving Trail to drive Texas longhorns in the late 1860s) fought Indians, facing the land and the elements, and taming them all single-handedly. Eventually he came to like the Indians more than the white men who moved in on his coattails.

My great-grandmother, a Goodnight, raised thirteen kids and a one-armed Negro named Tom, who could roll a cigarette in the crook of his stump and even rope cows. She cooked a mean biscuit, don't you know, with all those cowboys to feed breakfast to every day. Back then they all drank gallons of black bitter coffee with fresh cream and a lot of sugar. They raised longhorns and always paid cash. She didn't tolerate much foolishness, and she had a pretty serious cut due to her Germanic ancestry, as shown in all the old photos. She gave her daughters names like "Fern" and "Ola" and her sons names like "Lum" and "Tobe," who was my grandaddy. At eighteen years of age Tobe went to visit Uncle Charles Goodnight and was "about half-scared of the old man, even at ninety." Tobe said, "Goodnight had just married a twenty-year-old Indian girl, and ninety didn't seem too old on his rock-hard frame." That may not beat Michener, but it's all true.

I LIKED MAKING SPEECHES. Making a speech to me was akin to delivering a sermon, since that was the kind of "speech" I had grown up hearing. My mother told me that as a child I would stand up on a chair using the back for a pulpit and yell at my congregation to stop being bad and try to be good instead. In the sixth grade I was required to be in the music class talent show, and, stumped, I bought a cheap plastic trumpet and learned to play something very unimpressive on it. Then I realized I was about to make a complete fool of myself playing a dumb tune on a plastic horn. So, in a moment of life-changing revelation, I (or most probably my mother) came up with the idea of making a speech. I sat down and wrote a speech, ostensibly about the horrors of war, which in reality was a celebration of all the gory, terrible horrors of war as only a sixth-grade boy Civil War fanatic could. Another time, dressed as Lincoln, I recited the Gettysburg Address, and the headiness of standing up before that many people was exhilarating, even though I fumbled

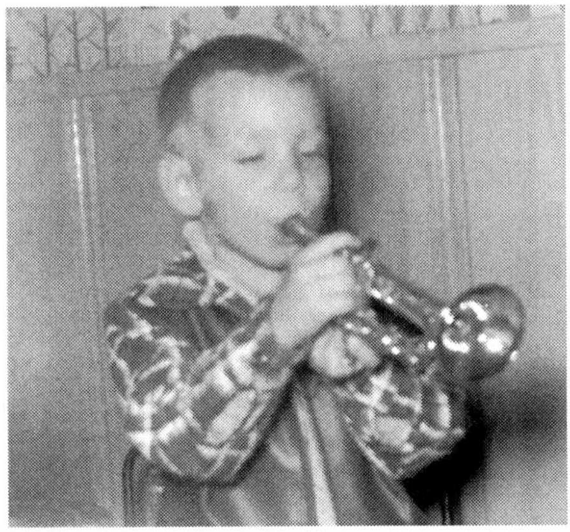

Gracey playing his toy trumpet.

during part of it. My speech was a great success in my own mind. I imagine that my classmates thought it was bombastic and weird, but I enjoyed the sensation and decided to do more of it. In seventh grade I enrolled in a speech class because I wanted to become a champion debater and then a lawyer like my father and my mother's father.

My voice at twelve began to be unusually low in pitch, to the point that I was a baritone by thirteen and a bass by fifteen. I was in every choir I could join. I loved singing and hearing all kinds of music. I got a little, cheap acoustic guitar at thirteen and began learning to play honky-tonk on it, which eventually led me to the blues.

My choir teachers despaired of me because I was a natural harmony singer and would try to slip into the third or fifth harmony chord parts to the melody, just for fun, screwing up the kiddie choir sound. I am convinced that harmony sense is something genetically wired. I had grown up listening to my mother and father sing harmony together in the car, one of my best memories of a very happy, sickeningly normal childhood. I thought it was palpable proof that my parents were in love, as, of course, it was. I could instantly hear every available harmony note to any melody and sing it on demand, which still comes in handy in the studio when producing background singers.

Most radio personalities have relatively deep voices. There is a reason for this. The science of measuring human response to audio tells us that the human brain responds favorably to sounds of increased complexity. This is why we like our concert halls to have a certain amount of reverberation. A completely "dead" hall creates a less interesting sound to our aural sense. It is why sound engineers add reverberations and echoes to the taped sounds we hear on records. A low human voice, whether male or female, has more overtones, the sounds that mirror the lower parts of any sound. For example, if you play a low A note on a piano, you will hear the reverberant overtones of that note all the way to the top notes of the piano. If you play a high A, you hear correspondingly fewer overtones because you are starting higher up on the scale and there are fewer overtones available to be heard. Consequently, we perceive the big, low A to be richer than the tinkly, little high A. A low-pitched speaking voice has multiple overtones and is therefore more pleasant and interesting to the human aural sense than a thin, unresonant voice.

IN ADDITION TO SINGING, I played football. Having enjoyed the sensation of having my face smashed in fifteen times a day about all I could, I ended my football career at fourteen. I joined a rock 'n' roll band to play bass. It was natural for me since I sang bass in choirs and could easily hear the low note of any chord in my head. It was also because they told me that if I had a bass I could be in the band but otherwise, forget it. "Can you play bass?" they asked. "Certainly," I lied. I had been a guitar player previously, but at that moment I became a bass player. This taught me something I have used many times since then: When a door opens, step through it. Even if you don't know what the hell you are doing, go through that doorway. You can catch up later.

I had been in a few little garage get-togethers in which we all banged on our cheap acoustic guitars, but no offers to play in real bands had come along before this one, which was one of two hot-stuff bands in our junior high, the big leagues finally beckoning. The Mods (the rival band was the Esquires) played at all of the school assemblies and a lot of the dances, and we had Beatles-esque haircuts. We were pretty damn dangerous characters, being musicians and all. I begged my mother to let me buy a bass guitar and amplifier, and she loaned me the money,

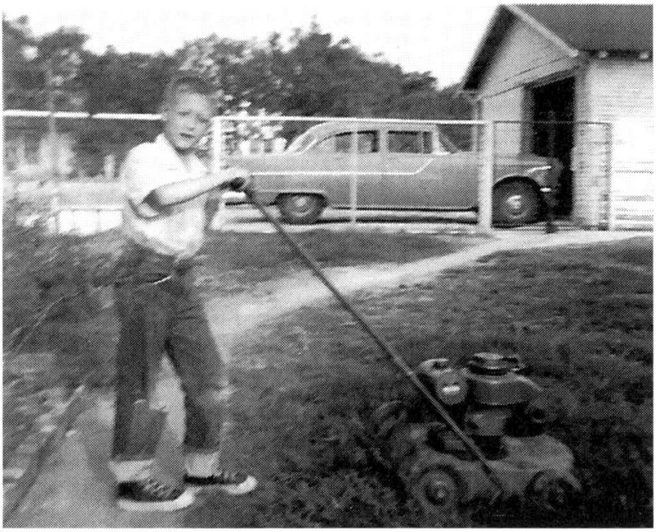

Gracey mowing the lawn.

which I agreed to pay her back by mowing lawns that summer. I learned more valuable lessons from this, which I am sure was partly her intent. The first was "Don't borrow money," because paying it back was a lot harder than borrowing it had been. The second was "Never go outdoors unless you are forced to by circumstances, like to get in the car." And finally, the third one was "Physical labor sucks, especially outdoors." I still borrow money, but mowing dog-shit-covered lawns in the Texas heat was the last "real job" I ever had.

THE WATERSHED EVENT of every '50s child came along when Elvis entered our lives. Elvis shook me up. I was fascinated by the sound of "Hound Dog" and "Blue Suede Shoes" and went around with it in my head nonstop. Elvis dropped out of the picture after he entered the Army, but he was replaced by the next god in my musical pantheon, Chuck Berry. There were the others, of course. Buddy Holly got a lot of play in Texas, but Chuck Berry, with his guitar that sounded like banging on a big glass bell and his sly, white/black voice, took me on down the road with him.

Then the music died. Chuck Berry went to jail. Holly's plane crashed. Elvis went to Hollywood. It seemed all we had were novelty songs like "Ahab the Arab" and "Does Your Chewing Gum Lose Its Flavor on the Bedpost Overnight," sappy Eastern Seaboard rock 'n' roll that was just recycled doo-wop, and terrible-ass girl groups, all Dick Clark and no Alan Freed, all white or very white-sounding. It seemed to be the final blow when "The Twist" came along and all you heard on the radio was twist songs. "Peppermint Twist," my ass! It was almost bad enough to make a kid listen to country radio, but not quite. To a city teenager in Texas, country music was hick music, low-class beer bar music for old white guys.

However, country music had already snuck through a backdoor to my heart. On Saturday, the independent Fort Worth television station that ran all of the cartoon and kiddie shows would start running local country and western shows around noon and would run them pretty much all day and into the evening. We would be sitting around and suddenly these weird, intense guys in funny suits with deep country accents would come on and start playing live music on TV. Before I learned to be prejudiced against it, I got a full education at the hands of not only the local luminaries like Cowboy Weaver and Howard Crockett but also from the great shows out of Nashville with Ernest Tubb and the Wilburn Brothers and Bill Anderson and Porter Wagoner and the Grand Ole Opry and Jimmy Dean. Not only did these shows have great stars, but they also featured guests from the country roster every week, so I saw Patsy Cline and Cowboy Copas and Johnny Cash and Lefty Frizzell and Ray Price and everybody else who was still alive, all singing live to me. Then, to top it off, there were two more live shows that were actually promos from legendary local venues—one from Panther Hall in Fort Worth and one from Big D Jamboree in Dallas. These live remotes would go on around six o'clock in order to give folks at home a chance to get fired up about the act in town that night. I'll never forget hearing Lawton Williams, who wrote "Fraulein" (and who would later be my boss), saying, "And now live from the Dallas Sportatorium, it's the Big D Jamboree!" over the sound of the steel guitar.

Panther Hall was a big dance hall that all of the major stars came through, and I remember seeing Bob Wills on one of those shows, in the twilight of his career but still vital nonetheless. I loved the music and the glitter, but I was fascinated by the fact that it was all live, a fact that would bear on my later life and work. My little brother and I would park in front of the TV eating El Chico frozen enchilada dinners (I wish I had one right now—all gooey and cheesy and the tortillas get all mushy and the rice is dry, but you mix it all up together into a glorious Tex-Mex mess). We would watch Merle Haggard and Buck Owens and Dolly Parton selling Breeze detergent. I got enough grounding in country roots to last a lifetime, but then I got too cool for country and swore that I would never, ever play country music in a band, which goes to show that you should never say "never." One day fifteen years later I was working for a Texas act at a Nashville function and I ran head-on into Doyle Wilburn and nearly died. It was like I was living inside our old TV in my head. Standing there at a bar drinking bourbon and bull-shitting with Doyle, my old Saturday afternoon companion, felt exhilarating but also normal.

At last the fresh air that was the Beatles swept through America and saved us from manufactured fake pop rock and endless girl groups and Lesley Gore and Andy Williams—a repeat of the early-'50s musical pause for breath. The Beatles had energy, soul, charisma, great songs, great style, rebelliousness. To an American thirteen-year-old, they were like a lifesaver to a drowning kid. We took the album home and put it on the big new console stereo and turned it up loud as hell and pogoed around the room, jumping up and down in goofy innocent reaction to the pure energy of it. Again, my life was made different by my reaction to a record. I wanted to be like that. I wanted to be in a band and grow my hair out over my forehead and smoke cigs and be cool. I wanted a guitar. I forgot about debate.

In a sense my father was probably right for saying that *Mad* magazine and the Beatles ruined the world. They seemed to attack the world that his generation had fought to preserve. However, I would say that the inherent problems of that world are really what destroyed it and that the symbols of that destruction were merely that. Racism and economic inequalities and ultimately the Vietnam War are what ripped the world apart and put it back together again differently.

It was then that I joined the Mods and played a few places and made a little bit of money. I had a beautiful red mahogany Gibson EBO bass and a Sears Silvertone amp, which I still have and play. I began to sing some songs in the band. Eventually I quit the Mods and started my own band, Clyde and the Cliffhangers, with some guys I knew. We could play pretty well and for high school kids made lots of money playing country club dances and frat parties and birthday parties. Being in a band was a good way to attain a form of independence that I might not have had otherwise. My dad had given me a great '57 Chevy, which he allowed me to paint red even before he gave it to me—a true sacrifice for a conservative lawyer like him. I could throw my gear in my trunk, pick up my girlfriend, and head for the gig feeling cocky and cool and free. If we were lucky we'd score some beer somehow and go out and neck during the breaks. It was fun. We'd have band rehearsals and go out and fight and then go in and rehearse some more. Being in a band and rehearsing always leads to fights, especially if you are all of sixteen.

I'll never forget the first time I had anything to drink before I played a gig. It was cherry sloe gin poured into some 7-Up, and by the time I got inside the pool lounge at Ridglea Country Club, I was a little bit high, just high enough to get up on top of the music and ride it, feel my big bass in my hands, feel myself singing and digging down into the groove. It was a transcendent experience. I learned that a drug could

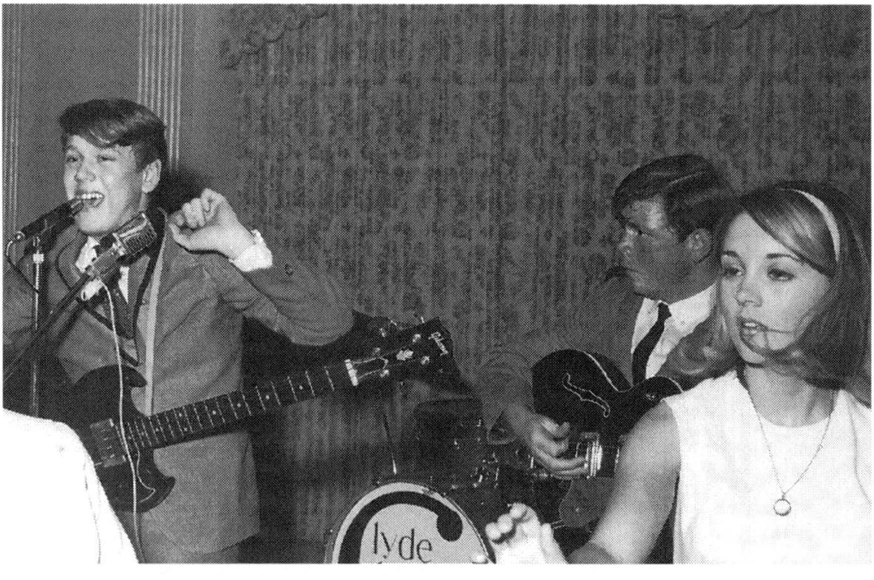

Clyde and the Cliffhangers, Fort Worth, Texas.

1 It's all over now
2 I'm a man
3 Shapes
5 Have Mercy
Freddy King
What a shame

Gracey's band set list.

be used to enhance and intensify the magical aspects of playing music, which would lead to all sorts of both good and terrible things later in my life, but which is an inescapable fact. Music is a form of calling down the magic, just as is dance or poetry or painting. Playing music is in itself a mystical experience, which is one reason musicians do it over and over. Sometimes it can be transcendent, and sometimes it doesn't rise above routine, but always you are calling on the muse. One reason so many musicians get into drug and alcohol troubles is that not only are they prone to be the type of person who is constantly searching for "The Answer" to some large, mysteriously unanswerable question, but for some of us, our drug of choice tends to become entwined with the act of playing music. It is an easy step from merely enjoying the experience of taking a drink before you play to saying, "I can't play unless I'm drinking/smoking/drugging." If you are an alcoholic or a dependent personality this inevitably leads you downhill fast.

But something else was tugging at me. Back when I was in my eighth-grade speech class, there was a kid whose dad was the manager at the local Top 40 radio station, KXOL. This meant that he had access to some cool stuff like concert tickets and being able to hang around the radio station sometimes and interesting things like that. So one day I went down there with him and we stuck our head in the door of the control room. There was a guy in there playing rock 'n' roll records, yelling his head off, and appearing to be having a great time. There was a palpable spirit of showbiz and energy and intensity in that room that I had not really considered as a kid, having listened to it every night with my little transistor. The room was dark, lit up only by the glow of the equipment dials and the tubes. He was screaming into an old birdcage Altec-Lansing ribbon mic, which was designed in a beautiful '40s art deco style. The darkness and the look of the mic, the loud rock 'n' roll, and the intensity of the DJ stunned me, captured me. I was hooked again and only dimly realized it.

My friend up the street was an electronics wizard. Sandy was one of those guys who knew how to build amps and speakers and radios, and one day he said, "I have this kit for building a radio transmitter that broadcasts on the AM band, just like real radio stations." He got me into doing that kind of stuff, too, and we built the transmitter, connected it to a turntable and a microphone. Then we connected that to a tall, old TV antenna and started pirate broadcasting from his bedroom, playing Beatles and Beach Boys and Nat King Cole and making up ridiculous ads for Aunt Grandma's Cookies. I was the copywriter, apparently. We even took it all, put it on a wagon, built a cardboard mobile unit, and went up and down the street doing "remotes" of yard football games and dogfights. I had been bitten pretty hard by the radio bug.

Later, my friend in speech class got us tickets to a Herman's Hermits concert. We went by the station to pick them up, and I felt the same sensation again—the loud, relentless music and the DJ all wrapped up into it, part of it, a minor god ensconced in a cocoon of beautiful old audio gear and big-ass speakers and softly glowing tube gear, in a darkened room behind double-glass panes. By this time I had been building electronics gear and I knew how good that was. The DJ was smoking. Everybody in the station seemed to be smoking. It seemed to be part of the gig.

Herman's Hermits were pretty bad. They could play, but the songs were happy, silly pop songs. It was beginning to dawn on me that not all British bands were created equal. Afterward we went with one of the DJs to the hotel to meet the band, and I talked to the bass player about his gear, asking him about recording sessions while he checked out girls over my shoulder. I got in trouble later because I had gone over to the hotel without having a ride home, so I had to call my parents to come get me. It was cool. Dangerous. Rock 'n' roll! I dug the hotel room scene with the girls and the scruffy English guys and everybody hanging out. Everybody was smoking there, too.

Another thing happened then. There was a recording studio downstairs from the radio station where everybody in Fort Worth made records. There was a producer who had an office there named Major Bill Smith. He had produced hit records by Paul and Paula ("Hey Paula"), Legendary Stardust Cowboy, Bruce Channel ("Hey Baby"), and others. Delbert McClinton, T-Bone Burnett, Stephen Bruton, and all of the Fort Worth music cats hung around there, making records and learning how to do sessions. The engineer was Phil York, who later cut Willie Nelson's *Red Headed Stranger* album. I was totally captivated by this scene. I loved the equipment and the look and feel of the studio and everything about it. If you can compare falling in love with a girl to falling in love with a place, I was in love. I was a kid, at that time just fourteen years old. I would catch a ride down to the studio, and Phil was kind enough to let me just blend into the walls and watch while he cut records on everybody in town. They had a four-track tube Ampex multitrack, a green Altec Lansing mixer (probably eight or ten inputs I'd guess), Voice of the Theater speakers, an Ampex 350 stereo two-track mastering deck, a lacquer cutter disk lathe, and a big Neumann U47 for vocals.

As far as I know, the only limiting device in the room was the peak limiter on the mastering lathe. The only EQ was a unit called an audio baton, which had little dials on it showing each frequency that you could move up or down; it was mono, very primitive, usually only used to fine-tune the final mix as it went to master tape. They probably had an EMI echoplate. This was the classic American recording studio up until around 1966, when things began to change quickly and radically—basic, straightforward, not much signal processing or tricks, just get in there and cut it and use your ears and your mic technique to make it work. I remember T-Bone was the most innovative of the group, always wanting to push the envelope and see what he could wring out of the multitrack and the gear. He made records that sounded like English records, like the Kinks or somebody. He wore his hair like the Beatles, and when he sang, he sounded English (to us). One of his songs got played on local Top 40 but didn't break out.

In the eighth grade I got a little tape deck and started to fool around with taping myself at home. It was all part of the pirate radio station Sandy and I were building. I bought a tiny little Radio Shack mic mixer and a cheap crystal mic (the one that looked like an RCA 77) and some headphones. There was an assembly at school where the Esquires were playing, and I asked them if I could tape the show for them. They said yes and then I realized that I only had one mic, no long mic cords, and no way to actually do this. I went down to the studios and begged Phil York to let me borrow some mics and cords and stands, and somehow he relented and I did the show. I gathered all of his gear up and took it all back to him, having told the school principal that I had to return it immediately. However, when I got back to the studio with the equipment and the tape, Phil and I started critiquing the tape that I had made. I stayed longer and longer until it stretched into a couple of hours, so it was three hours later when I got back to school, and I was in some deep shit. I was informed that it was in no way acceptable to be absent from class just because I was fooling around in some rock 'n' roll recording studio. In the back of my mind I was thinking about the Bible story where the young Jesus is missing from the camp and his anguished parents finally find him all the way back in town at the temple, carrying on with the learned men. Upon their expression of dismay (and probably the kind of anger parents exhibit when they are worried sick, then they find you safe), Jesus simply said something like, "Where else would I be but here?" I felt like my real school was down there in the basement of the radio station in a recording studio, surrounded by gear and tape and music. School seemed like an interminable jail sentence, long days filled with irrelevancies, social agonies, and mathematics.

There were parts of school I enjoyed, like English and history, but I was a socially awkward kid and in no way a true scholar. I would slog all the way through to a bachelor's degree from the University of Texas, but much of the reason for that was a worthy desire to please my family and not be a quitter and because I was proud of being an educated person. However, I was also doing what I was born to do the first time

I played a chord on a guitar, turned on a tape recorder, spoke into a microphone, or typed a word in my newspaper column.

I STUDIED THE LITTLE government pamphlet and took the test to get my Third-Class Radio Operator's license. I got my mother to drive me to my first radio job interview because I didn't have my driver's license yet. I talked to the people at KXOL, but they sent me to a little FM station where they knew that a kid with no experience had a chance of getting on the air. (This was when FM radio was beginning to become more prevalent. Most people at the time still listened to AM radio.) The program director had been an announcer in the grand old days of network radio and had one of those deep, oratorical kind of deliveries you never heard after the mid-60s. He sounded too old-fashioned to get a good job anymore, so he was marooned at this station. He had discovered tape delay echo—where you can run the output of the tape recorder back into the mixer in a delayed mode—and used much too much of it on all of his advertisement recordings. So, here was this guy doing ads for shoe stores, trying to sound like Peter Jennings, only with the kind of vocal effects like they used on Mexican stations. It was truly bizarre. He agreed to try me out on a Saturday night shift so that his regular announcers could have that day off. It paid minimum wage, which at the time was $1.65 an hour. Gas was twenty-five cents a gallon, and cigarettes were a quarter. I was doing cartwheels in the parking lot, out under the thousand-foot tower. I had landed my first job in radio.

I finally got my driver's license, got my '57 Chevy, which was painted fire-engine red, and on the way to my first radio gig I bought me a pack of Lucky Strikes. I had been fooling around with cigarettes before then, making myself sick trying to learn to smoke, buying little dumb-ass cigars with wooden holders. For some reason I was obsessed with smoking. My parents never smoked and were strongly against it, so part of it was curiosity. At twelve, my best friend, Kirk, would steal cigs from his mother and we would try to go off in the bushes and hide and smoke them. One day my mother figured out I was acting funny about where I was headed, came and found us, dragged me out of there, and lectured me all the way home.

I think I was partly trying to emulate Kirk, I was partly just curious, and partly responding to the deluge of ads showing macho cowpokes and beautiful people smoking. It was as if something inside me was driving me to do this thing and wouldn't let go of me until I did it.

I liked the way the Lucky Strikes and Camels looked like a living survivor of the '40s. The artwork was seductive to me, like something from a WWII movie or an old black-and-white Bogart film. I liked the non-filter cigs; it seemed more romantic or more real that way. For some reason, I sensed romance in tobacco. Words like "Balkan" and "Raleigh" and "Turkish" made me think of outdoor cafés and little cups of strong coffee and English explorers.

I had noted that everybody at the radio stations seemed to be smoking, so I decided that it would be cool to smoke, too. Armed with Lucky Strikes, I went to my first Saturday night radio show. I was so nervous and excited that it was a miracle I could drive at all. The college guy who normally worked one of the afternoon shifts stayed there with me for a while to show me the ropes. (He seemed friendly and I struck up a dialogue with him as the weeks went by.)

The sun went down, and you could see the lights on the thousand-foot-tall antenna tower come on, red against the blue Texas sky. The college guy left the building and shut the door, and I was alone on the radio for the first time in my life, flying solo with the big broadcast console and the industrial turntables and the big glass windows through which I could see the production room (a mirror image of the broadcast control room, where ads were recorded onto tape cartridges for airplay) and into the transmitter room with the seven-foot-tall array of dials and meters and huge final output stage tubes. I nervously pulled out albums and put the vinyl platters on the turntables and cued them up, turned on the mic to read the weather forecast (which was only for storms), and, in that instant, a sound like a bomb falling surrounded me. The lights went out. The radio station went off the air, and all I could hear was silence. I was sitting alone in a pitch-black room in a little yellow-brick building on the crest of a hill above Fort Worth, and for all I knew at that moment, I was dead. I could hear and see nothing at all. The crack had been tremendous, as the direct hit of the lightning slammed into the tower, ran down the wires into the transmitter, and blew me off the air before I had uttered a word. Some people might see this as an omen, perhaps even a bad omen. Maybe it was. I'm not sure, but it sure as hell scared me. The station would be off the air for a few days to replace parts, but I was back on my Saturday night shift the next week, ready to try again.

I found out some interesting things right away. One was that being in show business—even the low level of it that I was in at that point—turned you into a thing that some people related to in strange fashion. I had been on the air for a couple of weeks, doing nothing but reading the weather forecast and announcing the records and maybe reading a few ads, nothing whatsoever that called upon me to have a personality, when I began to get phone calls on the request line from a lady and her daughter. These calls became regular, and soon the lady asked if it would be okay if she and her daughter dropped by the station sometime to say hello. I said sure, and one night when I was on the air, she and her daughter, my age, show up in the control room bearing an apple pie. It became very obvious, even to me, a kid, that the lady was attempting to get me to date her daughter, with the pie as a kind of "dowry à la mode." I think that I became nonplussed by this, and, as I recall, the girl wasn't pretty and wasn't my type at all, and something about the whole thing felt creepy, as if these two women had been sitting around fantasizing about me all these weeks and conspiring on how they would entrap me with a pie. I have never been facile in these situations, but I must have managed to get rid of them or I guess they would still be sitting at my dining room table thirty-five years later. Variations on this theme would recur in later years, with cakes and pies and drugs and horoscopes and whatever the person had to offer being offered, but always in the service of a fantasy revolving around a me that did not exist. As a celebrity, you begin to have two of you: the public you that belongs to the people you entertain and the real you, which they all think they know but don't.

I also learned a shocking life lesson. There was an ex–pro football player who did a radio shift and who sold ads for the station. He was a big, rough, not extremely bright man who had played as a lineman for the Los Angeles Rams, had just left football, and was casting about for a career after sports. He had huge hands that looked like they had been carved out of wood. He reminded me of my old line coach in football, a guy who equated your worth with your physical ability and toughness.

A couple of times on my Saturday shift, he would come into the control room with his wife, and his eyes would be the most amazing shade of bloodshot I had ever witnessed on a human being. He looked like he was about to bleed to death any second. This was before Visine was invented, so he was either grotesquely hungover on whiskey (likely), or he was stoned on pot (possible). I made passing mention of this to the college guy I thought by now was my buddy, and I probably said something wiseass about the football player's IQ in the process, since I really couldn't stand the dumb bastard. Lo and behold, the next day the football player walks into my Saturday radio show, eyes red as hell again, and glares at me and says, "So, you little punk, are my eyes red enough for you today?" and gives me that look that only professional athletes who are truly dangerous can give. I thought he would just go on and take me apart on the spot, since he was 6'7" and wide as a barn and half drunk, but he left me cowering in my chair, the realization dawning on me that the college guy had been going around repeating every single word I had said to him for weeks.

This was bad news, because in my naïveté and my cockiness I had been making disparaging—or at least humorous—comments about a lot of the people in the station and the things that went on there. This was an odd place. It was owned by a wealthy fundamentalist type who would only allow us to play "easy listening" music. What this really meant was that the old announcer guy would go to the discount stores and buy all of the old cutout albums in order to save money on records. So instead of Sinatra, we had third-rate Vegas lounge acts that sounded like him, sort of. We had those terrible, terrible harmonica bands and Lenny Dromgoole on the Mighty Wurlitzer and Montovani knockoffs and horrible albums playing Broadway musicals, but never the actual cast soundtracks themselves. In those days there were record labels that specialized in doing cut-rate recordings of all sorts of pop music, so you could find really bad imitations of just about everything for fifty cents an album. So we had a radio station that played nothing but terrible knockoffs and has-beens and retreads. It was very dynamic, especially to a fifteen-year-old rock 'n' roller like me. I would dig for hours in the record bins just to find five decent records out of a thousand so that I could stand to hear what I was playing.

One day very shortly after the near-death experience with the ex–pro football player, I was called into the production room, where I had been hired. The old announcer put down his fried chicken (he seemed to eat nonstop) and said, "You know, none of us around here can figure out where you are finding the records you play on the air. All I know is your shift doesn't sound like the rest of the radio station." (I considered this to be a grave compliment but refrained from saying so.) "Also, I hear that you think my use of tape delay is corny and terrible sounding." (It was.) "And now you have insulted the pro football player's eyes. Therefore I am going to have to let you go. Why don't you just go on over to KXOL, where you really belong?" This would be a theme I would hear repeated from time to time in my radio career: "Why don't you just move on to XYZ and leave us alone?" He picked up his fried chicken and cranked up his reverb and turned his back on me and resumed his retirement. I felt relieved rather than upset. I did take it hard that the college guy, instead of being the friend I thought he was, had, in fact, just been a company spy and backstabber. I was horrified to think that he had repeated some of the unkind things I had said in jest to him. It is a bad thing to have to learn that you can't trust everybody you meet.

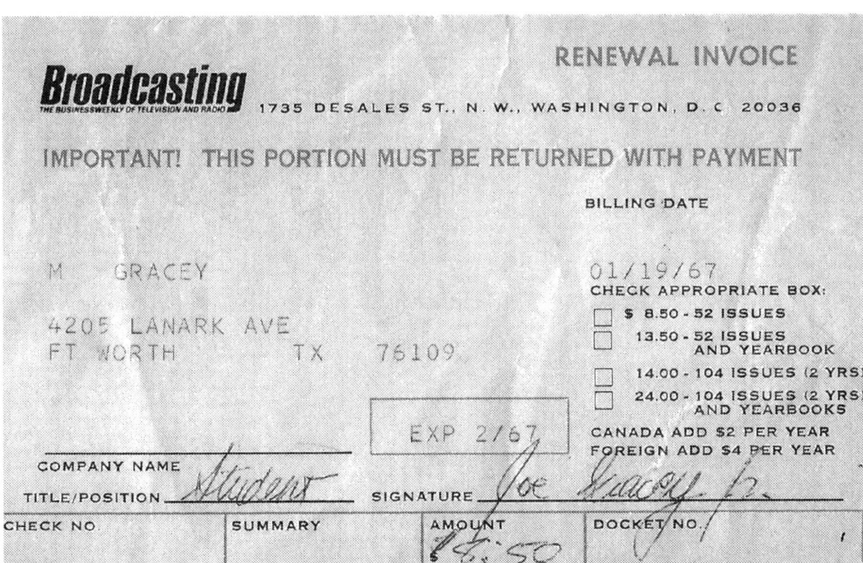
RENEWAL INVOICE

Broadcasting
THE BUSINESSWEEKLY OF TELEVISION AND RADIO
1735 DESALES ST., N. W., WASHINGTON, D. C. 20036

IMPORTANT! THIS PORTION MUST BE RETURNED WITH PAYMENT

BILLING DATE

M GRACEY
4205 LANARK AVE
FT WORTH TX 76109

01/19/67

CHECK APPROPRIATE BOX:
- $ 8.50 - 52 ISSUES
- 13.50 - 52 ISSUES AND YEARBOOK
- 14.00 - 104 ISSUES (2 YRS)
- 24.00 - 104 ISSUES (2 YRS) AND YEARBOOKS

CANADA ADD $2 PER YEAR
FOREIGN ADD $4 PER YEAR

EXP 2/67

COMPANY NAME
TITLE/POSITION Student
SIGNATURE Joe Gracey Jr.

CHECK NO.	SUMMARY	AMOUNT	DOCKET NO.
		$ 8.50	

Gracey's broadcast license renewal, 1967.

But I had the experience I needed to apply for a real radio job, and that's what I had come there for, so leaving wasn't bad at all.

The next weekend I was working on KXOL-FM—new station, new chapter in my life. The program director there was Lawton Williams, who was a country songwriter. He had written a huge hit song for Bobby Helms, "Fraulein," on RCA Victor. In the process of working with RCA, he got a record deal of his own and worked with Chet Atkins. He never made it as a singer, but he had several other songs recorded.

At this time, FM radio was little used and little listened to because people weren't really aware of its existence. AM radio was king; FM was the stepchild. Most station owners had an FM frequency that merely simulcast the AM signal, but the FCC passed regulations that forced the owners to start putting different programming on during a significant portion of the day.

So these owners had hired Lawton to try something new. Chet Atkins had been working in Nashville to broaden the appeal of country music, which drew a predominantly white, older (thirty-five to sixty-five) male audience, and, as a result, its sales were low compared to rock records, and the radio stations ratings were okay but didn't reach women or teens at all. Chet urged Lawton to do the same thing with the radio station that he was doing with RCA records—add strings and choruses and tone down the country fiddles and dobros to make it sound more citified and less about drinking beer and shooting deer. We started purposefully playing things like the new *Hank Williams, Sr., with Strings* albums and Ray Price and Eddy Arnold, who had both taken to wearing a tux onstage and singing in front of orchestras, crossover things like Bobbie Gentry and the RCA Bobby Bare records, which were very folky-sounding. We de-emphasized Ernest Tubb and the old Ray Price stuff and anything that was overtly honky-tonk or bluegrass. Middle of the road country. We called it "countrypolitan" and aimed it directly at women and city dwellers. Chet did station IDs for us and visited the station one day to urge us onward in this new direction.

Our format was really revolutionary because it presaged the whole movement of country music away from its male, middle-aged, low-income, rural, and transplanted-country-folks-in-the-city beginnings to a more female, middle-class, urban, younger audience. Chet started it, and it never stopped moving in that direction, because that's where the money was. Chet was tired of a big country hit being ten thousand 45s sold primarily to jukeboxes, when pop acts were selling a million LPs. Willie Nelson tried to do it Chet's way, putting on turtleneck sweaters and wearing sharkskin suits and Beatles boots and singing real jazzy and slick with zero vibrato and combing his hair real nice. "The Party's Over" had a whole string section on it and had a great arrangement.

One of the DJs there was a young George Carlin, and one of the news guys was Bob Schieffer before he went to CBS. I was just a teenager with a deep voice, had no idea what I was doing, and thought country music was dumb, but I wanted to be in radio so bad that I was willing to play literally anything just to get a gig. Working for Lawton was a trip because I had grown up listening to him on the Saturday afternoon broadcasts of the Big D Jamboree. He was a Nashville insider and big-timer, and he'd throw names around like "Chet" and "Willie" all the time. The way Lawton talked sounded like an old-time country person. He'd say "milyone" for "million" and he'd try to say, "I" in a more "refined" fashion than a hayseed "ah," and it would come out "Aaaeee"—sort of long and goofy. I think being around him was very eye-opening because it caused me to realize that the big time wasn't actually out of reach for a kid from Fort Worth, that it was something very real and there for the taking, if you were smart and tough and lucky and talented. He wore a Stetson hat sort of cocked in a jaunty angle, bigger than the Open Road style that LBJ wore.

They named me music director. A big raise with an office and a car and big responsibilities? Nope. My only responsibility was to open up *Billboard* and look at the Country Top 20 singles chart and put those singles into the rotation unless they were too down-home for Lawton. There was no raise for me. (I was making $1.65 an hour working every day after school and on weekends.) I had a little cubbyhole in the attic with unfinished walls and an old desk with a phone so that I could call the record promo guys and beg them for records since they never sent them to FM stations. One record they did send me and which we played was *Sweetheart of the Rodeo* by the Byrds. Another thing they sent me was all of the Willie Nelson records on RCA. I loved them.

Willie had always been an interesting story. He was from Central Texas and had lived in Fort Worth for a while. (I went to elementary school with his nephews.) He had become big in the Texas dance hall circuit, and Chet was spending the farm to try to make Willie a star on RCA. We played the hell out of Willie, particularly the album with "Turn Out the Lights," which I still say was a hit song. Willie struck me as someone special, when I was still ambivalent about country music in general. I was there because I loved radio, not because I loved country music . . . yet. He appealed to an aspect of me that had nothing to do with "country," but was more on a general pop level. I remember bringing one of my high school buddies into my little office and playing Willie for him and saying, "Listen to this! This is cool as shit!" He was just somehow different. This was before I knew anything about him or had seen him live. Once I realized he was the writer of those great classic songs and saw him a couple of times at Panther Hall, I was a confirmed Willie fan forever. It would be nearly thirty years before I would get to record a Willie Nelson record, and it was worth the wait. It was the highlight of my career. He's in the same group as Ray Charles and Bob Wills and the Beatles, not only a great talent but a great innovator who took the threads of the musical culture around him and drew them into a new synthesis all his own.

So, I learned the country music canon and the difference between Willie Nelson—who was obviously very, very hip—and say, Bill Anderson—who seemed like a cornball, whether he really was or not. Later I learned that even the cornballs in Nashville were usually pretty sharp operators who were a lot hipper than they let on. You don't break into "the bigs" by being a dumb-ass, and even if you do, you sure don't stay there long. One time, years later, I interviewed Willie for an Armadillo Texas tour after he moved back to Texas from Nashville and was doing his outlaw thing and none of the hippies knew who he was yet, and I asked him if anybody in Nashville smoked dope. This was how we distinguished the hipsters from the squares. His reply was, "Everybody in Nashville smokes dope." He was, of course, only half-serious, but he was also making a point. Nashville was never as square as the face it tried to put on itself for the benefit of the audience. If those moms and pops from Indiana who were making pilgrimages to the Opry to see all those clean, nice young people sing those clean, nice songs knew what kind of hanky-panky was going on backstage and on the buses and at some of those parties, they'd have had their minds blown.

By now I was getting too busy being on the radio to be in the band, so I stopped playing gigs and went back to playing acoustic guitar. I bought a brand-new Gibson J-45 for two hundred bucks with my first IRS refund check. I made a few halting attempts to become a lead guitar player but gave up when I realized I had no talent for it. I had a blues band for a couple of gigs but felt silly and white doing B. B. King. Radio was my love now. I could sit around the house and play blues on my Gibson all day, but nobody was going to pay me to do that. Radio paid me so much. (By that time I was making thirty-three dollars a week!) I could go out and buy a new pair of shoes (the highest-quality men's leather shoes cost thirty dollars in 1967) or a record or take a girl on a date without even thinking about the money. I started to hang around Record Town, the shop near my school that was owned by Stephen Bruton's parents. They had turned me on to my first blues record and my first jazz record and pretty much educated me on American musical culture. It was a salon atmosphere there, in fact, with all of the writers (Bud Shrake and Gary "Jap" Cartwright and Dan Jenkins) from the paper and all of the jazz and rock musicians hanging out all the time.

My last fling with a band was with Stephen Bruton and T-Bone Burnett. We got together and called ourselves the "Loose Ends," and I played bass on my Gibson EBO. We did all the old Fort Worth dives for a while until T-Bone and Stephen went off to seek their fortune, leaving me behind to grind through high school and be on the radio every day.

Lawton eventually left KXOL for another job, I think perhaps at KCUL, where Bill Mack and some of those guys worked, and I never saw him again. When Lawton left they put a guy in charge who was more of a typical radio man of the day. He had one of those really nice voices and spoke very clearly and rapidly, and he had very set ideas about what was good radio and what wasn't. He had gone to Texas A&M but was forced to drop out, so he was even more radical about his Aggie attitude than a normal Aggie who graduates, as if to prove that he was as tough as any of them. I was from a long line of University of Texas graduates and was headed there myself, so he and I were polar opposites on every possible subject. He disliked me as much as I did him. However, his radio boot camp was good for me. He taught me valuable basics about being a good air personality, stripping away my bad habits and green gaffes. He also taught me how much I loved radio.

I had done something really stupid one day trying to impress the AM program director and had gone out of my control room and just let a Bobbie Gentry album play through several cuts in a row, which was verboten. I was so desperate to get on the AM side and play rock 'n' roll records that I risked my job that day. I was headed out with Alan Schutts that evening to go coon hunting, but as I got off the air, my boss took me into a room and said, "I heard you playing that whole side of that record this afternoon. What were you doing?" I made some lame excuse, not wanting to admit I was bullshitting with the AM boss. He said, "I'm going to have to let you go. That was something I can't allow here." I was stunned and horrified, expecting a tongue-lashing but not this. I began to do something I haven't done very often in my life. I begged. I was on the verge of tears. I pleaded to him to please, please, please not take this thing away from me that I loved. I would do anything to make up for this mistake, just don't throw me out into the cold. He let me go on pleading like this—probably enjoying his power over me, with the relish of all sadists—for a while, then finally relented and let me keep my job. I know now that he was merely torturing me and probably had no intention of firing me. I was too good and too cheap to fire.

I was incredibly scared and relieved. I realized how deeply I loved this thing, and in that way it was a valuable lesson. However, our relationship was scarred by this ugly, pointless episode, and it would not be very long before the AM boss, taking pity on me, got me out of there and offered me a gig on the big station, which I gleefully accepted. He and the news director, seeing my plight, agreed to let me do a six-hour shift as a newsman and a six-hour shift as a DJ, using two different air names. As a newsman I was "Joe Gracey"; as a DJ I was "Robert W. Morgan," which, of course, was stolen from a real West Coast DJ. I was exultant. This was the real thing! I had to give up some of my hours, but I had gotten away from my Aggie tormentor. I was the Saturday night rock 'n' roll DJ for all of Fort Worth and the Sunday afternoon newsguy. I also got to do all of the summer vacation fill-in shifts, so I did okay.

2

WEST TEXAS HEAVEN

KIMMIE RHODES

MY FATHER, Ray Willingham Jr., was an abandoned child, an orphan, a self-made boy with a second-grade education who became a mathematics whiz on the sidewalks of Wichita Falls, Texas. We were never allowed to ask about his past, but one Sunday morning just before he died, he roused me while the rest of the family was still sleeping, led me onto the front porch, and told me everything. The story goes like this: At the tender age of seven years, his father, who was evidently a *Grapes of Wrath*–era preacher-cum-alcoholic type character, took him to a tall bridge and tried to push him off of it into the treacherous muddy waters below. Fortunately, he struggled free of his drunken father's grip and was able to escape. He had plenty of siblings, but having been singled out for some reason, his beatings had become so unbearable—by then anyway—that he realized he could never return home after that.

Heartsick, I sensed the emotional pain of his trapped inner child longing to be cut loose by this long-deserved, howbeit embarrassingly

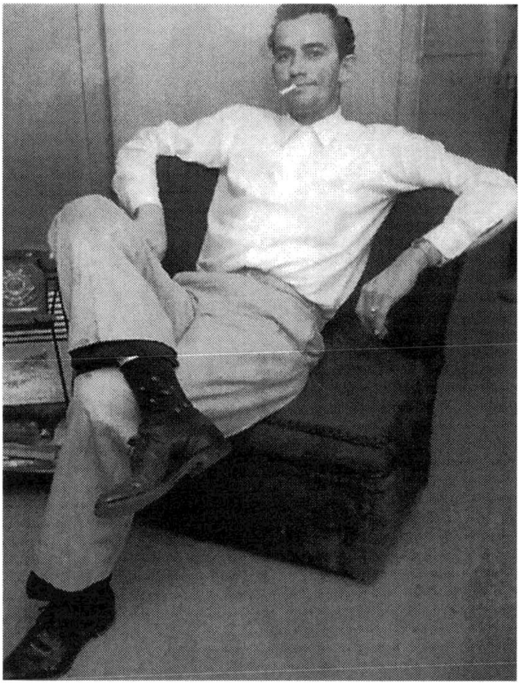

Kimmie's father, Ray Willingham.

pathetic, confession. "Oh, Daddy," I consoled, "That must have been so awful for you. I'm so sorry!" He shrugged, "No, Baby. It was good because after that things got a lot better!" Then he looked me square in the eyes and smiled. This is the essence of who he was—forever strong and positive. And above all, Daddy Ray was fun.

I was never given much information about my grandmother either, except that she was one of those odd women who in the olden days "took to bed" and refused to get up ever again until her death, seemingly at a rather early age. I suppose the world was just too much for her to bear, so she stubbornly refused to participate, but who knows? Maybe she was ill. For these reasons I never knew either of my grandparents on my father's side. I'm told they were Cherokees, so they were probably ancestors of those who settled in East Texas rather than walk the "Trail of Tears" to the Tahlequah, Oklahoma, reservation in the winter of 1838, when President Andrew Jackson decided to give their lands away as lottery prizes.

Anyway, bravely, little Daddy set up shop across the street from the window of the drugstore where his much older sister, Gladys, a small-town Marilyn Monroe, worked behind the counter. As testament to his perennially optimistic character, he bragged that he made more money during the Great Depression than most adults by selling Gladys's phone number (for a quarter, which really was a goodly sum in those days) to passing men after making sure they also purchased a newspaper while he was "spit shining" their shoes. He claimed to be able to sell "an Eskimo a refrigerator" or "a man his own hat." He taught himself to read and achieved beautiful left-handed penmanship but was awful at spelling.

He said his greatest challenge was having business interrupted by truancy officers who would haul him into the police station. When nobody showed up to claim him, he was repeatedly taken to one of those horrible boys ranches for juvenile delinquents, where he was treated like a criminal and forced to pick cotton. (He loved Lead Belly's song "Boll Weevil" and taught me the words: "Just a-lookin' for a home, just a-lookin' for a home." Now I know why.) During one of the uptimes in a series of escapes from and returns to the work farms, he was rescued by a hoochie-coochie dancer named Rose Grace, who found him on the street and took him to live with her at a traveling carnival. She dressed him in a suit and bowtie, and his job was to introduce the "voluptuous exotic dancing girls." Allegedly, according to my mother, this is where he received his early sex education and why she was inclined to forgive his blindly unapologetic penchant for womanizing. Soon he had advanced his career to become a full-blown barker, someone who rustled folks into the sideshows and worked the arcade games. He was the only dad I knew of who could pull a nickel out of your ear and find it by making it drop out of his nose while jabbering a constant stream of carnie jargon. He also played the spoons and percussion on the phone book with his elbow. Luckily, my mother worked for Bell Telephone Company because Daddy also liked to demonstrate his masculinity by tearing the Lubbock phone book in half. Really.

After Daddy Ray's unexpected autobiographical revelation, some of my own youthful mysteries began to unravel. When we'd made our annual trip to the South Plains Fairgrounds, Daddy had shown a suspicious knack for knowing how the games were rigged, so I always

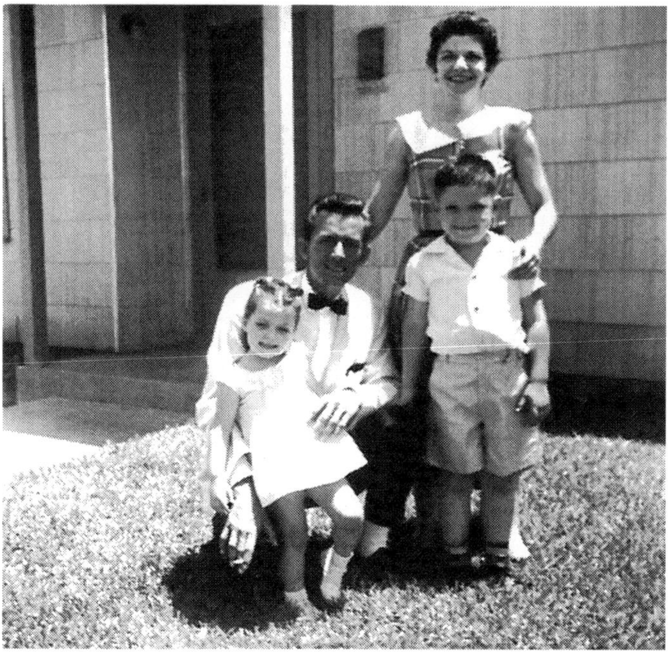

Kimmie and family, Wichita Falls, Texas, 1957.

walked away with the impossible-to-win giant stuffed animal. He could never pass a “gumball prize” machine without filling it with change to win worthless junk because he was a natural born speculator who lived to test his luck at every opportunity. To him they were like “playing the slots.” Once, when we were at the State Fair of Texas, in Dallas, he led us down a dirt path through the midway to a makeshift shanty covered with a ragged canvas and introduced me to a hunched-over old woman sitting on a stool. As vivid in my memory as yesterday, I recall the curious crone who cocked a sideways glance and studied me through intense steel-gray eyes, and, finally, in a gravelly cigarette voice, rasped, “That’s a real cute little girl you got there, Ray.” I’d had no idea at the time that the woman to whom he’d proudly presented me was none other than the faded Rose Grace, who had sheltered my father and allowed him a childhood . . . of sorts. (In the end she took up with a professional wrestler who didn’t want him around, but by then Daddy had grown enough to pass for someone old enough to be out of school, so he easily returned to the streets of Wichita Falls.)

Eventually Daddy Ray met my marvelously unique mother, Bettie Lee Grbavace, who was the daughter of two immigrants from Eastern Europe. Her mother, Stella Ruth Piva, committed suicide when Mama was a very young girl, so she had also been treated to a brutal upbringing during the severe economic slump of the '30s, howbeit with a father who kept a shabby "roof over her head" as a consolation prize to her weekly beatings, but not much else in terms of food and clothing.

As a boy, Mijo Grbavace, my grandfather, stowed away on a ship sailing to from Yugoslavia to America because he mistakenly believed he had killed his brother by way of a blow to the head with a shovel but in reality had only knocked him unconscious. After working for a while in a bicycle shop in New York City, he returned to Yugoslavia and came back to the United States legally at seventeen. He was a master tinkerer and made his way to California, where he became an auto mechanic. He spoke seven languages and became one of the first people to make the journey from the West Coast to Texas in an automobile. He and Mama's short-lived new stepmother, Gladys, settled on what later became "the family farm" in Sunset, Texas, just north of Fort Worth. I sort of knew Mijo when I was a kid. He made moonshine, even after Prohibition, as his drink of choice, ate dried armadillo meat, and was bent toward paranoia and delusions of grandeur. Not knowing he was probably dangerous, I observed him with an innocent curiosity and liked the way he called me "Lily Monkey" in his weird almost Italian-sounding accent. I can't say I loved him and don't recall ever sitting in his lap or such things one usually does with a grandfather. I had once survived an extremely frightening ride in the cab of his pickup truck across a plowed field on the way to "run a trap" one afternoon, so I was not terribly shocked when he died in a fatal head on collision . . . on Father's Day. So, understandably, we were not allowed to ask about my mother's girlhood either.

I marvel that my parents could be so loving and good to me, given the unspeakable traumas of their upbringings. They were, of course, not at all like the "ideal" parents my friends had, but they owned extraordinary strength and resilience and were true believers in life itself, and I feel blessed to have been their girl and to have inherited the courage and dumb blind faith one needs to be an artist. Relatively, normal life

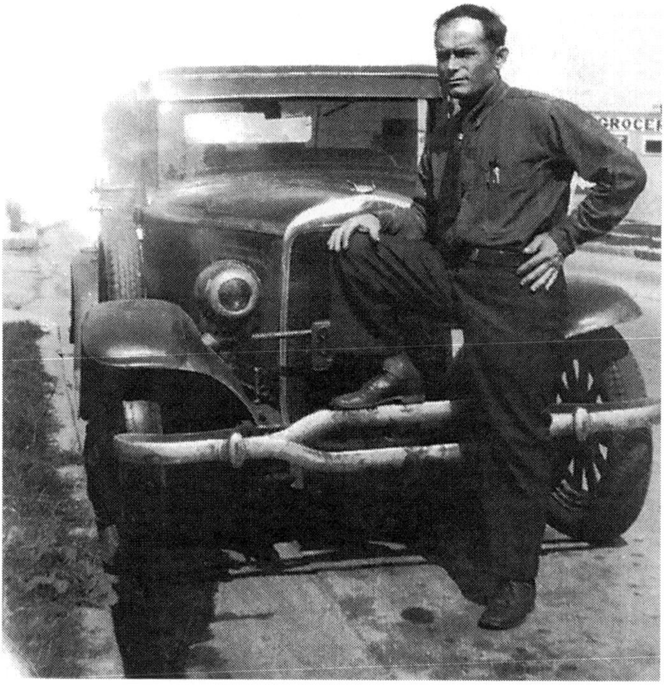

Kimmie's grandfather, Mijo Grbavace.

seems abnormal. I was allowed more freedom to run absurdly wild than any of my friends, and I never had to eat anything I didn't want to, like squash and spinach. I could walk as far away from home as I wanted, by myself and barefoot, as long as I was back by dark. Later, when I questioned my mother about how she could possibly know how to be such a good parent, she always said she knew exactly what kind of mother she wished she'd had, so it was easy. She would stay up all night sewing a dress for me to wear to school the next day and then head to work having had little or no sleep. She never ever—ever—let us down. She bailed Daddy and brother Mike out of trouble many times. She was our angel.

One Christmas when times were tough and Daddy was enjoying the holiday spirits so much that he forgot to come home for a couple of weeks, Mama showed extraordinary faith by wrapping rocks in the boxes under the tree because we liked to shake our presents and try to guess what was inside. Just before Christmas, when the money (and

Dad) arrived just in the nick of time, she unwrapped them on the sly and inserted gifts but forgot and left a rock in one of mine. When I opened it on Christmas morning the rock rolled across the floor. I looked up at my parents, puzzled. Daddy improvised, "Oh, that's a magic rock so you can wish for anything you want." That moment has become a shrine by the wayside in my memory. Our existence depended on an undying belief in things we couldn't see. I still believe that you can have what you want in life if you keep the faith until somehow you reach what you envision.

Unlike my mother, Daddy honestly didn't have a clue about how to be a parent, so he just made sure to "look out for us." He maintained an interesting dichotomy of generosity and self-indulgence that kept us all conveniently confused most of the time. He referred to life as a "rat race" and, sadly, his self-worth was ceaselessly bound to winning

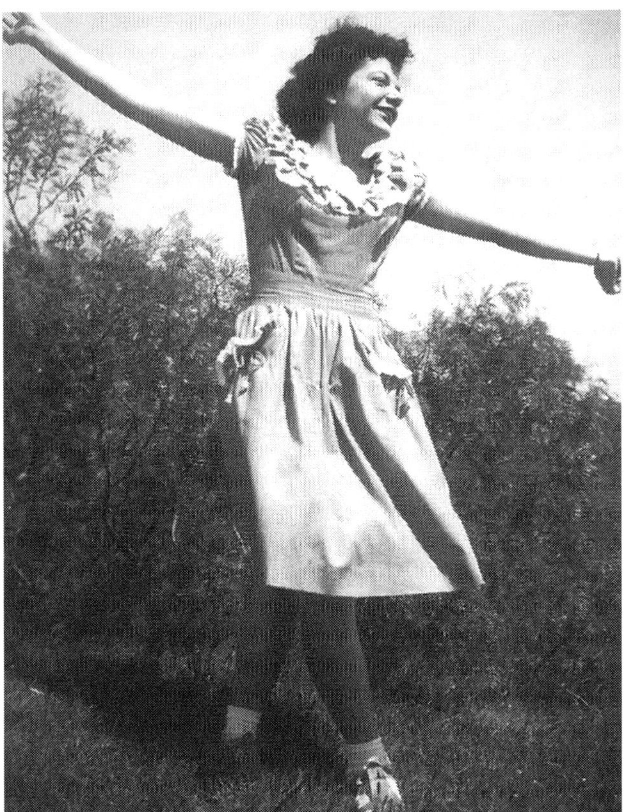

Kimmie's mother, Bettie Lee Grbavace.

it. He would quickly build our life to the brink of success and then disappointingly destroy it overnight so he could begin building it back again. It was like a game of Monopoly in which you constantly "pass Go just for the sake of collecting the two hundred dollars." He was such a genius at survival that he never learned the joy of security. He toggled easily between church choir leader and hustler, Boy Scout master and gambler. He had a selfish heart that was made of gold, and I saw him do a lot of crazy things, but I never saw him "cheat an honest man," and he was never violent or abusive toward us. He was a terrible husband and drove my mother nuts, but he had endearing ways that kept their marriage alive for almost thirty years. However bizarre our world might have been, it was certainly never boring, so I guess in that way maybe he was irreplaceable. And again . . . above all, Daddy Ray was fun.

One evening our family sat down to dinner and we realized we needed bread, so he volunteered to "run down" to the neighborhood store a couple of blocks away and didn't come home for three weeks. But when he did return he brought a damn loaf of bread! He had a boyish sense of humor, was incredibly quick-witted, was a champion bowler who could roller-skate backwards, and with him by my side we achieved our goal to break the Hub City sales record on Girl Scout cookies year after year.

Daddy always took chances, believing things would work out, and most times they did, because they had to. Every year at Christmastime we would hit the road for California to visit his half-brother Oran and my favorite aunt, Aunt Francis. I remember one time we had a car with a huge trunk, half-full of our luggage and the other half-filled with bundles of plastic flags. Along the way, when we would run short of gas money, Daddy would stop and persuade a car dealer to purchase the flags and pay him to hang them from the nearest tall pole. We would carry on in this way until we reached the land of palm trees, where Daddy secured the cash for the vacation from the blackjack tables on a quick AWOL to Vegas, then sold the car we had been driving at a profit and bought another one for the journey home, which he then "flipped" to buy groceries . . . and so on.

By the time I was five years old, Daddy, because he had curtailed his drinking somewhat, had managed to work his way up to owning

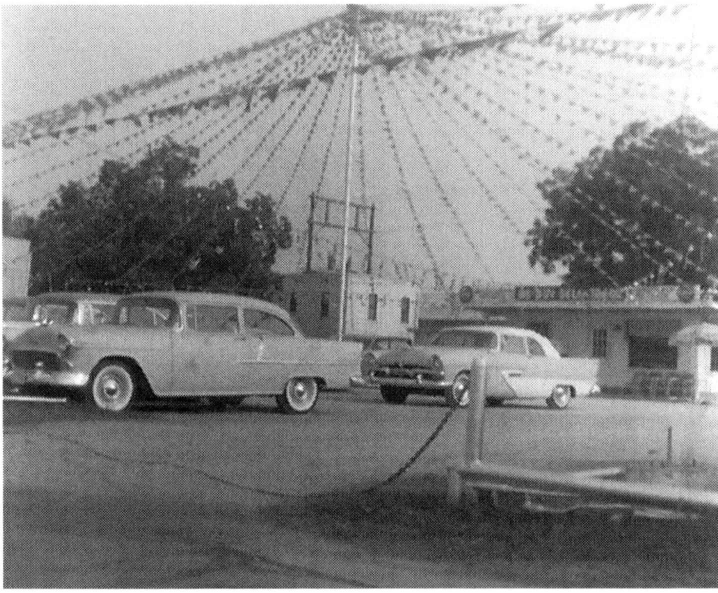

Willingham Motor Company with Ray's flags flapping in the breeze.

a brand-new used car lot! He took great pride in the row of "slick one-owners" and "cherries," with prices and sales slogans cleverly sponged onto the windshields in white shoe polish. (He also brought in money at Christmastime by painting candy canes, reindeer, and Santas, etc., on store windows with tempera paint and canned snow.) Our glistening "spotless," "previously owned," "low mileage" automobiles lined the front of the lot, which was covered by a grand open-air tent made of colorful flags that flapped crisply against the backdrop of a blue sky. Then one day that sky turned a toxic shade of green and a twister spun down from a darkly looming cumulonimbus and blew the hard-earned cars away, rendering our family penniless in the short space of one afternoon.

Quickly, the decision was made to pack and move farther up Tornado Alley to Lubbock, Texas, where my Uncle Les owned a pool hall, the Golden Cue. I've always thought it was a strange decision on Daddy's part that he chose an even more hostile climate, but looking back, it becomes clear that he was naturally lured by the hustling opportunities, and, besides, Lubbock is a peculiar backdrop where strangers go to be friendly with other strangers and prove that a life can be cobbled together out of nothing. So, really, it was perfect.

As luck would have it, Uncle Les was hands-down the most feared and revered pool shark on the Great Plains, so everyone was inclined to put their money on him when bets went down. Since nobody knew that he and Daddy were brothers—initially—Daddy would bet against Les winning so all that was required was for Les to "throw the game," which he was equally skilled at doing. There was no way to lose . . . almost. Daddy came home beaten up pretty badly one time when their hustling was found out. He also came home one Christmas Eve without his shirt and shoes because he had been handing out presents with the Optimist Club and kept giving his clothes away to prove he was "the kind of guy who would give you the shirt off his back." Seems like I can count on one hand the times Daddy ever arrived home in any normal way!

Aunt Gladys and a few other ragtag friends soon followed us to Lubbock, and before long we had another new world of our own. Daddy sold advertising by presenting samples from a leather case, hustled pool, offed the occasional used car, took illegal football bets in backrooms and bars, and studied in the evenings for a real estate license. My mom worked at the telephone company, and I began my longed-for first year of school at Dupre Elementary.

WHEN I WAS A GIRL, my mother, the bedrock of my reality, would take a yearly trip to Dallas for a three-week Bell Telephone Company training seminar. A disturbing insecurity crept into my young soul as we steered down the windblown stretch to the Lubbock Municipal Airport. As I rode quietly in the backseat beside my brother, I gamed a means to distraction by turning my head in sync to row after row after row of cotton plants, discovering that, if perfectly timed, you could see straight down each line. Once we'd reached the tiny airfield I clung to the chain-link fence watching Mama's thick but shapely legs in patent noir stilettos click down the tarmac and mount the stairs to disappear into the hull of a silver plane. She was so beautiful, clothed in

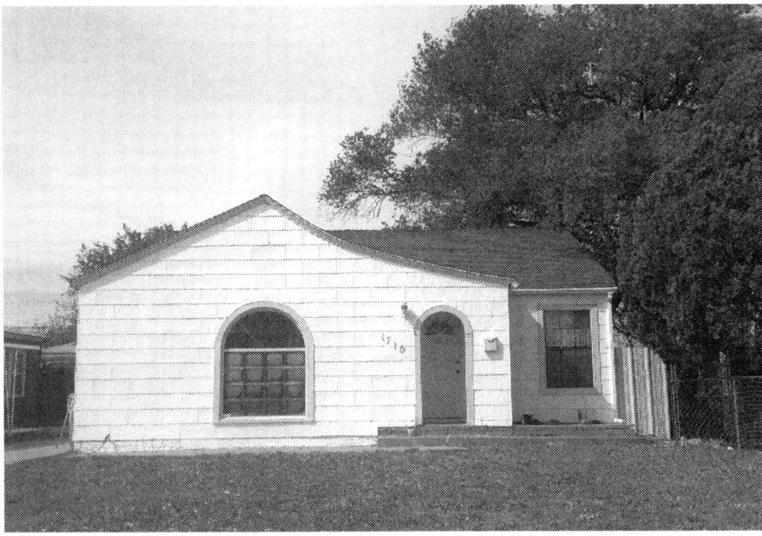

Kimmie's childhood home in Lubbock, Texas.

her excitement, impeccably fitted business suit, jet black curly hair, red lips, sexy silk stockings, and never-quite-voguish-but-well-organized purse. I loved my mother so very much.

Back in the car her scent still filled the air, although the world seemed to have taken on an entirely different atmosphere, one of danger and intrigue. My father's anima was suddenly on holiday, signaled by a loosened necktie and a dreamy face with a Lucky Strike dangling from the corner of his lips. Riding shotgun in the front seat, I watched with a slightly raised brow as he switched on the radio, allowing a '60s country croon to enter the smoky air. We arrived back to a home now void of a chaperone. Mama had instructed me to be the woman of the house while she was away. At six years of age I had no idea how to "be a woman," but I was working on it in the back of my mind, determined to stand and deliver, once I had it wired. Hamburgers and french fries were eaten, and I cleared the greasy bags responsibly. Then unexpectedly, Daddy, the sole heir to my safekeeping, kissed me on the forehead and left.

My memory skips past most of however my brother Mike and I must have filled the evening hours and zooms to one magical moment that usually happened around 3:00 a.m. all of the nights until the relief

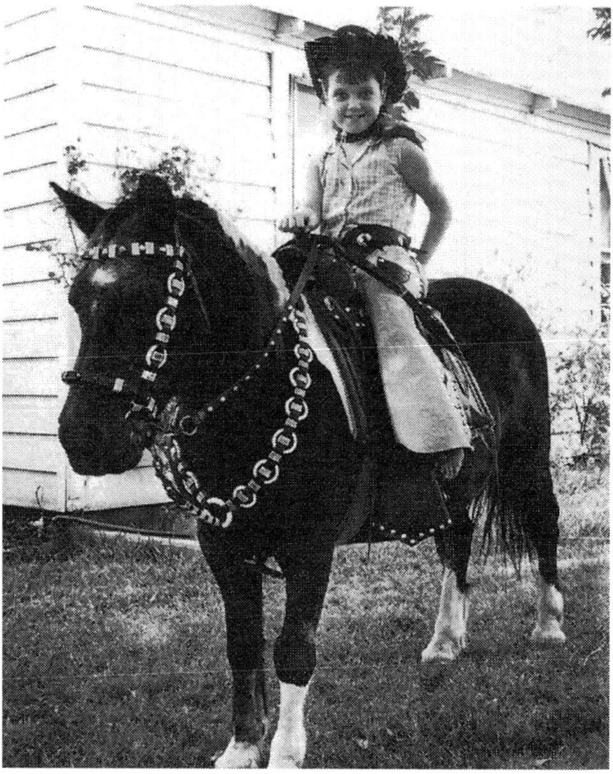

Little Cowgirl Kimmie.

of Mama's return. Mike would eventually put himself to bed in our shared room in the back of the house, but I was frightened, so I left the too-vividly bright ceiling light burning and took to my hiding place between my parents' bed and the wall to stare, facing the fan-shaped window of the exterior door to await Daddy's safe return from the honky-tonk on the edge of town. Lubbock had synchronized trains that rocked through, whistling the passing of each hour, so if you kept track you would know the time. It was a sound for which there is no good word, so much deeper and more lucid than "so lonesome I could cry." I kept count, understanding nothing of bar time, of course, but some internal clock trained me to know when it was okay to surrender to a dizzy, knowing that Daddy would soon be home. Sitting in silence, listening as the night trains passed, wonderfully alive, autonomous, and almost painfully self-aware, I witnessed my own ageless mystery to the ticking by of the stars outside the glass. I hummed and thought and hummed and watched the white door and came to know my heart as I slipped through the mystical space between wake and sleep.

In what eventually turned out to be forty-three years of faithful service to the company, Mama received a grandfather clock as a reward of perfect attendance, which still stands beside my front door, testifying to the uncanny fact that she was never once late and never missed a single day of work.

HAVING NEVER HAD A ROLE MODEL, my dad had to rely on basic instincts for parenting skills, so when I was around six years old, about the same as he had been when he was orphaned and living on the streets, he studied me to see what strengths I might possess that could be relied upon should the same fate befall me. (To his credit it worked, because I rely on those strengths in my job to this day!) I was constantly chirping hymns and old folk songs and making up my own tunes about whatever was happening in the present moment. So Daddy polished a couple of the favorites in my young repertoire, one being the traditional gospel song "Old Rugged Cross," and started taking me with him on his rounds to car lots, which were also fronts for illegal bookmaking establishments. I was placed outside as a foil to distract and charm salesmen and their customers, singing for ten cents per song, while he checked gambling bets in the back office. My career status soon grew into lead singer for a gospel trio with Daddy and Mike, performing at nursing homes, civic events, and church gatherings. I sang in the choir at church and school and learned to read music and sing harmony parts.

I stumbled into my first paid gig at a bank lobby in Lubbock. My third-grade choir was rehearsing for the Christmas show, and I burst into full alto harmony at the end of "O Come All Ye Faithful," having learned the part in church. I thought I was in trouble because the teacher asked me to stay after class, so I was really surprised when she cut a slit in a sequined reindeer covered tablecloth, dropped it over my head "poncho style," and whisked me away to a bank to sing

"Little Drummer Boy." Back in those days people still smoked cigarettes indoors. (Even the doctor might be smoking during an office visit!) The picture in my mind of that event is like a smoky movie set, as, singing, I gaze through a layer of drifting smoke past the red velvet bows on the office Christmas tree into a roomful of admirers. Orphans in attendance from a local foster home are presented with gifts labeled "girl" or "boy." I'm given a gift labeled with my name, so I count my blessings. I count the five one-dollar bills I'm given for performing a single song, when my price up to that point has been ten cents per song. I'm told I can keep the wardrobe and am given the rest of the afternoon off of school with no make-up work. It was my first taste of how suddenly, magically, life can turn on a dime. It was my first taste of stardom.

WHEN I WAS AN INFANT, barely two weeks old, my mother, the breadwinner of the family at that time, had been forced to hand me over every morning so she could go to her job. One of my earliest memories is of a large, plastic, yellow radio that sat in the pass-through window between the kitchen and dining room of the humble but comfortable home where I spent weekdays with my babysitter, Bobby Carol.

I was extremely fortunate to have fate land me in her arms. Bobby was a paradox, a magnificently uncomplicated person with an ocean for a soul, one of those rare spirits so centered in her desires and beliefs that she could manage to have the same basic temperament everyday—neither moody nor morose nor overly dramatic. Whether happy or sad as she dodged "the slings and arrows of outrageous fortune" that life fires at even a lowly wife and mother of two young boys, she was never knocked from her horse. Bobby Carol sang the popular tunes of the day while baking homemade pies and biscuits. From the speakers of the yellow radio, Buddy Holly—who had already died in the fateful plane crash by then—immortally sang along with her to "That'll Be the Day" and "Peggy Sue." She had a rich alto voice, and I followed her lead, parroting the harmony parts as if they were melody.

I didn't play house with my dolls. I didn't fantasize that I was their mommy, and I quickly lost interest in the mundane tasks of feeding, burping, and changing the diapers of an inanimate child. I spent lots of time sitting on the kitchen floor at Bobby's feet (which she referred to as "in her hair"), threading needles with colorful spools from my sewing box, piecing together scraps of fabric, fashioning dresses for my dolls, and singing along with Bobby and Buddy. I studied her hands and methods as she picked the purple Concord grapes from the backyard fence and made jelly, cooked meals, and burned trash in a strange little kitchen fireplace. I loved to watch her tackle the piles of ironing she took in to earn a nickel per piece, sprinkling them with water from a coke bottle and making them sizzle until crisply perfect, before hanging them on metal hangers.

Her domestic chores were endless, and I mimicked her characteristic way of brushing her bangs aside with the back of her hand to wipe the sweat from her forehead as she worked. Once a month she would curl her hair, put on lipstick and perfume (purchased from the Avon lady who would visit the house from time to time), slip on a homemade flowered cotton dress with a full skirt and belted waist, and load me into the blue T-bird convertible, which she named "My Pride and Joy." We would drive downtown to several local businesses—the gas, electric, and telephone companies—because oddly she preferred to pay the bills in person rather than mail them. I lived for this day and sometimes came home with a new toy from the drugstore or got to have ice cream in a waffle cone.

I don't recall my role model sitting to rest, although she would pop up and down, sort of putting in an appearance of having a meal while waiting the table at breakfast and lunch. Bobby's husband, Clyde, was the good-humored, warm-hearted, hardworking, well-respected master of the household. He worked as an operator at the oil refinery down the road in Wichita Falls, the smallish North Texas town where I was born. Clyde was delightfully playful and fun to be with at breakfast, but mostly he wasn't around much on weekdays because he was either at work or often sleeping from having worked the night shift, which they called "the hoot." Not often, but some days, he would stay home and build grandfather clocks in his woodworking shop and let me hang out and piece scraps of wood together with excessive amounts of Elmer's glue.

There was, as in most houses of that time, a formal living room, oddly named because it went unoccupied for the most part unless one was perusing the *National Geographic* magazine collection, decorating the Christmas tree, being seen by the family doctor making an occasional house call, or greeting the rare guest who was too special to be invited into the room off the kitchen area, where all the real living took place and where cartoons were watched every morning. Sometimes, out of the blue and always when just the two of us were alone in the house in the afternoons because the older kids were off at school, a rare and beautiful hour would occur. Bobby would finally take a break, seating herself on the swiveling stool of the ornate pump organ, which was the centerpiece of the room.

I would prop myself against the wall and watch quietly and in awe as she transformed from the hardworking substitute mother in a home-sewn apron into an angel who brought down a curious and powerful magic by way of the tones exhaled from her chest and the bellows of the fascinating instrument. As she rocked back and forth, pumping with her feet, manipulating the keys and stops with her elegant work-worn hands, she and the organ became one, and I followed her as we drifted into a time continuum that was very different from the usual task-based routine into a place where everything—the timbre of her voice, the overtones from the organ, and the air that surrounded each note—hung absolutely still in the vibrating air that filled the room. It was a truly holy experience, although the pieces she played were not always hymns.

Show tunes and campfire cowboy songs were decoded from the curious math, black-and-white spaces, lines and circles, and sophisticated symbols scripted inside paper sheet-music folders decorated with colorful and clever covers. I would practice drawing G and treble clefs, notes and rests on black lines intermingled with crayon daisies, and houses and sunshines with faces and rays for hair and eyelashes. "What a Friend We Have in Jesus," "Tumbling Tumbleweed," "Pennies from Heaven," "Stardust," trippy and wonderful words and melodies took us far away from anything ordinary and normal, songs and songs and songs! So I discovered that this new hidden realm existed and began to make up my own songs and found that by singing, whatever was happening—whether playing or bathing or even drifting off to sleep—innocently I could filter reality back into that magical, still place where what is happening can be named and better understood by way of a childhood form of alchemy, where the metal of lower-middle-class life becomes gold.

My mind developed and learned to work in this way as a child, and to this day when I am off in that place, people tell me they say things to me several times before I hear them. My own children laugh and tease me about how they became accustomed to having to bring me back from there to tell me something by finally yelling, "MAMA!" I've heard it referred to as "having your head in the clouds." I call it "writing," although there are no pen and paper involved. To write poems you have to dig under the surface of thoughts and find an irony that's buried slightly beneath the obvious, and I'm hooked on thinking in this way. Somewhere on a level just below every single thing, the meaning of life is hidden, and it's a poet's job to find it and bring it into the daylight and show truths to the world. This is the stuff that real songs are made of. That's why the simplest lyrics can have such profound impact: "Row, row, row your boat, gently down the stream, merrily, merrily, merrily, merrily, life is but a dream" or "let me take you down 'cause I'm going to Strawberry Fields, nothing is real" or "his clothes are dirty but his hands are clean and you're the best thing that he's ever seen."

One day my birthday came, and Mama, who was always observantly in support of where my little heart was headed, gifted me with a prized possession called "The Magic Mirror Movies." Produced by a company called Red Raven, this contraption—a faceted, mirrored carousel with a wooden red ball finial on top—when positioned on the center of special records, displayed three-dimensional, full-color movies based on illustrations of songs that were especially written and recorded and labeled for the cool toy. A red raven always showed up in the scene in subtle ways, along with frogs, ducks, trains, boats, teapots, soldiers, cowboys, Indians, and any other fantasy that the songwriter might have imagined in the lyrics of the tunes. The dining room just off the kitchen had an unattractive paisley gray-green floor covering that was cool in summer. So, I suppose, much like a dog does, I migrated to a spot in the dining room next to an electrical outlet and lay there all afternoon listening and watching these "before their time" music videos to the smell of Bobby Carol's southern-fried cuisine wafting over the yellow radio in the pass-through (now silenced by this new gadget), while Bettie Lee worked at the telephone company as an operator to earn more money for delightful things.

The music from the radio, the pump organ music sessions, and the songs we sang in church were the first songs to which I was exposed, but what was more affecting about these records is that they were composed especially for children my age and with the same imagery and themes that had been occurring in my own imagination as I sang my little reality into the atmosphere and beyond, joyfully expressing and unwittingly moseying into a foggy future. There could not be a heaven more lasting or meaningful than the days I spent with my face pressed to the refreshing linoleum, learning songs and watching as drummers drummed, ballerinas pirouetted, chocolate rabbits danced with little girls while fishes swam and cowboys lassoed mooing cows, all just beyond the fourth wall of the looking-glass world inside my wonderful Magic Mirror record player.

Bobby had two sons, Jack and Billy, and I had my brother, Mike. They were all quite a bit older than I was and were usually in school. There was a darkened boyish room (think Roy Rogers bedspread) that belonged to Billy, just off the dining room. As part of a strategy to keep me out of his room, he had warned me that there was a boogeyman lurking behind the curtain that covered the door of his disheveled clothes closet. I guess Bobby was unaware that said beast was living in there because she started putting me down for a nap on the bed in that room. I lay quietly with the open window at the head of the bed and stared through a peephole in the bedsheet at the curtain, afraid the horrible man would do I knew not what (because I had not been told) to me if I dared sleep. Mostly I think I dreaded having to see what he looked like, whether he actually did me harm or not, as I planned my screaming escape out the window to the neighbor's house next door should it ever happen. Some days it would rain, and I watched giant dancing drops hit the dry street outside the window, gracing the room with a heady scent that I would imagine drove him back into the darkest corner of the closet. Eventually, I decided that if he hadn't by now,

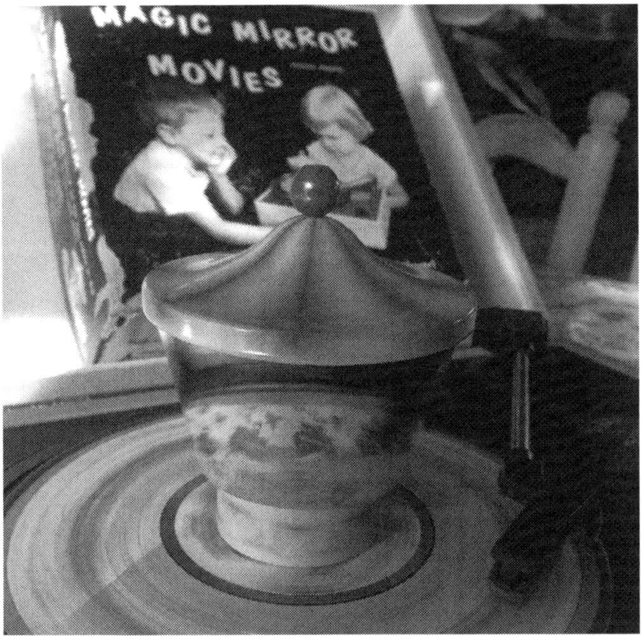

The Magic Mirror record player.

he wasn't ever coming out of there. Bored but still on guard, I became brave enough to have a look around the forbidden zone.

Hidden between the mattress and springs I uncovered a cartoon magazine called *Mad*. It featured this funny-looking fellow named Alfred who could transform his face to look like different people but still somehow manage to look like himself. He was obviously making fun of people, but he always had a not-so-mean, big, toothy smile on his lumpy face. I'm not sure what it was about the magazine that held my interest but I flipped through all the pages, studying the drawings of cartoons that were too sophisticated for me to understand.

One day I wandered into Billy's room and there was an acoustic guitar lying on the bed. I was too small to hold it the way I had seen singing cowboys on television do, so I sat beside it and plucked a string. I did it again, noticing how long it took the sound to disappear back into silence. I experimented with plucking different strings with various intensities, gauging the time. I plucked two at a time, discovering that some combinations made pleasant sounds and some didn't. I hummed along, making different notes with my voice that either did or didn't fall into the sound correctly, adjusting until it sounded good to me. I started plucking the strings in patterns I memorized and without really realizing it, practiced the tunes I invented, enjoying the way the sound of the notes drifted around in the air before disappearing back into the empty space from where they had come. Later I would understand that this is the place from where life itself like a note plucked from a string slips forth and then returns.

Instruments, including the human voice, which is the most soulful of all because it is filtered through the heart, are like tarot cards or Ouija boards, a way to unlock the realm beneath the veil and momentarily release secrets about the mystery, whether named in poetry or in feeling tones that speak just as loudly (think *Moonlight Sonata*). I sometimes wonder if we are already born who we will eventually grow up to be and if birth places us exactly where we are supposed to be at exactly the perfect moment in time to accomplish some cosmic back room bargain reached just before we were born.

Whatever choices are made that shape the world, is there is something numinous going on all the time that plucks the strings as the deal goes down, making it impossible to irrevocably "screw things up" so long as we learn something? The question "What is the meaning of life?" in scientific terms is not even a well-posed question because no thing can ever be proven. Why do we even have a thing called life? Do we live many lives in infinite time, each time taking away one small concentrated notch on our soul for a lifetime spent chipping away at it? Do we live to learn to love over and over and over? Thankfully for me, music is the trick that keeps the monster in the closet so that I am forever safe to explore the room.

I FIRST HEARD ABOUT HEAVEN in Wichita Falls, Texas, attending worship services at 23rd and Grace, the Church of Christ, where my babysitter took me as a child. If you were "good" during your lifetime, then on some undisclosed day, a shout would unexpectedly come from the sky and angels would begin playing harp music to awaken your and others' spirits, which could then rise up from their graves and drift to

"The Promised Land," where heaven was located. Once you had arrived at "The Pearly Gates," you were screened by a saint named Peter, who checked "The Book of Life" to be sure you were where you belonged. If indeed you were on the list and gained clearance, greatly relieved, you were welcomed through the gates onto gold-paved streets into the most beautiful place you could imagine, where you could then spend eternity in a blissful garden setting among departed loved ones and docile beasts. Once I had gotten my head as best I could around a time continuum with no end—ever—my small mind moved forward, delighted and amused by trying to picture paradise.

After we moved to Lubbock, our religious denomination changed to Southern Baptist, Mama's preference. Then the sacred hymns we sang could be accompanied by the funky sounds of a Hammond organ, but the tone of the sermons became threatening and grim. One Sunday morning the preacher chose "The Judgment Day" as his topic. Repeatedly slamming the Holy Bible on the pulpit in dramatically timed intervals and screaming in rehearsed vocals that rose and fell like Beethoven's Fifth Symphony, the scary man with the wildly flailing pompadour spoke not of a land of hope and wonder but of a hell, where there was "weeping and gnashing of teeth" and a "brimstone fire" that mysteriously never quite consumed your melting flesh completely so as to wrench you with pain for (again) . . . eternity . . . meaning forever. To make matters worse, the Devil, a clever, mean guy who tricked you into going there, stoked the furnace. The day when this hell was to begin was apparently the same day as the shout and harp music one that was to send the good souls drifting off to heaven, but now it had a name: Judgment.

Having been uprooted and moved to the Texas Plains less than a year before by the destructive results of tornadic winds, I was immersed in fearful contemplation as we left the church that day. During the two-hour drive to Aunt Gladys's house in Odessa, where we were to dine, I vowed to myself never to do one bad thing ever again that might anger God and his son, Jesus, whom up until then I'd always thought loved me.

While the meal was being prepared, I wandered outside onto the covered back porch of the house, which faced a vast expanse of plowed flatland that would have stretched all the way to the horizon had it not been interrupted by a roiling black cloud peculiar to arid regions and known as a haboob. Driven by cold fronts from the easterly winds, these dreaded monsters overtake a sunny day like a freight train gathering every grain of stray dirt that has been kicked up by cultivation for the springtime planting of cotton, which is the mainstay of the Great Plains economy.

Staring in quizzical amazement at the rapidly approaching phenomenon, it began to dawn on me that I was standing directly in the pathway of something biblical that was about to happen. The fact that I'd been deeply pensive for the past several hours was not lost on my big brother, who was a professional opportunist when it came to torturing me. Lounging on the porch swing, he nonchalantly remarked, "Oops! Looks like Judgment Day is here!" Mobilized by the shocking realization that I wouldn't after all be having the time I'd counted on all afternoon to repent for my sins, I hit the screen door to the kitchen and began circling the table, which had been set for lunch, crying in horror, "The end is here! The end is here! It's the end of time! It's Judgment Day! We are all going to hell!!! Run!!!!!"

My parents, unaware of the approaching calamity, tried to calm me, but by then the storm had begun hitting the house. Cracking lightning bolts rattled the windows as gigantic mud globs mixed with golf-ball-sized hail pummeled Gladys's vulnerable rent house, smacking the roof with a vengeance that only God could rain down on us wicked people trapped inside. Hiding beneath the table, eyes closed in prayer, and shaking uncontrollably, visions of ghosts rising from nearby graveyards underscored by haunting harp melodies rendered me inconsolable as I waited for the earth to open and receive us all, especially my dad and brother, into the fiery depths.

Mercifully, and most probably because my repentant shrieks were heard on high, we were spared, and soon the sun was shining again and the few trees that existed in the Panhandle glistened with raindrops as we headed home, leaving the past stretching safely behind us. Monday morning, the first day of the rest of our lives, was just a short night's sleep away and there would be all the time in the world to try to be better people.

In the days following my divine forgiveness, as we drove down Broadway Street in downtown Lubbock, I imagined a magnificent

"West Texas Heaven," because that was the only landscape I had ever known. The bricks that paved the street (which I had been told were laid by prisoners) were solid gold, and the park at Buffalo Lakes was lush with flowers, like in the Garden of Eden. My favorite place in the city, Prairie Dog Town, was running with lions that would gladly and peacefully lie down with the tiny mound-dwelling creatures, as well as any lambs that might come along.

This became the inspiration in later years for a love song I wrote about leaving those innocent days behind. It became the title track of an album that featured duets with Willie Nelson, Waylon Jennings, and Townes Van Zandt, recorded at Willie's Pedernales Studio, just outside of Austin, Texas, and Jack Clement's Cowboy Arms Hotel and Recording Spa in Nashville, Tennessee. It was the first recording session my son and producer, Gabriel Rhodes, ever played with me, and the signature guitar part that he created for the intro set the tone for the entire track and made the song unique. One day out of the blue, my publicist received a call from the producer of David Letterman's show asking that I play "West Texas Heaven" on the famous *Late Night* show at his request, so I took Gabriel with me to perform with the stellar house band.

As I stood singing my song on the stage of that famous theater in New York City where the Beatles had played their American debut on the *Ed Sullivan Show*, I remembered the night I sat cross-legged on the floor in our little house on 27th Street in Lubbock watching. I realized I was standing in roughly the same spot John Lennon had stood crooning, "She loves you, yeah, yeah, yeah." Thank heaven that now "the most beautiful place I can imagine" looks more like somewhere along the French Riviera!

WEST TEXAS HEAVEN

I left West Texas Heaven, it was the only one I'd ever known
I've been on the road down here driving with my blinders on
All life was to me was like a truck stop where you want to stay
I never even saw it when you built your dream right in my way
No, I just passed on through like a lonely town

Playing in my head I heard this music like a radio
In another town somebody turned on somewhere down the road.
Everywhere I turned I tuned in something that you had to say.
Your signal never cleared so I guess it matters that you're so far away.
So, I just kept on going like a lonely town.

I left West Texas Heaven, no, I guess I'm never goin' back that way.
Did your love get lost, or, Baby, did your love just get misplaced?
Everywhere I go the ghost of you just follows me
And everywhere I go I hear you whisper down my empty streets
And everywhere I go looks like a lonely town.

MANY FAMOUS AND INFAMOUS musicians have come from Lubbock, Buddy Holly, of course, being the most celebrated, but also Waylon Jennings, Roy Orbison, Delbert McClinton, Joe Ely and fellow Flatlanders Butch Hancock and Jimmie Dale Gilmore, Terry Allen, and Natalie and Lloyd Maines, to name but a few. In my song "Windblown," I sing, "Why anyone lives on the plains, there ain't nobody knows." Why the Great Plains has given rise to a constellation of songwriters there also "ain't nobody knows," but there has been a lot of speculation. One of my favorite theories is that when we were children, we were encouraged by our mothers to run and play in the spray from the massive DDT trucks that constantly trolled the streets spewing forth toxins.

Encephalitis lethargica is a disease, which described medically "attacks the brain, leaving some of its victims in a statue-like condition, speechless and motionless." Between 1915 and 1926, an epidemic spread around the world, so my mother's generation would have still been reeling with fear from legends of how even one tiny mosquito bite could instantly take down a frolicking child. The potential to arouse excitement in our community incited by the hiss of one of these virus busters approaching from the distance was second only to the musical sounds of the ice cream truck on a summer afternoon. The more logical explanation for talent coming from the area during the '50s–'70s might also be attributed to not only the pre–video game battle against pubescent boredom but also the delightful abundance of good programming across the dial in all genres during an age when rock 'n' roll had just been born and radio had yet to lose its innocence by way of the commercial hijacking that took place once it came to be considered a viable "product" by big business.

I grew to be a quite street savvy teenager, having been well mentored by Daddy Ray. I was proud to have the rare "cool dad" who was willing to score alcohol for my underage friends. The devout Southern Baptists in the community had arranged it so that no alcohol could be legally sold within the city limits, so anyone who wished to imbibe had to drive outside of town (through a deadly traffic circle that had been strategically placed) in order to finally arrive at a location where beer, barbeque, and sinning did abound at a joint called Pinkie's.

Once the liquor for the weekend partying was secured, payback always began with the statement, "I need to check my crops, Baby," although he was by no means a farmer. The local economy depended entirely on agriculture, meaning hours had to be spent drinking and driving past miles and miles of the monotonous rows of cotton. It was during this seemingly wasted time that a priceless education in country music appreciation was forced upon me. I was a hippie chick geared up and ready to get back into town and dig to the Stones and Zeppelin et al., but song after song after row after row after song after song, Hank Williams, Lefty Frizzell, Johnny Cash, Loretta Lynn, Charley Pride, Ray Price, Buck Owens, Jerry Lee Lewis broadcast incessantly across the plains through the dashboard's blown speakers. Daddy would plead, "Just listen to this, Baby! These songs have words that say something!" as we listened to George Jones croon, "Take me to Siberia coldest weather of the wintertime. It would be just like spring in California just as long as I knew you were mine." Sigh . . . what would I give to be back there now to cruise along listening to a great country classic and have the chance to thank him for ignoring my tragic hipness and preparing me for the unimaginable life that lay ahead?

WINDBLOWN

Written by Kimmie in memory of Daddy Ray

It's too hot for the corn and the grain
And the cotton's not gettin' much rain
And why anyone lives on the Plains there ain't nobody knows
Winters that seem not to end
Go out like a lion and then
Springtime comes stragglin' in all windblown
And it's a welcomed sight for sore eyes but it's all windblown

Do you think it's unkind to suppose
That a desert's no home for a rose?
I guess I'll always wish I could know things that you never told me
Sometimes it's so real I could swear
That I can see you standing right there
With the sand in your eyes and your hair all windblown
What a welcomed sight you would be tonight all windblown

There's a whisper I hear on the breeze
It's like a ghost and it drifts through the trees
And oh, it's like a song that somebody sings and nobody knows it
A dust devil danced down the street
It gathered the trash and the leaves
And like a gift it just fell at my feet all windblown
What a treasure your memory is even if it's all windblown

3

GROOVER'S PARADISE

JOE GRACEY

I HAD PLAYED IN BANDS, worked on the radio, produced records in my free time, and written a column for the high school paper by the time I enrolled as a freshman at the University of Texas, in the School of Communication (since I had already been on the air for three years at that point and was now a DJ on an Austin rock station and the rock music writer at the *Austin American-Statesman*). When I made a C in Communications 101 because it was so incredibly deadly dull and pointless, I became an American Studies major. At the time, I didn't have enough snap, and nobody ever counseled me to consider changing my major to Cultural Anthropology so I could study folk music, which would have at least made sense.

I tried so hard to do the frat thing, but it was just awful. When they started talking about hazing and how three days in the basement being paddled and egged and diapered and "pushupped" to death would make us "bond as a pledge class," I just said, "You know, I have this really cool gig on the radio every day and plenty of girlfriends already, a rock 'n' roll band, and a convertible T-bird, and I don't think I need you guys to make me cool. You'll just have to go on without me, I guess. They sent an older guy up to my room to try to talk me out of de-pledging, and I just sat there and looked at him like he was crazy. When he left I went out, got in my car, and drove out into the night, feeling free for the first time in my life.

Obviously, there were good people in that scene. I really dug some of the girls I met at the mixers, or whatever those parties were called that we had with all the sororities. They always put me with one of the older girls, I guess 'cause I seemed more serious or something, and the girl would always be taken aback and insulted that I was a freshman, but I would work hard to loosen her up and we'd end up having fun.

I think what I finally recoiled from was the artificiality of the thing. I am just not a person who can "network" or look forward in time to a day when it would be useful to know somebody for that purpose. I understand the concept and the reason for it all, but I am just too much of a loner and a free-floater to care about that kind of thing. I was almost physically incapable of doing it.

My parents had a fit. I was dashing their dreams. It was as if they had become "well off" lawyers so that I could enter the elite cadre of Texas high "muckety-mucks," and I shook it off to slink back into the gutters and play music. It was a problem that would not be solved until I got cancer and nothing else mattered at that point.

So, I'd come to Austin in 1969 to attend UT, which I did. I also worked in Top 40 radio at KNOW-AM and then album rock at KRMH-FM. I was the first DJ at KRMH-FM to play the *Shotgun Willie* album because when the station got a promotional copy, I was the only DJ there who had any idea who Willie Nelson was. And then I fell in love with the people at Armadillo World Headquarters and became their radio producer and "voice." Eddie Wilson, the head honcho there, conceived of a plan to pair Willie Nelson with Michael Martin Murphey for a tour of Texas after Willie played the Armadillo to great response. At this time I had the rock column in the *Austin American-Statesman,* and I used it as a bully pulpit to preach the virtues of Willie to the hippies and to challenge the local media to air more Austin music, which resulted in my being hired as talent coordinator for *Austin City Limits.*

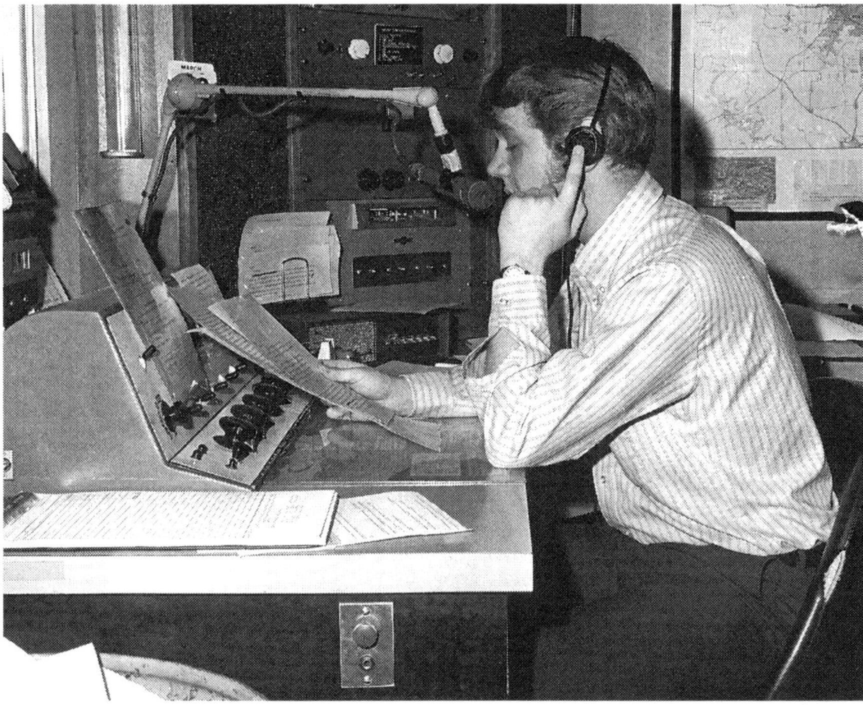

Gracey at KNOW-AM, Austin, Texas.

Austin in '72–'73 was a place of incredible ferment. We had the sense of reclaiming a part of our musical heritage, which had been "taken" from us during the war/hair/politics schism between the Texas rednecks and the Texas liberals. We more or less refused to let Merle Haggard keep us away from our rightful Texas music roots, that is, Wills, Tubb, Jones, Lefty, Thompson, et al., and bands like Freda and the Firedogs and Greezy Wheels were doing country through a hippie filter, taking a cue from Willie, who insisted on being both hip and country. Sociologists have a name for what we were doing. It's called Hansen's Law of the Third Generation, I believe. The first generation does things a certain way—maybe they are immigrants or new arrivals to an area—and things get done in a sort of basic and soulful way. The next generation wants to distance itself from the old ways and generally screws everything up and you have stuff like frozen dinners and Melmac dinnerware and all that awful '50s and early '60s nonsense. The third generation realizes that something precious has been lost and tries to revive and preserve and renovate the positive things in the first generation's lives. We truly believed that we were on a kind of holy mission, or at least I did.

There were many nights in Austin dives where Jerry Wexler would watch from a wobbly table as Doug Sahm and Marcia Ball and Willie traded the mic and literally created a new Texas music out of the fabric of the '50s and '60s sounds we grew up with. Nothing was left out or ignored—the blues, Gulf Coast, T-Bone, Wills, Hopkins, Lipscomb, Flaco, Lefty, Jones, Houston Cajuns, mariachi, Guthrie, Holly—it all went into the mix. What emerged was roots music, which we were trying to preserve against the barbarians who will always try to tear down, disown, and downplay the roots of their own culture.

Anyway, Wilson and I and several other people met and came up with a radio format that would model itself after what was already happening in the Austin live music scene with Freda, Greezy Wheels, Willie, and many others. Wilson pitched this idea to the management at KOKE-FM in '73, where there was an FM frequency being wasted on miscellaneous trash programming. (This was still before anybody played country music on FM.) They liked the idea, but they didn't especially like us, since we were sort of uppity hippies with pretty firm ideas on how we would do things, and they grabbed another guy who was more malleable (to put it charitably) and told him to do it. I later joined KOKE-FM as the midday DJ and resident bad boy who was a real pain in the backside but had too good of ratings to fire, even though I deserved it many times.

Eventually I became program director, but by then I was itching to get out of radio and do something else. In addition, they turned the station into a normal country outlet, and that was that. I realized then that I had no business being anybody's boss, period. KOKE-FM was not only the first progressive country station; we were also the most free-form one, and I was playing everything from Lightnin' Hopkins to Bob Wills to Willie to the Rolling Stones and somehow getting away with it. After it died, radio pretty much all went to formats and those weird groups that sit around wired up to a machine that tells the radio people whether a song is a hit or not, garbage like that, which has clearly ruined radio and caused it to become a grisly wasteland, playing pre-chewed phony music and being run by payola, which is now legal, by the way. Not all stations mind you, but most of them.

So KOKE-FM was the radio reflection and embodiment of that attempt to enshrine our roots and combine all the various Texas sounds into a new synthesis. I was on the radio for four hours per day, being as outrageous as I possibly could. I was a local celeb in the clubs and eating joints. I ate chicken-fried steak or enchiladas every day. I was the emcee at Willie's picnics and would hang out in the studio with Doug Sahm and Roky Erickson and Ry Cooder. I wrote for *Picking Up the Tempo* and the *Austin Sun*. Everybody was into free sex; good, cheap Mexican weed; cold Pearl and Shiner beer; and swimming naked together. Girls loved me. Musicians loved the fact that I would play them on the radio just because I thought the record was good, if you can imagine that. Armadillo was hosting everybody that I was playing on my radio show, and we were making tapes of a lot of it in a studio there and broadcasting it, too. People got to see Sonny Terry and Brownie McGhee and Emmylou with Gram Parsons, and it was just completely wonderful and perfect and glorious. Leon Russell played, Willie and Waylon, and Jerry Lee, and all of them got a shot at a whole new audience there. Freddie King had a second career there.

DOUG SAHM CALLED AUSTIN "Groover's Paradise," and he hit it right on the nose. For one little moment there, Austin was about as close to heaven on earth as I imagined it to be. Willie wasn't actually the "leader" of the scene yet, but what he did was kind of mosey around the joints so he could figure out what was going on. He'd show up at a Freda and the Firedogs gig and just kind of be there, and then they'd ask him to sit in and he would, or he'd show up at a Doug Sahm gig at the Split Rail with Wexler. He was unobtrusively obtrusive. However, because he was the biggest songwriter any of us had ever seen, he was clearly the most important industry figure here. But there were a lot of people here, and they each had a sort of crowd or favorite bar and that kind of thing. It wasn't until after Willie began to hit it bigger and do the picnics and stuff that he became the overarching star here.

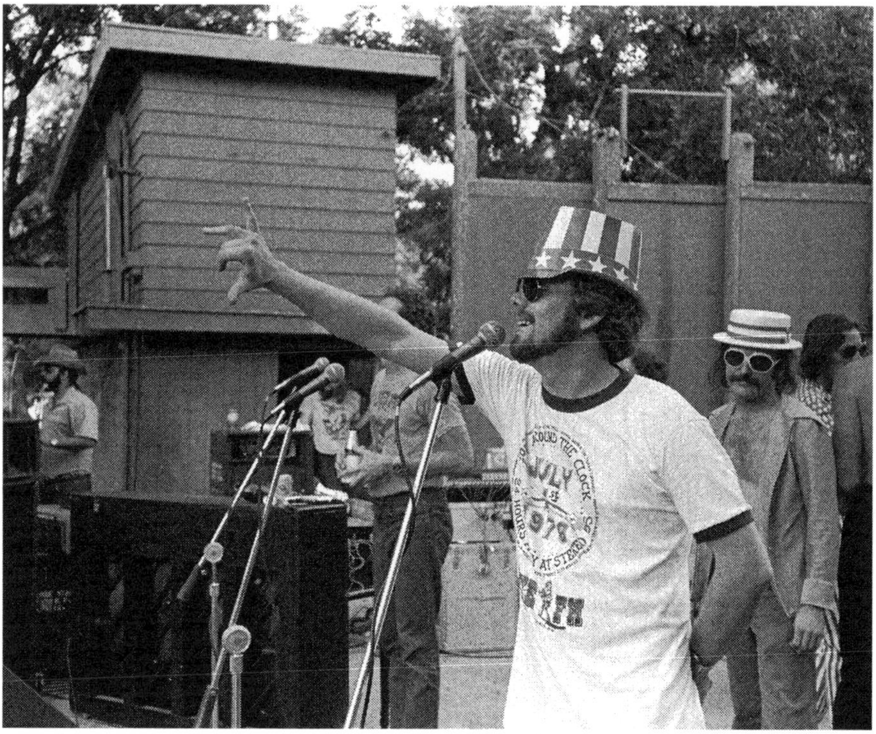

Gracey at Bull Creek, Austin, Texas. Photo by Gary P. Nunn.

I didn't hang around him much in those days, outside of a couple of parties and gigs—lots of gigs. He had a kind of circus going on around him all the time, and I always felt a little bit on the outside of that, but that was probably just my own choice at the time. Paul would come sweeping in, dressed in his devil drag, black cape, and red velvet, all that stuff, and Bee had a rooster that would perch on the head of his bass. Interesting times . . .

I'll admit when I first listened to *Red Headed Stranger,* I thought, "Uh oh, Willie has screwed up this time. This will never sell to the country audience." And of course, "Blue Eyes Crying in the Rain" went on to make him the biggest country star of his generation, which shows what I knew. After that, it was easy to see that he had carved out his own special niche in the world and that he could do just about anything he wanted to then. The huge pop success of "Stardust" was, again, a little bit surprising, but nobody can predict that sort of huge mega-stardom, so I was not alone. By then we all admired Willie almost to the point of worshipping him, in the sense that he had really done it his own way—no more compromises with the industry—and he had continued to stick to his guns. He didn't just talk it. He was doing it.

KOKE-FM DID OKAY IN THE RATINGS, but I have always felt that the Arbitron (ARB) method automatically ruled out most of our audience, because it requires a methodical, stable, orderly life and rather a lot of time on a person's hands to be able to fool with the damn diary at all. We did much better in the other survey, a random phone survey, but the ad agencies used the ARB, and we just didn't get the big national accounts. We got a lot of support from local businesses and Lone Star beer and the clubs. This was when the ratings were still rather

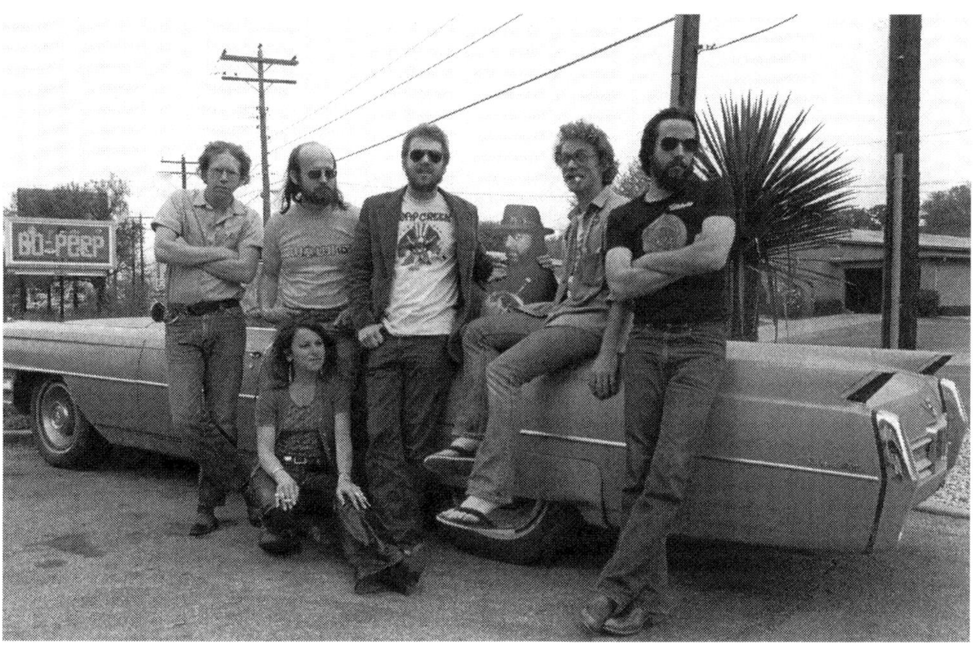

KOKE-FM 1977 staff. Left to right, Nick Spitzer, Dr. Dinger, Kandy Kicker, Ol' Blue Eyes, Chuck Mangione, Marty Manning, Steve Jaxon, Gracey's '62 Cadillac.

monolithic. Anything less than a ten or fifteen share was worthless, and we never rose above six or seven. In narrow demographics, like men eighteen to thirty-four, we were pretty spectacular, but this was before the day of narrow target buying. The ratings eventually killed us off.

Other factors in our demise include burnout (by '77 I was totally worn out from battling management) and loss of format focus. We couldn't quite decide whether to be a rock station that played some country, or the obverse; I opted for the former, but management never liked it, and the sales staff hated it. It became a battle and a general cooling down of the whole progressive country scene here. I went off to pursue a producing career, and KOKE-FM went straight Nashville and cleaned up on the next ARB.

We did many live broadcasts from Armadillo and elsewhere, which we sponsored. (Some of that was taped by Hank Alrich in the studio there.) We also did hundreds of other live broadcasts, some of which were taped and some weren't. Those tapes may or may not exist now.

I can't tell you how demoralizing the KOKE experience was for me. In between all of the great things we were accomplishing, there was a continuous bloody struggle for decent pay, decent treatment (we were treated like some sort of weird animal), decent equipment, more artistic freedom, more promo budget, etc. When I quit they were still paying us some miserable amount, like a hundred fifty dollars a week, and we were all starving to death, blah, blah, blah. It's the old radio story. At least in the '70s it was.

I am not cynical because I still believe there is a place for this format in the world, but I have had painful firsthand experience with being too adventurous in a square world. One reason KOKE ultimately failed was that we demanded too damn much from the audience. We were too diverse and too off-the-wall and just too weird to succeed as a mass market station.

The following is a transcription of an interview conducted by Robert Hall for KUHF radio with Joe Gracey at Steamboat Springs at an Alvin Crow and Leon Rausch show just after Gracey left KOKE-FM.

It all began at a station called KRMH. It was about 1973. At that moment in cosmic time, the Jerry Jeff Walker album came in, the first one on MCA. The Willie Nelson *Shotgun Willie* album came in. The Asleep at the Wheel album came in. I was the music director by some happy accident, nuthin' but a punk, twenty-two years old. It was essentially a rock station. But I said, "Wow, this is great music." So, we started programming Jerry Jeff on MCA, Willie on Atlantic, and Asleep at the Wheel on United Artists. Everybody started howling and puking and mewling as babes in arms and saying, "Oh my God. What is this?!" We got phone calls out the ass! I was working the afternoon drive shift. We had a storm of protest. But I knew, not because I'm smart, but because of my cultural background in country radio in Fort Worth, I sensed this was an occurrence, an event, just like San Francisco in the Psychedelic Era. Just like when Basie and the Boys went to New York in the '30s. I knew this was an event.

I said, "There's something going on here." We started playing progressive country music on a rock 'n' roll AOR radio station, KRMH ("karma"), which at the time was very bizarre because there was no such thing as progressive country. We had no label for it. At that same time, Willie Nelson put on his Dripping Springs Festival in the summer of '72. Willie had also played Armadillo World Headquarters that summer. I played Willie and Asleep and Jerry Jeff during the fall of 1972. Fall of '72 led up to January of '73. So, those records all came out and we got this howl of protests from the listeners, but we knew we were right! Eventually, I was fired because of the inevitability of radio politics. It had nothing to do with the music or the way we were playing it or the "revolution" or any of that stuff. It was a political thing. KOKE went on the air in January of '73 so I went over to KOKE-FM and went on the air.

At that point, the Byrds had made *Sweetheart of the Rodeo*. Crosby, Stills, and Nash had recorded their first album. We had Waylon and *Ladies Love Outlaws*, and Willie had just made his *Shotgun Willie* album.

There was a whole idea going on, where you had people who had previously never considered playing anything but rock 'n' roll now playing country with seriousness. The Byrds' *Sweetheart of the Rodeo* was a great and early breakthrough. KOKE-FM was the first time anybody said, "We are going to create a niche of our own. There's rock 'n' roll over here—AOR as it came to be called—there's country over here, but there's nothing like where we are." It's like the Grateful Dead and Jefferson Airplane and Creedence Clearwater Revival later and whoever else was out there in that thing. And they said, "There is no label for us." It's precisely what happened when Dylan came out and the Byrds played Dylan's music. They had to make up a name for it in *Billboard* magazine. They called it "folk rock." Well somebody has to call what we were doing something, so they called it "progressive country." Well, unhappily or happily enough, that's what they called it.

KOKE-FM rocked on from '73 until the summer of '77, a four-year life, during which we were arrogant enough to believe we could create a niche of our own. Austin had venues—the Armadillo, Castle Creek, Soap Creek Saloon, the Split Rail, the Rome Inn, and the Ritz Theater. At the Ritz, we did many live broadcasts without being able to see the stage! I was up in a little tiny booth in the balcony saying, "Oh my Lord! I can't see the stage!" We had decided the only hope was to create a "place of our own." It happened to be called progressive country.

KOKE-FM was the first neo-revival of Texana. Do you know that in 1935 in Fort Worth, Texas, there was a theater called Casa Mañana . . . with no roof? Under the stars! They had Billy Rose come down from New York and produce a review that was as good as anything that ever happened on Broadway or in L.A. or Chicago . . . a review! With transvestite dancers and girls and feathers and songs and a big band, and Glenn Miller played there!

Texas has always been there. . . . Bob Wills was there. . . . Texas always had boots and hats and bluebonnets and mockingbirds, but they had faded somehow. But that all came back for one brief shining moment. We said, "Wait a minute; we're not going to let it go." Eddie Wilson had more to do with it than anybody else. Eddie convinced the whole world that Texas was back with the Armadillo World Headquarters. So, all of a sudden, we had the revival of bluebonnets and armadillos and boots with high heels and long white tops (like the one I'm wearing right now) and leathers that came from Texas calves and chicken-fried steaks and the appreciation of the things that we have down here! We have a unique culture here in Texas.

The people who pander to the pop culture thing would have you believe that everybody is alike in America. But they are NOT alike. Texas is completely different. As is Tennessee . . . as is Georgia . . . as is California . . . as is Seattle. We are all different. And we will continue to be different. It was merely a search for identity, a search for roots. In 1970 in Texas, we all said, "What are our roots? Where do they lie?" We started trying to find them. KOKE-FM and progressive country and Willie Nelson and Bob Wills and Alvin Crow and fiddle music (like you can hear in the background right now) are all merely the attempt to get back to our Texas roots because they are there and they'll never go away. I'll never be anything but a Texan! I can't help that. I could go through a thousand superficial changes, but I'll never be anything but a Texan.

Now, the second half of that is that, like all movements, just like San Francisco, an energy like that cannot be sustained. Hemingway, in *The Sun Also Rises,* wrote about a Paris that only existed for a brief period of time. Paris in the '20s was a magnificent collection of artists who were all so intense that they all got together and helped each other out. From 1968 until 1976, Austin was the same kind of thing. There was a gathering of the forces. That was "breath one."

Now we're talking about Chapter 2. . . . It couldn't possibly last. There were hippie bands playing country music and a catalyst like Willie Nelson who brought people like Charlie Rich and Kris Kristofferson and George Jones and Waylon Jennings and Leon Russell together in the same place. There was no possible way that that kind of intensity of energy and creativity could last. Everybody gets tired. Everybody wears down. So, as of 1978, the first wave on the beach had worn down.

What you have in Austin now is a bunch of people who have retrenched and pulled back to the point where they say, "The business of making music consists of publishing, writing, recording, and managing. So, you'll see these mundane, day-to-day business activities take place. The important thing is that the creativity is still there. It's not as intense, but it is there, and the spirit of KOKE-FM lives on. The overlords of the music scene would have us believe that all Americans are all alike. The television consciousness, the mass media consciousness would have us believe that we're all alike . . . but we're not. This is Texas. This is the South. We have something to say, and we're going to say it. So we are all consolidating our cultural gains now. We're gonna drop back and we're gonna make records, write music, copyright the music, and make money off of it. I'm sure we'll see as big a renaissance of Texas music as we saw in the days of the Big Bopper and Buddy Holly and Bob Wills.

Alvin Crow is the most incredible, populist symbol of the current Texas common man. We have Townes Van Zandt, Clifton Chenier, Delbert McClinton, Janis Joplin—praise God and bless her heart—who grew up in Port Arthur. The idea exists and it's up to all of us to keep it going. Progressive country was a misnomer. The real name was something like . . . Texas Music . . . or Our Music.

In his own time, Bob Wills was the symbol for the people of the southwest. He was a symbol for the man, the guy who worked his ass off all week and finally on Saturday night he could finally let go of the traces and put the mule in the barn and have a dance. Right now, in Houston, there are a million people who work a job they probably don't like, and on Saturday night they can come in and dance and drink and get high and go crazy, and this cat here . . . this crazy, weird "Okie" playing here tonight is their symbol, their ideal.

And when the intensity of Austin faded a year ago, this being 1978, KOKE-FM folded. It was a beautiful, incredible, impossible dream that crossed all the traditional boundaries of blues and rock and country and conjunto and Cajun music all across Texas. Out of that is the most fertile thing I've ever seen in my life. Somehow out of all this is going to be a synthesis that is going to rock the world. And it becomes the duty, it becomes incumbent on anybody who has anything to do with it to see to it that it happens and that we don't lose the faith.

JOE GRACEY—"BEFORE THE NEXT TEARDROP FALLS"

Doug Sahm, who had been a tireless promoter of this obscure guy, Freddy Fender, for years, had convinced my radio station that this guy, who at best was just a vague memory to anyone by then, was a star. So we brought Fender up here to Austin from his regular club gig in Corpus Christi in 1973 (where he was the local somebody) and had him play at Soap Creek Saloon. We promoted the gig, and Soap Creek went all out and I played the hell out of Doug's version of "Wasted Days and Wasted Nights" (which is itself a classic work of Texana), and I dug up some old album of Freddy's from before his pot bust, and we all figured, "Oh, boy, what has Doug gotten us into this time?"

The gig rolls around and we had the crowd there and this very handsome and gracious charismatic Tejano gets up there, blowing his bass with Doug's band as his backup, and just proceeds to knock the doors and windows out of the joint. He floored us. Soap Creek Saloon, which was like a smaller, more intense Armadillo World Headquarters, was rocked to the limestone!

I went back to my radio station in my ragtop '61 Caddy and played "Before the Next Teardrop Falls" for six months nonstop until *Billboard* finally gave in and picked it up and it became Number 1 in January. We got him on *Austin City Limits* that year, too. It was the radio equivalent of a filibuster. I have never had a more satisfying experience in the music business than that. Well, none that I can talk about here . . .

JOE GRACEY—MEETING COWBOY JACK CLEMENT IN AUSTIN

Cowboy moved to Austin in '72 to escape Nashville and married Waylon's sister. I had followed his career on the back of all the great records he had produced, and I heard he was in town. So one night at the Armadillo Beer Garden I saw this guy who I swear had a sort of aura around him, like he wasn't like all the other people or something. I walked up and asked, "Are you Jack Clement?"

He adopted me as his Austin Boy. I drove him around, procured weed and coke for him, introduced him to all the bands, and generally

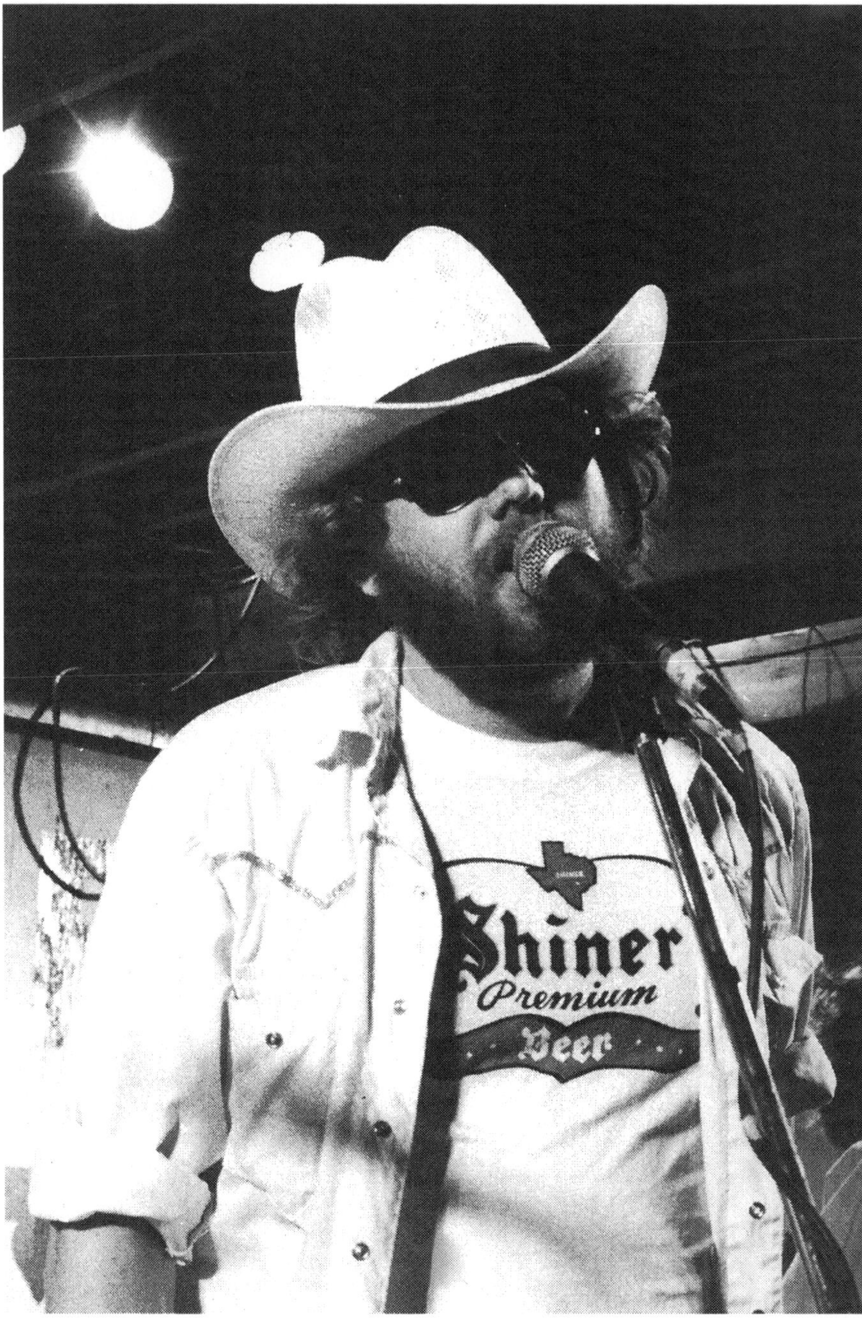

Cosmic Cowboy Gracey.

soaked up every word that came from him. He decided he liked my radio voice and that since I could sing, he would turn me into the next Don Williams, who I actually did sound like.

He'd call my radio show and sing long, goofy songs over the phone. Finally, he moved back to Nashville, and I used to go see him a lot up there, and we were planning to record me and make me a star. I even found myself slipping into his mannerisms. That's how serious his impact was on me. A rare American indeed! Hell, he even produced a hit on Louis Armstrong, "A Wonderful World," during which time more dope got smoked than in the entire state of Oaxaca, Mexico, on a good day!

ROCK BEAT: ARMADILLO GETS NEW FAME
AUSTIN AMERICAN-STATESMAN, 1972

Austin gets famouser and famouser by the day. Not only are we now known to have the prettiest, calmest, friendliest, funkiest, and most musical city this side of Berkeley, but now we have appeared in *Rolling Stone*.

Rolling Stone, the "*Time* magazine of the counterculture," features a very fine article about Armadillo this week. They even have a picture of Jim Franklin, looking weird, and one of Eddie Wilson, looking promotional. Ah, Fame, your fleeting twine across the glade . . .

ROCK BEAT: COVERING THE NOW SOUNDS
AUSTIN AMERICAN-STATESMAN, 1972
ARE ROCK CONCERT FANS BEGINNING TO LISTEN?

Rock 'n' roll lives somewhere near Tulsa these days. In Disney, Oklahoma, to be more exact. For in Disney lives Leon Russell, along with friends and hangers-on, in a motel, which he has commissioned local artist Jim Franklin to paint. That's right, Franklin of Armadillo fame received the summons from Disney and went to "muralize" Leon Russell's motel and swimming pool. For an example of Jim Franklin's work, check the covers of Freddie King's albums *Texas Cannonball* and *Woman Across the River*.

What all this means is that Russell came down through San Antonio last week and just flat tore things up. I generally leave giant concerts kicking myself for going, but this was the exception. Leon brought three new girls and had another piano opposite, which was manned by an incredible black gospel singer. The total effect was gorgeous. The band was tight and rock-steady, and evidence of mastery was rampant, as well as welcome. Russell not only moved the crowd with sheer power but also displayed his grasp of theatrics and satire. His stage lighting actually seemed part of the concept of the concert, and his spoof of "your favorite rock star" was hilarious. It reminded me of Elton John, the difference being that Leon knows it's funny.

I believe that Leon Russell's concert marked an important point in rock's development analogous to the same time in the history of jazz. At some point the audiences stop dancing and start listening to the performers with their minds as well as with their bodies. Bad or good, it is happening to rock.

One could not help but be aware of the complexity, artistry, musicality, and brilliance evidenced by Russell's group. It is rather sad to me that we have left the days of simply feeling a response to a sound, but people like Russell take the sting away with their dedication and love of "the black man's music."

If you didn't see Dan Hicks and His Hot Licks last week you may get another chance soon. Unconfirmed rumor has it that he may be back for a weeklong gig. We don't know where yet. At the risk of treading on Townsend Miller's boots, I would urge you to come out to Armadillo's Garden tonight and hear Willie Nelson. Willie is genuine Texas-size talent and is a real fine guy besides.

Back when I was a country and western disc jockey, I used to look forward with great anticipation to the chance to play a Willie Nelson song. He writes and sings some of the most listenable music in any category you can name. I'm looking forward to the concert for another reason, too. Austin is one of the few places in the world where a traditionally "country-western" performer can play in a traditionally "rock" hall and attract both types of crowds at the same time with lots of good feeling and good beer and none of that polarity or fear encountered elsewhere.

We have a unique and wonderful town here, all credit to its people. A sign saying "Willie Nelson at Armadillo World Headquarters" could only happen here, and I'm proud to see it.

JOE GRACEY—*AUSTIN CITY LIMITS*, NOVEMBER 23, 2004

As for *Austin City Limits*, my small contributions to that program began when I was a disc jockey at the first progressive country/Americana radio station in the United States, KOKE-FM, and when I was the rock music columnist for the *Austin American-Statesman*. John Bustin was my editor. Several Austin progressive country bands, I believe including Freda and the Firedogs and maybe Michael Murphey, had gone up to Dallas and appeared on TV on the PBS affiliate there. This lit a fire under me (which wasn't hard to do in those days), and I wrote a column decrying the fact that the Austin music scene was getting more respect from a Dallas PBS station than it was from our own media outlets, and how come KLRN didn't do a show featuring the burgeoning Austin music scene? Bill Arhos was then head of KLRN and I think he had been mulling over an idea for some sort of musical show already, and when I threw down this gauntlet in the papers, it helped galvanize him into action.

He got ahold of Willie Nelson and shot a pilot for the show and used that to sell the concept at the PBS programming convention, where it was successful enough to produce a full thirteen-week season of hour-long musical shows centering on Austin and Texas music. He then realized that he needed some sort of guidance in deciding on who to book on this show, and decided that since I thought I was so damn smart he'd just give me a call and see if I wanted to be his talent coordinator and make recommendations as to who to book and then try to book them for the rather untidy PBS-scale sum he was able to offer in those days.

I jumped all over this. It was nice money for me because disc jockeys in those days made horrible, pitiful salaries, which encouraged things like moonlighting, payola, and prostitution of all kinds. I also felt that I had a sort of personal mission to help not only preserve Texan culture before it was homogenized away in a wash of bad TV and degenerate outsider culture in general, but to preserve Texan music and food as well. This would give me one more way to help do this, I thought.

So I got me a briefcase (and went around looking stupid until I threw it away one day) and started trying to figure out who to book on this TV show. Arhos had a few people he wanted, all of whom I recall agreeing with, like Willie and Michael Murphey. I added Doug Sahm, naturally. I was also writing features for a little rag called *Picking Up the Tempo*, and I had written about how I'd taken Ry Cooder to meet Flaco Jimenez and hooked them up to do Ry's next record, *Chicken Skin Music*, so I booked Ry and Flaco to play a show together. I had written a story about Clifton Chenier, who was actually a big act in Houston and the Golden Triangle, so I booked him. He kind of kicked about the fee, which in those days was only six hundred dollars, but I begged him to do the show because I knew it would be a great career move for him, and it turned out to be, both for him and for Flaco.

I didn't realize that Bob Wills's widow had forbidden anybody to do a Wills band reunion, so being thus blissfully ignorant, I put together a reunion of as many of the original Texas Playboys from the '30s up to the '60s as I could find. That band included Leon McAuliffe, Sleepy Johnson, Johnny Gimble, Jesse Ashlock, Leon Rausch, Smokey Dacus, Tommy Allsup, and several other Playboys who would do an absolutely stunningly good show together and then go on to have a great career for the next few years. The only way I could afford to get them all down to Austin was to promote a gig with them at the Broken Spoke. Bobby Earl Smith and the owner of the Spoke, James White, helped me put it all together. Micael Priest did a now-legendary poster for that show.

James agreed to donate every penny from the door to the Playboys so they could go home with a little bit of money in the end. I was naïve enough to put them all in a hotel without telling the desk that any room service, phone usage, etc., was to be paid by them, and I got stuck with a gigantic bill afterward with no way to pay it! I honestly didn't care because I felt proud of what I thought was probably the most significant thing I had ever done in the music business, the bringing together of the Texas Playboys for a second career, so that they could get the recognition they deserved and so that my generation could see what brilliant music they could make. And it was an accomplishment that sprang directly from my love of Texas music. Even Mrs. Wills gave her blessing to the project after she saw that it was being done in a respectful and honest fashion. Somehow, the best things you do are almost always the ones you do the most sincerely, ya know?

I had a few acts forced on me that I disagreed with, but I won't name names, since it doesn't matter now. The producer, Paul Botsford, and I tended to clash, a matter of personality and style. He would go out and get all pumped up over an act that I thought was utterly banal, and I'd tell him that, so he disliked me more and more as the year went on, I thought. So I did the best I could to get what I considered to be the roots acts—the soulful acts—on the show while I still had the power to do so. After that year was up, he didn't renew my contract, which I expected, but I still feel a great sense of accomplishment and pride in the acts I was able to book that first year. It actually helped the careers of some of the artists, and those tapes are valuable now purely in terms of historic and cultural importance, which, after all, was my original goal. Some of the artists that I had lobbied hard for but didn't get, like Ernest Tubb and Lightnin' Hopkins and George Jones and Waylon Jennings, would eventually appear on the show, to my joy.

And, of course, the day came when I got to see my wife, singer-songwriter Kimmie Rhodes, and my son Gabriel Rhodes appear together on *Austin City Limits* many years later. This was a kind of bathing in pure happiness, to see something I had a small part in creating play host to the artist and human that I believe in above all others. What could be better than that?

JOE GRACEY, JOHNNY GIMBLE, AND FLACO JIMENEZ

Flaco and Gimble are like trees that when you poke a sap spike in them, they flow perfect music really fast. You'd better have the mic level set and the mix in the cans right because they are gonna nail it the first time, Buddy, and if you want it again then you may have missed it.

The first time I saw Flaco Jimenez, it was in 1973 out at a club south of Austin called the Rockin' M with his conjunto band, and he was the best-looking man I had ever seen. I wrote a story about it and called him

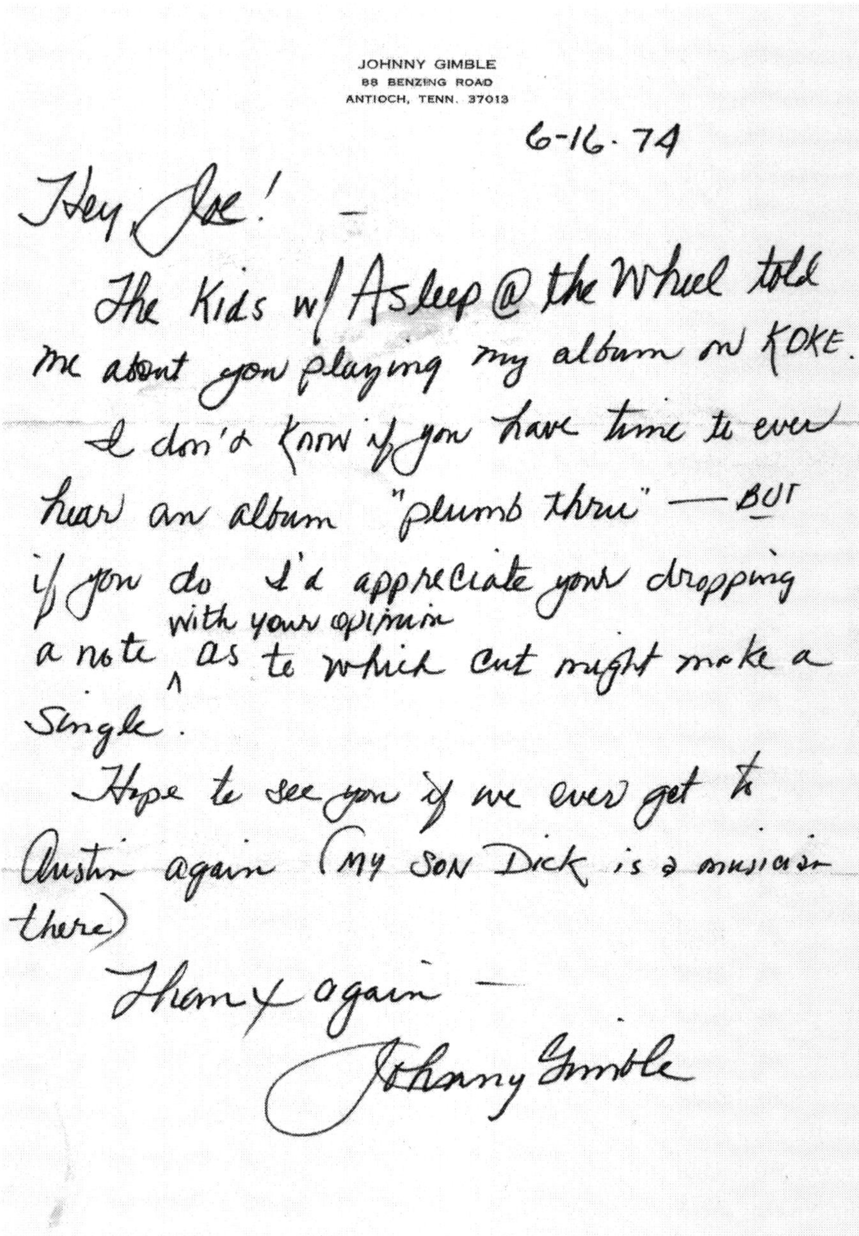

JOHNNY GIMBLE
88 BENZING ROAD
ANTIOCH, TENN. 37013

6-16-74

Hey, Joe! —

The Kids w/ Asleep @ the Wheel told me about you playing my album on KOKE.

I don't know if you have time to ever hear an album "plumb thru" — BUT if you do I'd appreciate your dropping a note with your opinion as to which cut might make a single.

Hope to see you if we ever get to Austin again (MY SON Dick is a musician there)

Thanx again —

Johnny Gimble

Johnny Gimble letter to Gracey.

"The Chuck Berry of the Conjunto Accordion," in an effort to describe both his astounding beauty and his revolutionary use of the button accordion to play things that sounded nothing like anybody had ever played before.

Johnny Gimble was twenty years old when he joined Bob Wills's Texas Playboys, and he is the greatest swing fiddle player I have ever heard. He has hands that my wife, Kimmie, would describe as "pretty hands." I played him a rough mix last Saturday and he sat there in the chair beside me, and I put my ear about four inches from his fiddle while he bowed out the most gorgeous licks to the tracks as he was learning them.

When Sir Doug shook this "mortal coil," it reminded me and Bobby Earl anew about how you'd better make that music count and call "them boys" on the phone and get them down to do that stuff they do so well, for, as Sister Terry said at Doug's memorial service, "You'd better be ready. . . . We'd all better be ready." Yesterday one of Doug's old bandmates and compadres said to me, "My captain is gone."

Indeed. Learn that guitar. Learn that damn recording board. Learn all those chords. Lay that shit down so that in a hundred years, if you were any good, it will still be here. It matters. It really does matter.

ROCK BEAT: NOW SOUNDS AROUND TOWN
TOWNES VAN ZANDT: UNIQUE TALENT
AUSTIN AMERICAN-STATESMAN, 1972

Townes Van Zandt is a contrast when viewed against the backdrop of smiling lies and averted eyes and glitter that exists in a great part of the performing and recording world. When somebody like John Denver comes along and jabs his lukewarm little poker of a song into your ribs and whines through the echo about the miserable Colorado winters, it makes one thankful for the likes of Townes.

Subtlety is what he's all about, and if you're careful he'll slide right by; he doesn't demand your attention, he quietly proceeds to deserve it. I know few people, pickers or no, who are quieter about themselves and less concerned with superficial impressions. Unless you're careful, you'll miss all the drama and the pain and the searching questions put to a silent universe. In some ways he reminds me of Hank Williams—the planed surfaces of his face and the plaintive long notes held as if by tension stretched by pain.

However, there's something else. Townes Van Zandt is an observer, and when he sets things down to memory, they are usually bizarre, or amazing, or unusual, and always howlingly funny, if the viewfinder in your perception is tuned just right. His world is the same kind of incredible palace that Chaplin and sometimes W. C. Fields lived in, one where daily occurrence gets puffed up and looks hilarious, like the face on a balloon after you blow it up. When you look at things his way, sad and happy merge into each other in a new way. The same thing happens in Hank Williams's and Bob Dylan's songs. (Try "My Bucket's Got a Hole in It" or "Talking World War Three.")

JOE GRACEY—DOUG SAHM

The thing I always come back to on Doug was what an incredible voice he had. The vocal on "She's About a Mover" was the closest thing any white man ever came to sounding as good as Ray Charles.

In '72 or so, when I had moved over to KOKE-FM and Doug was starting to hang around Austin, he would come down to the station when I would do a night shift, and we'd lean on the balcony overlooking Lamar and smoke a fat joint from Mexico and I'd soak up his wisdom and vibrant goofiness and righteous take on things. Doug had the peculiar quality of caring about you when you didn't expect it. He saw in me a person who would drink in his tales of the old days with real thirst, and so he would fill me with stories of Lefty and Hank and Bob and his incredible range of experience with blues giants, country giants, rock legends. He was cool. Texas cool. South Texas cool. I learned a lot from him about a lot of things.

There are too many stories—most of them only half-remembered now—of the big show down in Houston for KPFT-FM in '73-ish, a giant arena full of people with him and Freda and the Firedogs (Marcia Ball, John Reed, Bobby Earl Smith, et al.), when I saw him go out in front of those many thousands of people and really turn on as a "big star." He had that in him when he wanted it.

Doug saw himself as part of the Texas tradition of combining and assimilation. He straddled eras because of his precociousness. He could be absurd (but likeably so) or self-centered (but all artists are), but his generosity and brilliance overshadowed everything else. He had the best voice in a white body that I ever heard. He loved to live and reminded all of us how much fun life could be and how important it was to uphold our Texas traditions in an increasingly single-faceted world.

JOE GRACEY—WAYLON JENNINGS "LIVE"

I remember Waylon and Willie's live shows as being the sort of high-water mark of the progressive country movement, with Waylon bearing the standard, poking fun at Willie with the Bob Wills song and prowling the stage like the hero that he really was.

Those recordings capture at least some of the exaltation of that wave of alt energy. Listen to it really, really loud, please. Texas country was rock 'n' roll and was music heaven there for one brief sweaty shining moment. There really was some guy who was screaming during all the intros, and at one point it started to irritate Waylon during the intro to "Bob Wills Is Still the King," and he kind of stops and starts over or something. That guy was slightly overserved.

That was Waylon's best, most simpatico band and the point where his sound really came together, and he had just made his greatest studio record with Jack Clement. He was getting pretty high, but it wasn't messing up his music yet, and he was just riding the crest of that whole scene. Man, that band cooked. Ralph Mooney almost redefined the steel guitar in that band.

In 1974 Waylon was certainly the best-looking, toughest stud in all of country music and was as cool as anybody in rock, too. He literally prowled the stage and zapped out solos like shooting sparks out of the end of his Telecaster, with the leather cover on it "à la Holly." The band was into that groove, and they would just sweep you away with it for hours.

Then there is something really powerful about an incredibly rough-looking guy with a deep voice singing a soft ballad. Clement had gotten Waylon to use the lower part of his voice more and relax his vocals more, and to hear him sing that slow, soft stuff was real magic. It was as good as any Stones or Springsteen or T-Birds thing I ever saw, and it was incredibly real, not a pose or anything false about it. I actually long to go back in time to one of those shows again, just to see it happen once more, but it won't now.

JOE GRACEY—ROY ACUFF, BROTHER OSWALD, AND JOHNNY CASH

I saw Roy Acuff once in the flesh. I was unprepared for his blend of energy, humor, goofiness, and kick-ass singing. It was an eye-opening experience for me. He ran around onstage balancing his bow on his nose, and then he would literally rare back and belt out one of those bone-chilling songs from somewhere down around his toes, with Brother Oswald back there playing the dobro.

I went over to Cowboy's one fine morning, and Brother Oswald was sitting there in the office playing the dobro with Jack, who was strumming a rhythm guitar. Oswald looked old and frail but he sure could play that thing. It was mighty fine. Goddam, it was beautiful.

I went over there another morning and there was Johnny Cash, in the flesh, dressed in black. Jack introduced us and they started playing songs together, and it was almost more electricity than I was able to engage in, I swear, when Jack said, "John, this is Joe Gracey." Cash leaned over and stuck out his paw and said, "Hello, I'm Johnny Cash." Couple of silly bastards, those two . . .

JOE GRACEY PLAYLIST

Numbers 9–12 are missing because the notes were never completed.

1. Waltz Across Texas, Ernest Tubb
2. A Smooth One, Wills Tiffany Sessions?
3. Charlie Christian w/ Benny Goodman
4. Papa Ain't Salty, T-Bone Walker ('40s–'50s Imperial or Capital version)
5. Night Life, BB King Live at the Regal

6. You Don't Know Me, Ray Charles
7. Crazy Arms, Ray Price ('50s Version)
8. Bloody Mary Morning, Willie Nelson
9. Undo the Right, Johnny Bush
10. King of the Road, Roger Miller
11. Let's All Help the Cowboy Sing the Blues, Waylon Jennings
12. Contrabandistas, Kimmie Rhodes & Willie Nelson

Introduction to Playlist

One of the interesting things about Texas music, and what made it so vital, was the cross-fertilization that took place there. Texans were exposed to southern white church music, African American sacred and blues songs, Mexican folk songs and mariachi orchestras, and Appalachian fiddle tunes. I have chosen this playlist as a way to illustrate my point and to tell a few stories about the relationships between the songs and the people playing them.

1. Ernest Tubb was one of my heroes for several reasons. He was a Texan who managed to join the country music establishment in Nashville while maintaining his artistic integrity and remaining true to his Texas roots. It was he who negotiated the deal between Bob Wills and the Grand Ole Opry. When Bob got there and set up to play, the Opry manager told him that drums were never allowed on the Opry stage, as if it were some sort of sacrilege in a holy shrine. Bob said, "Okay, pack it up, boys; we're going home." Nobody ever, ever told Bob what to do. Ernest was horrified and finally managed to get them to let Wills set up his drums, as long as they were behind a curtain onstage. Silly, but typical of the Opry. Bob never went back. This song has always been one of my favorites, and Kimmie and I always played it in our sets at Texas dance halls. I got to interview Ernest Tubb several times when I was a music writer, and he was a true gentleman and a great musician who always had great bands. He bridged the gap between his hero, Jimmie Rodgers, and the honky-tonk style, which he pioneered and which would eventually become the commercial Nashville style of music for many years.

2 and 3. Bob Wills was a dance fiddler who loved African American music. His idol was Bessie Smith, the great blues shouter. He also loved the New Orleans sound of Emmett Miller, who wrote "Lovesick Blues." When he lived in New Mexico for a short time, he joined a mariachi orchestra and learned that style, too, which is where he picked up his famous "Ah-ha!" yell, which was his version of the Mexican "grito," or shout. In the '30s and '40s it was forbidden for black and white musicians to appear onstage together in the South, but after hours, the guys in Wills's band and the black musicians would jam together in the clubs, and you can hear the licks crossing over from band to band, if you listen to the next two tracks. The second track is the black guitar player Charlie Christian, who was from Oklahoma, with the Benny Goodman band. Listen to how similarly he and the Wills guys are playing, as Wills does a Christian song. This is a great example of how white and black players influenced each other, even if they had to do it in secret.

4 and 5. T-Bone Walker, from Dallas, was the first great combination blues singer and electric guitar player. He straddled the line between Texas-style jazz and blues, and used the electrified guitar as a solo instrument, like a horn. Every guitar hero since Freddie King to Chuck Berry to Clapton to Stevie Ray Vaughan owes his licks and his style in some part to T-Bone Walker. I follow him with one of his many acolytes, BB King, doing a song written by one of the greatest Texas songwriters, Willie Nelson.

6. Ray Charles loved country music, so when he became popular enough to stretch out, he made two albums of country songs done in a very pop style. This is by another one of the great Texas writers, Cindy Walker, who wrote hugely successful hits for Bob Wills and many other popular stars. This song demonstrates how beautifully her material could cross over from country to pop when interpreted by an African American blues and jazz singer.

7. Ray Price was another Texan who went to Nashville seeking fame. He began fronting the Hank Williams band, opening for Hank and then doing the whole show when Williams was unable to go on. After he left them, he made records in the same 2/4 style as Hank and even sounded much like him, but at some point in the '50s he made a revolutionary change in his sound, one which would totally change country music for many years. He developed a 4/4 beat with a walking bass and a characteristic fiddle sound, and had a string of huge hits, including "Crazy Arms," "City Lights," and "My Shoes Keep Walking Back to You." He also found his own voice and began singing in a dramatic operatic style with lots of vibrato, and the recording engineers used a lot of the new-fangled reverberation in his records. With the great Jimmy Day on steel and Willie Nelson on bass, Johnny Bush on drums, and Roger Miller on fiddle, he lit up the dance halls in Texas like nobody ever had. One of the most euphoric moments in my recording career was getting to do a Grammy Award–winning CD with him and Willie Nelson.

8. Willie Nelson is a towering giant in the Texas music pantheon because he broke the mold every time he stepped forth. As a young songwriter, he changed the way country music sounded (think "Crazy"), he challenged the conventional pop fluff that had become Nashville, and he then turned the whole thing on its head by recording an album of pop standards that stayed on the *Billboard* pop charts for years.

4

DUCK AND COVER

KIMMIE RHODES

MUSIC IS VERY SIMPLY MADE for the most human of reasons and is a pure and ancient art form. A man with a leftover leg bone from dinner hits an animal skin stretched over, oh, say, a couple of tree limbs and wails in sorrow because his heart feels near breaking. Relief is found so the moaning and beating continues falling into a pattern and rhythm in a workout akin to crying, except less painful and more physically satisfying, and even damn enjoyable. Others who share the airspace understand, because the sound informs them, and soon the man is not alone. Maybe he chants words found to express his feelings so the others relate even better now and join the man and soon they are all singing a song and the whole wacky primitive village finds momentary delivery from the shared pain and knowing, and something beautiful happens.

This soon becomes a therapeutically healthy addiction, and others have begun to cobble together noisemaking devices and join in, and the villagers find that they are dining and engaging in the creative ritual frequently because of its mystical, holy, healing quality. Time passes.

Soon the music evolves to become a form of communication expressing all kinds of feelings, like excitement, joy, fear, sorrow, anger, freedom. This music becomes the centerpiece of celebrations. More time passes. Slaves in the fields moan, calling out, and answering repeated phrases—not just saying, "Get us out of here," but collectively pleading, "Help us make it to the end of the row."

The blues are born and morph into jazz. And so on, until the '70s come along and a brotherhood and sisterhood of hippies looking for meaning return to the well of their roots to invoke the gods of love and joy and then, voilà, one day a guy named Townes Van Zandt shows up to write "For the Sake of the Song." This process is simply the nature of a beast that *will* be fed. People can show true genius for taming, feeding, labeling, and marketing it, but nobody—be they rock star, country legend, zydeco or blues king, symphonic god of the universe, the Rolling Stones or Jimmy Reed—ever truly owns the thing that exists as a true force of nature and will outlive all who participate in its keeping, proving once again the inarguable ecclesiastical truth that "a living dog is better than a dead lion."

ONE WOULD NEED to be the offspring of horrified parents who had endured the Great Depression, borne the consciousness of the mushroom clouds over Hiroshima and Nagasaki, witnessed the Holocaust and fought the war that brought down Hitler, loved a young man with a draft number standing between him and the inexplicable carnage of the Vietnam War, borne witness to the aftermath of slavery and the war for civil rights that was raging in the streets of America, and the public assassination of those in power who defended freedom, including the president of the United States, to even begin to try to describe the unstoppable rumble of the times and the cry for change. A man walked on the moon, and a race of well-educated, middle-class children were born into very hard-earned good times, like bees born into too much honey.

Sigmund Freud and Carl Jung had let the psychological "cat out of the bag," and a disillusioned generation learned to take its emotional temperature daily and wonder how our parents could honestly support the potential deaths of their children in a war economically complicated. J. Edgar Hoover died suddenly during the night, the assassinations strangely ceased, and President Nixon lied to us all on TV.

Cancer was beginning to rear its ugly head, but with no cure anywhere in sight, and treatment still in early stages, the "C word" was whispered in hushed and fearful tones. Although cigarette ads targeting youth continued to run, the surgeon general announced to the multitude of smokers who had been seduced by the advertisements that smoking was suddenly "hazardous to your health."

Modern medicine had begun to achieve all sorts of miracles, and pharmaceutical delicacies were abundant, although still in the experimental stages. Some were made available by prescription, and some were rejected as not useful. Mothers who were first-generation descendants of the snake oil–cocaine era took and dispensed pills with hopeful anticipation of results, trusting without question the doctors who prescribed them. Mick Jagger sang "running for the shelter of her mother's little helper" and Bob Dylan had already told us that "the times they are a-changin'" and "a hard rain" was falling on the jungles in Vietnam, as we watched the bodies come home. Indelibly marked by the lyrics from the civil defense film *Duck and Cover* (a little ditty sung to us by Bert the Turtle to prepare us for the ever-looming event of an atomic bomb, which would most likely occur on our walk home from primary school), we followed the advice that the "establishment" had unwittingly given us, and it finally backfired, so to speak.

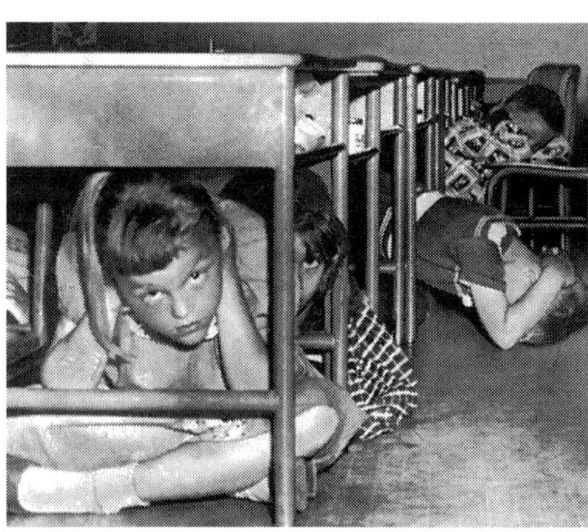

Duck and Cover. Civil Defense photo.

DUCK AND COVER

He hid beneath his little shell until the coast was clear
Then one by one his head and tail and legs would reappear
By acting calm and cool he proved he was a hero, too
For finding safety is the bravest, wisest thing to do
And now his little friends are just like Bert
And every turtle is very alert
When danger threatens them
They never get hurt
They know just what to do

Good advice. We knew just what to do. "Fuck you and cover" became the rewrite from a generation of children who felt abandoned, confused, and angry, sensing that they would soon inherit a society badly in need of reinvention.

The traditional street drugs, marijuana, the opiates, cocaine, had been tossed aside by a technology bound for the glory of the nouveau synthetics. Then, a powerful newbie, rejected for having failed to cure schizophrenia but still in use by the military to extract information from POWs, surfaced on the streets. LSD, a micro-tablet made from fungi growing on grasses, promised instant enlightenment. Just one hit and the spell of the unremarkable threat to utopia would be forever broken! So, we bit. It was fun until it wasn't.

LUBBOCK WAS STARKLY VIVID and just too weird of a place for a virgin adolescent female who had been "raised by wolves" to find herself in the midst of all of the global flux of the late '60s. I'm not sure exactly at what point things began to shift inside of me. At around fifteen years of age, I surrendered to a sad knowing that just about everything I'd been taught was clean and good about life had taken a back seat to one big lie or another. The loss of innocence is, I believe, the most painful loss there is. The more I became aware of the underbelly of human nature, the more my innocence slipped away, bit by bit, until no Santa Claus,

Easter Bunny, fairy princess, or Bible stories were believable anymore. It was like somehow, overnight, all the magic had been sucked into a black hole. People were even reporting that God was dead. Wow. That's big.

Home life got worse and worse until finally it became unbearable. My parents were unhappy and barely spoke to one another anymore. My brother, Mike, had fallen off a cliff and sustained serious head injuries during a Boy Scout retreat, and although he had always been the kind of kid who would set the fence on fire and torture the cat, he had become insufferable and violent, and I was afraid of him.

Looking back, Mike taught me more about unconditional love than anyone I've ever known. When all was said and done, despite his troubled soul, he was a really sweet ol' boy. We loved him because we were supposed to, not because he was lovable, but because he was ours, and we covered for him as best we could. He had an invisible disability, which I later learned had a name: sociopathy.

Mama was a natural-born survivor. She always found solace in the security of her job, which kept her out of the house most of the time. Experience had helped her develop an instinctive ability to deny what she could not change, so mostly, I think I learned to play along with that and try to keep her from knowing a lot of what went on when she wasn't around. One night the police came to our door and took Mike away for brutally beating the poor nerd who was the focus of all the school bullying. From the den I observed Mama pleading with the officer at the front door to, please, just let him put his shoes on before they took him away in the squad car . . . barefooted.

So I avoided Mike as best I could, but it was difficult, seeing as we still lived under the same roof. Once he learned to drink he became extremely volatile. One afternoon he broke my dad's ribs in a drunken scuffle while I sat in the living room and watched, too scared to intervene. Nobody could control him anymore, so like a prisoner who'd best just lie low, I made myself scarce when he was around by staying gone from the house as much as possible or by hiding in plain sight.

I'd had a grade-school teacher who had this delicate little live chameleon with a tiny gold collar and chain that she wore as a broach. The amazing creature would scamper about on her shoulder and change color to blend in with its surroundings for protection. I loved it on the days she wore it, and usually when I asked her to, she would. I became like that chameleon.

IT FINALLY DAWNED ON ME that nobody was really protecting me from anything anymore. Every night from the same tube that had invited me to *Meet the Beatles,* world-weary anchorman Walter Cronkite would take off his glasses, wipe his brow, and conclude, “And that’s the way it is.” Trapped inside the time machine of Lubbock, I imagined the future from a town that’s present was far in the past of exotic places like New York and Paris.

I felt about the same as poor old Walter Cronkite did by the time I reached my junior year in high school. My formal education was running completely off the road because I had simply lost the will to navigate the social atmosphere. All of my friends were older and had graduated, and I felt like I didn’t belong, which I didn’t. Biology class was the high point in my day because I liked the subject and the teacher was a kind woman. I enjoyed art class. For some reason (many years before it became stylish), I decided I looked good in black so I started wearing it every day. I pretty much stopped eating and smoked cigarettes instead, which killed any appetite I might have had. I began dabbling in the mélange of street drugs that were flowing through town. Clusters of jocks from the football team started cornering me in the hallway and making fun of me, and much to my surprise one day, two upper-class girls pulled me aside and offered to “kick my ass.”

I had a boyfriend who was drafted, and when his number was called, he stopped by my house to say goodbye, but I wasn’t home. He left a note. I never saw him or heard from him again. Soon after, I caught wind of a “Moratorium Day,” with massive demonstrations taking place across America in protest of the war. People were encouraged to support the movement by wearing a black armband, so I wore one to school that day, and shortly after arriving to my first class, I was sent to the principal’s office for the first time in my life.

The principal was an authoritative figure who represented everything my father wasn't. Daddy Ray dressed "to the nines" every day—tailored suit, starched shirt, tie, matching hanky, nice haircut, manicure—but somehow this guy was cleaned up in a horrible, too-polished way, with a lot of sharp edges and angles to his navy-blue suit and a haircut and shave that was overdone and off-putting, as if his compliant squeaky-cleanness had somehow earned him the right to dominate. This was the first time I recall ever having been one-on-one in the presence of this type of man, in an office, behind closed doors, and soon to be engaged in a conversation in which I was "in trouble." He was brief but clear in his request, no questions and no negotiation. The two options were . . . a) I was to remove the armband and be allowed to return to class, or b) I was to go to my locker immediately, return with my textbooks and be expelled from school. I took option b, which surprised him because I was just a quiet, skinny girl, a brunette with blue eyes who made good grades, so he probably, up to that point, didn't even know I existed. When I returned a few minutes later with my books and placed the stack on the desk before him, he said, "Okay. Now you can come back in three days, but we won't expect to see this kind of behavior from you again." Not being used to being told what to think, I removed him from power by calmly replying with the kind of stubborn autonomous logic that has always been my saving grace, "No, thank you. I can get my own books, so anything I need to learn from now on I'll just read and teach myself."

Looking back I suppose there should have been some fear that my parents would be furious and march me right back up there to straighten things out or something. There should have been some fear that I wouldn't graduate, would be a failure, couldn't get into college or would be forced to live a life of shame . . . blah, blah, blah . . . but there had never been a conversation in my household about anyone attending college, and it had never been an option or a requirement or even a suggestion. My dad was a Depression-era hustler with a second-grade education. I guess we weren't normal.

All I felt was relief the day I left that miserable place behind, right in the middle of a school day, having made my own decision about my own future, without counsel or dissent from anyone. My mother, who had received a high-school diploma against all odds, was probably quietly disappointed, but by then we were off in our own worlds, and she didn't encourage me to return to school, or if she did, I ignored it, so I don't remember.

Oddly, I felt secure in my plans for the future because somehow I had always known I would be a florist "when I grew up." Back when I had loved going to school, on my walk to Dupre Elementary, many times I'd taken the long way, down the busy street that I wasn't supposed to go near, to spend my lunch money at the flower shop, just to watch a pink or peppermint carnation being wrapped in green wax paper and tied with a soft satin ribbon. The heady clove smell of the flower was intoxicating to me, and I marveled at how such a thing like a flower could possibly exist. One way or another, before I reached the school, I had usually given the flower away to someone, or sometimes I would take it to my teacher. If I didn't have the money, because I was "taking my lunch" that day, I would sneak flowers from beds along the way. I had to be clever because there was one woman who would knock on her window and yell at me to stop, until finally one morning I gave my carnation away to her, so she liked me after that. Once, a student teacher saw me walking home and pulled her car over, rolled down the window, and amazingly asked me if I would like to go to the garden shop with her. I wasn't supposed to take rides with strangers, but, figuring she wasn't a stranger, I gladly accepted the invitation. She must have noticed how much I loved flowers because when we got there she bought me an apricot-colored geranium in a clay pot. I was in love with my new first plant! I sat it on the front porch and lay with my face pressed to the cool concrete, marveling at how the sunlight passed through the petals, turning them every possible shade of apricot imaginable. I watched it grow and contemplated growth. I could find no explanation for how something so exquisite could possibly come into being from a tiny seed and some dirt, as if by magic. So pretty soon after I became a hippie "dropout," I got myself a job selling carnations from a white plastic bucket on a street corner very near that flower shop, and I was happy.

ONCE I'D OUTGROWN my juvenile hunger for Aesop's fables and mythology, what I believed to be true came mostly to me through song lyrics. The conversation in the music I was listening to had changed from magic dragons, or how it was fun to surf or drive around town in a Chevy on Saturday night to revolution and rebellion and psychedelia. With a page torn from my nursery book, Grace Slick of Jefferson Airplane wailed, "One pill makes you larger, and one pill makes you small, and the ones that mother gives you don't do anything at all." So with my newly found freedom, I jumped feet first down that rabbit hole.

Time's a funny girl, an illusionist, who can appear to both creep and fly by simultaneously. Einstein put it like this: "Put your hand on a hot stove for a minute, and it seems like an hour. Sit with a pretty girl for an hour, and it seems like a minute. That's relativity." Time allowed a lot in that foggy stretch, fondly, if vaguely, remembered as "the missing years," but ten summers quickly disappeared nonetheless. I found myself living on a truck farm/ranch in North Texas, married with two healthy and beautiful young sons, operating a small greenhouse business, dryland truck farming as a cover for growing marijuana and wrangling a herd of thirty horned and gestating Brangus heifers (which I figured made me a cowgirl, despite the fact that I had no horse) until we finally, mercifully, went bankrupt, and all the exhausting hard work went away. Thankfully, I'd achieved my childhood goal and had begun working a day job as a florist, so I was able to feed my kids and make ends meet.

I had taught myself to play guitar using chord songbooks and had even taken some music theory lessons from a friend who was completing his master's degree in guitar at North Texas State University in Denton, Texas. I took some oil painting and watercolor classes from an art graduate student in nearby Bowie, Texas, and checked books out of the library in order to study poetic device. I would write poetry and then make notes on which of the devices I'd stumbled onto without knowing what I was doing, sort of as a hobby. Without realizing it, I was in a very creative time of my life, writing poems that would later become songs—one of which, "Be Mine," would later be recorded by Waylon Jennings. I got a two-track tape recorder and learned how to operate it, and I would play Beatles records and record myself singing all the various harmony parts. I figured out how to work a small PA and would drag it into a nearby café and play a solo repertoire of cover songs to a polite roomful of people eating. I was delighted by the easy money I was able to earn doing something I was already going to be doing for fun anyway. As new guitar chords were added to my collection, I started to make up melodies, but I didn't assume that that elevated me to the unimaginable status of "songwriter," believing that that pantheon was reserved for Dylan, Neil Young, Leon Russell, Elton John, Joni Mitchell, Jimi Hendrix, and the like, but during my afternoon practice, eyes closed and singing to two birds that had started showing up on a regular basis to sit on the wire outside my window, visions of an audience began to appear in my daydreams.

LIFE GOT HARD AGAIN. Mysteriously, but seemingly connected to the "war on drugs" being waged by the bureaucrats in Washington, DC, cocaine was suddenly absolutely everywhere and had become the recreational drug of choice. Everyone from street rats to business executives was quickly getting hooked on it, and soon every single one of my friends had fallen under the spell, except for me. I still smoked some pot, but my experimental drug days were long over by then. So, being the only one not using, I wasn't on the same wavelength and therefore couldn't help but notice that coke seemed to give people an elated sense of self-importance and pseudo-power, even more so those who normally suffered from low self-esteem and/or felt insecure. Lord knows we've all got our checkered pasts, and it wasn't that I felt like I was more righteous than anyone else or judged them, and I really did try to just hang out and keep marching, but it was really awful to watch. Finally, I felt like I was living in a world that didn't look like mine anymore. Once again I felt like I didn't fit in and because I loved my kids and had hope of a better life for them, I just wasn't willing or able to "drink the Kool-Aid."

However dramatic, it's really unpleasant and boring to go on and on about such things, but suffice it to say it was certainly not a great environment for child-rearing anymore. Because we married young, we grew apart, and, sadly, I fell completely out of love with my husband

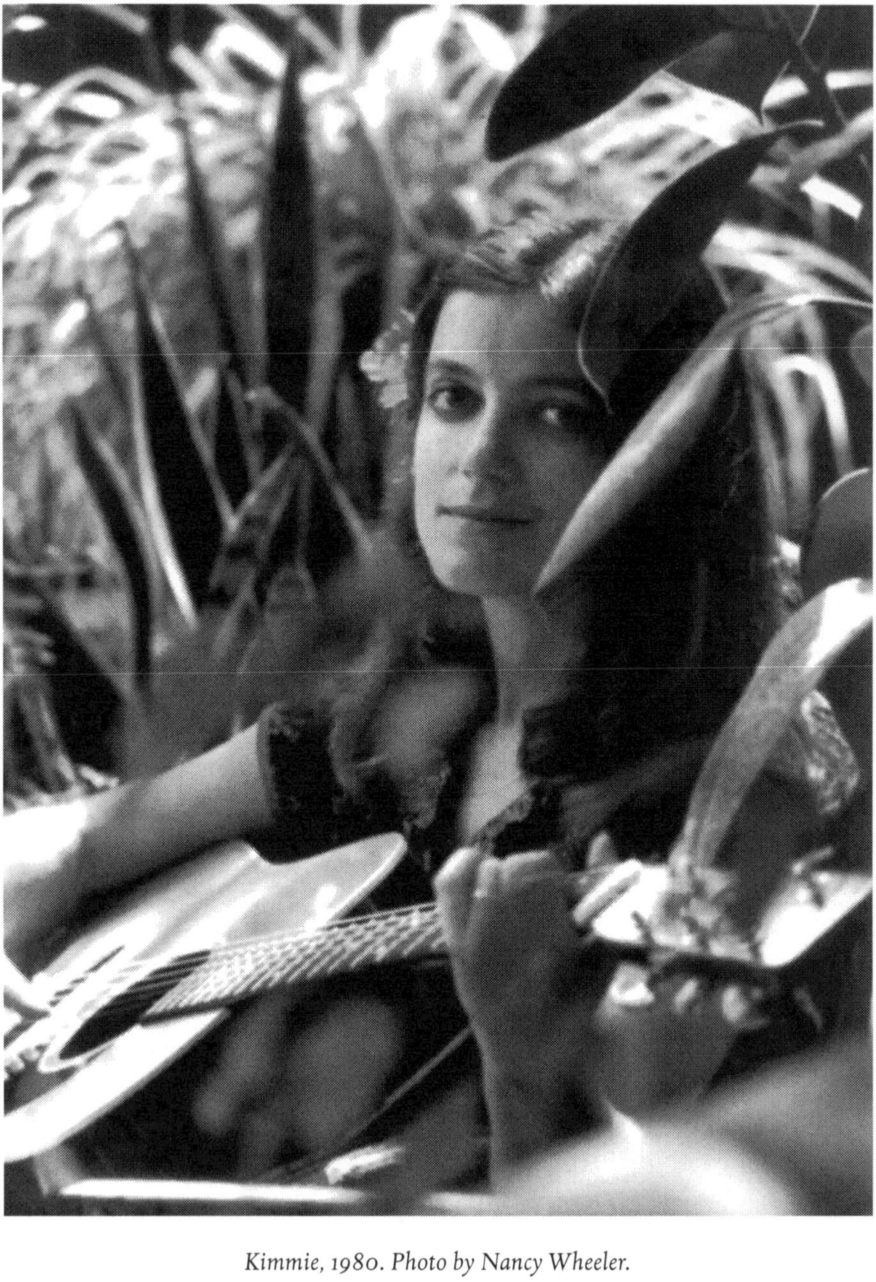

Kimmie, 1980. Photo by Nancy Wheeler.

and felt trapped and knew a new life was in order . . . quickly. I began to contemplate how one might suddenly change an entire life with the rapidity one might change, say, their socks. Strangely, one afternoon I discovered that out of sheer weariness and desperation and some fear, I was suddenly on my knees praying for deliverance. I prayed for new friends and fun and love. I prayed for vision and new direction and a miracle, and, surprisingly, because at that moment I became aware of a song playing on the radio, "Don't It Make My Brown Eyes Blue," I prayed to hear a record of my own playing on the radio, because I thought to myself, "Maybe I'm at least that good these days when I'm daydreaming and playing songs for the two birds on the wire."

I HEAR THE MUFFLED SOUND OF MUSIC, and I clearly see the face of a beautiful stranger that I am aware I am married to and in love with standing in a room behind a very thick window of glass. For some reason I'm sitting in a chair in a separate room, alone, looking at this man, who has begun making movements with his hands like someone conducting an orchestra, and I'm hearing indiscernible tinkling, chiming, distant music on the other side of the glass. My heart begins to pound, and everything becomes so real, more real than my waking life has ever been. I wake suddenly in a cold sweat, crying and breathing hard. Everything is still and dark, and I feel comforted by the creaking sound made by the old Aermotor windmill outside the bedroom window. I realize I will miss that sound when we leave the farm.

BE MINE

When the green green spring is waiting for the sun to shine
It knows the sun will shine . . . in time . . . in time . . .
How long until you dawn?
Is there any sign?
How long until your love will be mine?
Be mine . . . Be mine . . . How long until your love will be mine?

I've heard it said that 1,000 years is like a day,
Just a twinkle of an eye in time . . . in time . . .
Are you ever gonna wake up from the sleep you sleep?
How long until your love will be mine?
Be mine . . . Be mine . . . Oh, how long until your love will be mine?

5

CONTRABANDISTAS

JOE GRACEY

A PILGRIMAGE TO MEMPHIS

I JUST GOT BACK from a pilgrimage. While in conference in Nashville with a New York executive I became highly incensed at one of his comments about our production of Alvin's records, so I stood up in the silly bar, hollered, "Bullshit!," and stomped out the door. I got in my Cadillac and roared down the freeway trying to figure out what to do. Whilst thinking, I also received a ticket for speeding. Then I figured I would go to Memphis, but I realized I wouldn't stay mad long enough to make it all the way there driving, so I turned around and went to the airport and got on the first plane for Memphis instead.

Upon arrival I called a girl I knew and said, "I wanna go to the old Sun Studios." So we went by there. It is sort of like the Alamo. It's been a car repair place and all kinds of things since the '50s, but it is still there, so I stood out front and thought about Sun Records and old Sam Phillips and Jack Clement and how they merely single-handedly created rock 'n' roll without any advice from any goddamn record company idiots about the way to record—by God—Jerry Lee Lewis. Then I made her drive me over to Elvis's place. It's absolutely huge and very eerie. He was actually a king. The house impressed me with the absolute isolation the man lived in.

Then I went back to Nashville and listened to Jack Clement's new record that he just finished for Elektra Records. It's great. I returned to Austin somewhat inspired.

RECORDING IN 1965

When I first started hanging around the studio in Fort Worth in '65 (I guess it was '65, it all blends together now), they had a shiny new big Ampex tube four-track, like four 351s stacked up on top of each other, running one-inch tape. They had a shiny new green Lincoln Altec Lansing stereo mixer with big, black, round knobs, probably had ten or twelve inputs, two VU meters (not dumb-ass peak meters, which don't tell you anything worth knowing), a newfangled item called an "Audio Baton," with little thumb wheels at each of eight frequencies (so's you could EQ all of the balls out of the vocals), maybe one Altec compressor, a bunch of tube and ribbon mics, and a mastering lathe with a peak limiter in it so you wouldn't make the grooves too wide to track. They had Altec "Voice of the Theater" speakers that could blow your hair back and a bottle of Everclear to clean the smoke off the heads.

Everybody would set up in the room together; they'd put out a few Birdcages and 77-DXs with a U47 on the singer and then hit the "record" button and make a record. (As Jack Clement says, "Remember, it only takes three minutes to cut a hit record.")

If Major Bill Smith liked it, he'd have Phil cut an acetate on the granite-ass lathe and take it up to KXOL-AM upstairs, where I was the weekend kid DJ, and play it for the program director, and if he liked it, he'd put it on the damn radio to see if the kids liked it, on the night shift. If the kids liked it, Major Bill would press it up and have it on the streets in a week or two, and if it sold, he'd peddle it to a label, like he did with "Hey Paula" and "Hey Baby" and "Last Kiss" and a bunch of other hit records.

The only way you could fix a bad part in a song was to lift it out of an alternate take and splice it into the final mix, which happened a lot on hit records, actually. Any engineer worth a shit had to be able to take a guitar solo or a chorus and splice it in where the mistake had been made and have it not be noticed. I still take pride in being able to do this, although the chances of anybody asking me to do it are about two thousand to one nowadays. This was the '50s and '60s equivalent of overdubbing, so you don't get too romantic about pure recording techniques—everybody did this; they had to. When four-track came along, everybody still just cut the band track live in stereo and put the vocal on its own track so you could fix flubs, and saved one track for harmonies or hand claps or something, or cut the band in mono and have two extra tracks. When T-Bone Burnett discovered the joys of the new Ampex four-track, there was no holding him back. He used that baby like nobody else around Fort Worth had, doing triple-track vocals and adding weird shit to his tapes and singing through his nose and stuff. He cut a bunch of records on that thing that sounded like Texan Kinks or Beatles or something, and he didn't have anybody to ask how, either. He was a born producer and was only seventeen.

There is, in fact, no substitute for a group of people in the same room playing music together at the same time, listening to each other through the medium called "air" and not over some shitty headphone mix (which is like watching yourself have sex on a TV monitor, at best). In the quest for control over the process, we have lost much of the magic intrinsic in the act of making sound waves by striking things and singing and moving your butt to the groove. In the good old days, which actually were good in this case, nobody had phones, only a floor monitor maybe, in the fancy studios. Everybody mainly used their ears.

I have made good records in all kinds of ways, including the exact opposite of the way that I am describing, but I will always love the physical feeling of having a live band and a live singer all set up in front of the glass, a twenty-four-track two-inch tape machine with the ready lights on and heat waves rising from the deck, and that tiny little instant of dead air when the tape rolls and the band takes a deep breath before somebody counts it off. Roll the tape. Play the song. Magic—all at once.

The following is the original draft written in 1980 by Joe Gracey while preparing the liner notes that appeared on the back cover of the Best of Electric Graceyland *album.*

I was program director for KOKE-FM in Austin from 1973 until 1977. We had pioneered the progressive country format since 1973, but when KOKE-FM changed its format from progressive to Top 40 country, I decided I'd had enough of radio for a while. I was ready for a change and so were the owners of the station, so I took a walk down the circular stairway to the basement office of Bobby Earl Smith.

I noticed Bobby Earl was having a hard time, screaming at the record company in New York, because Alvin and Slappy were screaming into a cassette recorder in the corner of his office. I figured I could be of real service to Bobby Earl if I took Alvin and Slappy somewhere else to record. Alvin needed a place to work out material for his upcoming second album, for Polydor Records. I rented two small offices across the hall and set up my TEAC 2340 tape recorder, and thus was born Electric Graceyland. Eventually Alvin and Bobby Earl broke up their partnership and we converted the larger office into the studio, but not before we recorded two albums in the original room, which was eight feet wide and fifteen feet long. It was tiny.

In that little room with blankets on the walls, we cut an album by the hottest new wave band in town, the Skunks. We then cut an album by the hottest blues band in town, Double Trouble, with Stevie Ray Vaughan (Jimmy Vaughan's brother) and Lou Ann Barton. The room was so tiny that the musicians could play at thundering volumes, which they liked, and I think the albums have a great feel. We eventually released the Skunks album, which is currently out of print. The Double Trouble tapes never came to light, which is a damn shame.

During this time we also recorded *Freda and the Firedogs Live at Soap Creek Saloon* and mixed it at Electric Graceyland. Four-track, no equalization, no compression, a lousy reverb unit, no Dolby, just tape and mics and musicians.

Bobby Earl and I were using the room to make demos of our original songs. It was so much fun and relaxed. The music had a wonderful feeling to it. We eventually decided we liked the tapes so much that we wanted to put them out. We made no claims as to their technical quality or musical virtuosity. We just liked them and thought you would, too.

These songs were recorded between 1978 and 1980. None of them started out to be on a record. They were recorded mostly because we loved to make music and listen to how it sounds when it bounces off the walls. Out of all those miles of tape and those two hectic years, these are our favorite songs. I hope you feel the same tender affection for them that I do. Bobby Earl and I sincerely hope that the music on this album communicates the great feeling that went into the making of it.

I would like to thank all the musicians who put their hearts and souls into the music, Bobby Earl for getting everybody in the right place at the right time, my grandparents and parents for believing in me through thick and thin, and Jack Clement for teaching me that if you believe in magic, you have the universe at your command.

Joe Gracey

RECORDING STEVIE RAY VAUGHAN AT ELECTRIC GRACEYLAND AND AT THE COWBOY ARMS HOTEL AND RECORDING SPA

I was a regular at the Rome Inn, the club where a lot of the better bands were playing, just down the street from Electric Graceyland, my studio in the KOKE-FM basement. Stevie and them were playing there all the time, so I heard them a lot.

Stevie and I never had a contract, just a mutual attempt to get something good on tape and see what we could do with it. I never took session notes, and I doubt if there are even any track sheets, etc., from those days. The basement sessions were great fun because there was no money involved, just my studio and the band in two tiny little rooms. I had an old Shure SM55 mic that Stevie loved because it sounded so lo-fi on the vocals, and we would record for hours and hours just for fun. I'd be at all of his gigs then, just hanging and listening. He and I got to be great friends, and our girlfriends ran around together. We got to be like a couple of brothers, just running around having a blast together all over Austin.

All I had in that studio was a little TEAC four-track, quarter-inch tape deck, a terrible little cheap mixer, and awful mics, but we made some great tapes. Those tapes were later destroyed, as I understand it. I never made a dime out of any of that. In fact, I lost quite a lot of money on Stevie in the end. If I hadn't been so dedicated to Stevie and, therefore, dutiful in my dealings with him, I would have made a copy of those tapes and hidden them away, which I should have done. I wish now that I had done that, but I didn't. Stupid, yes, but karmically the right thing to do, since he didn't want them floating around after he got famous. We all knew he was about to be famous. I knew it all along without any doubt at all.

The Nashville sessions we did were much more complicated because suddenly we had this investor. I had my hands full . . . recording at my mentor Cowboy Jack Clement's place; he approved, and I put on about a B performance as a producer, considering the trying mismatch of Austin blues band and Nashville Jack Clement environment. Jack believes in getting up at 6:00 a.m. and recording during the daytime, while Double Trouble doesn't wake up from their Scotch stupor until 3:00 p.m. But Jack was happy to see his newest star pupil in the studio doing a straightforward album without overdubs or silliness about perfection. The engineer was a real asshole. The band was nervous and exhausted from the drive. So yes, between them and Jack's ghostly presence (he appears out of nowhere, listens intently, and disappears), I had my hands full indeed.

I had to get the band to Nashville and house them and feed them and keep them all happy. I also had to keep Jack Clement happy, which wasn't all that easy since he became worried about a blues band blasting his neighbors to death at 11:00 p.m. One day I came up to the studio to find him hammering three-quarter-inch plywood panels over the windows, which was his way of telling me they were playing too fucking loud, but there was nothing I could do about it. Unfortunately, the band had gotten ahold of some crank, and a lot of tempos to those tracks were too fast because of it, but, all in all, they sounded great.

The engineer made Chris tune his snare head down so it sounded more like an L.A. or Nashville snare, which was a mistake, but so it goes. Those tracks ended up being mastered by me on my last day in

Nashville. I only saw Stevie a couple of times after that and congratulated him on his Epic Records deal and wished him my best.

GETTING AND LOSING CANCER

In June 1977 I resigned from my job as program director at KOKE-FM and became Alvin Crow's roadie and front man. In July I was eating at Jorge's Mexican food restaurant in Austin with my parents, and I noticed that the cold sore on my tongue, which had been bothering me for a few months off and on, was starting to prevent me from eating large quantities of hot sauce. Hot sauce is like beer: you have to build up a tolerance for it over the years, until you can safely drink beer and eat jalapeño peppers all day with out crying. I had built up a pretty good head of steam on both accounts until this day, when I noticed the especially piercing burn on my tongue. I resolved to eat more hot sauce and burn the bugger out!

By October I was in Nashville for Fanfare Week, staying at the Nashville Hyatt House in a big, fine room, with Bobby Earl and Brother Bill, and I started griping about the place on my tongue hurting all the time. Someone joked that it was probably herpes and that I should stop worrying and fucking so much. We were there for Fanfare Week, where the Country Music Association sells tickets to all the fans that come down to Music City USA to spend money and gape around and see a few stars in the downtown auditorium. We were there with Alvin Crow because he was on Puppet Records at the time and they wanted him to play the Exit Inn for some of the Nashville folks. Not a bad idea since none of the people at the record company had ever seen, heard of, or given a shit about Alvin, or ever would.

Tommy Allsup was playing in the Columbia show over at the auditorium for all the yahoos. Tommy was our producer and one of the hippest, nicest cats in the music business. He had played with Buddy Holly, Bob Wills, and a host of other rock and country artists, and was currently the hottest tic-tac bass guitarist in the business. He let me carry his guitar into the backstage area so I could hang out. After a while I needed to get back out to use the phone or something so I went up to the security guard at the backstage entrance and asked if I could be let back in when I returned. Standard reply . . . "No." I said I was working for Tommy Allsup, carrying his guitar. "No."

Then this little, short, fat guy in mirrored shades who has been listening says, "Son, who did you say you are working for?" and I told him again and he says, "Well, let me see what I can do." "Thank you," I said. Then he took off his glasses and I noticed it was Doyle Wilburn, of the Wilburn Brothers. Doyle and Teddy used to be on Channel 11 in Fort Worth on Saturday afternoons before studio wrestling and Porter Wagoner. They used to have Loretta Lynn on the show, too. I was pretty impressed to see ol' Doyle in the flesh. He grabs my hand and says, "Let's see who we can scare up." We set off and who do we run right up on but Loretta herself! She's about 4'9" and pretty, but she has on enough makeup to fill the wrinkles in the palm of my hand, and she looks sort of permanently tired. We moved on outside, and a cop came up to Doyle and said, "Haw Haw! Guess what just happened to that old white caddy you were driving!" And Doyle said, "Did you fuckers tow it off again?! Jesus, Donnie! Where the hell is it?!" Cop says, "You know where it is . . . in the pound again." Doyle says, "Jesus! Why'd you have to do that!?" Cop replies, "Hell, Doyle, you parked it right in the middle of the driveway to the backstage and we had three Buffaloes lined up and waitin' to unload." Doyle just laughs and we walk on up the street to a tiny bar in a hotel lobby. They apparently know him, and he calls out for four double bourbons and water, two for him and two for me. I'd heard Doyle and Teddy had split up over Doyle's alleged dipsomania and now I thought I knew how he could be so jolly over his Cadillac getting towed away.

Back at Fanfare later it was absolutely the pits, like being on another planet. Everybody was decked out in the most amazing colors and styles, and lots of them looked sort of intense around the eyes, with funny-looking little kids, and lot of 'em looked like they had been eating too much pork, like they ate big southern breakfasts three times a day and maybe attended the "Primitive Church of the Airport Freeway." The fan clubs and record companies set up booths at the civic auditorium, and the little Jerry Lee Lewis ladies had an astoundingly gaudy velvet and glittery booth and giant pictures of "The Killer." Somebody would announce that Conway Twitty is now in the MCA Records booth signing autographs and they'd all rush over in a herd and surround little tiny Conway with his huge hair, and then when Charley Pride was over at the RCA booth, they would surge over there and surround him.

Alvin was on Puppet Records, which is a subsidiary of a huge German corporation and is run by guys out of New York who are fairly nervous. Puppets' only achievement is that they own the rights to all of Hank Williams's records. They had taken the original records and added orchestras and choirs and fake echo and drums and guitars to them in order to sell them to the yahoos. It would be roughly the equivalent of painting bigger tits on the Mona Lisa in order to draw a bigger gate at the Louvre. The man who was responsible for this amazing desecration was our main boss of the Nashville office of Puppet. He had an ulcer, drove a little pale blue Rambler, and was scared silly that someone in New York would somehow find out that he didn't know shit. All of the artists he had signed to the label were in some way flawed. One of them made records by reciting these catchy little poems he wrote about his dead mother, and driving trucks, and CB radios. The others were so nondescript as to boggle the mind. To be there, Nashville seemed like the tackiest, dumbest, luckiest town on earth. When the Austin scene started happening, they'd signed Alvin just to be on the safe side. They had never heard of him and didn't like his music, didn't like him or give a shit about his career. It was obvious that Alvin would go far on Puppet.

Their booth at fanfare consisted of some nice eight-by-ten glossies of their unknown artist taped up on the curtains and a folding table with some Xeroxed flyers on it and nobody there to man it. It was truly dynamic. About a dozen steps away, RCA had four giant video screens showing color tape of Charley Pride and John Denver and Dolly Parton in concerts around the world and three cute little numbers in hot pants handing out autographed photos, and every half hour a new superstar would be there signing programs and kissing the ladies.

So anyway, everything was just lovely, and back in the room at the Hyatt House later, I was looking in the mirror at my tongue again, remembering that the night before at the restaurant there I had been unable to eat my Steak Diane because it hurt so much. I was literally in tears from the searing pain that shot through my tongue every time any substance touched it. Booze, cigarettes, cocaine, toothpaste—everything hurt like crazy. I pulled my tongue out of my mouth and looked in the mirror and noticed a dime-sized white patch of skin with a little hole in the middle. It was a nasty-looking thing, like dead skin on the side of my poor tongue. Bill handed me some stuff that was supposed to help herpes sores and told me to put some on there three times a day. So I did, thinking, "Maybe it will go away."

At this point in my life I didn't know there was such a thing as cancer of the tongue. If I had, I still wouldn't have thought about it being on *my* tongue. If you get a big boil on your ass do you start wondering if you have cancer of the buttocks? See what I mean? So I put this pasty crap on my tongue and it got absolutely none better whatsoever. In fact, it got worse. So, like every intelligent American, I waited until it became unbearable and then went to the doctor.

He was the local benefactor of the music scene. Musicians are forced, by the hours they work, to sleep most of the day and work most of the night. We all know how happy doctors are to see anyone after 6:00 p.m. Musicians live incredibly stressful lives. They literally sell emotions, writing them down when they feel them, recording them, and then emoting every night in front of audiences. It is an incredibly wearing life, where the food is a never-ending stream of highway grease. Sleep is hard to come by in a world that doesn't make any exceptions for day sleepers. Imagine sleeping in a Holiday Inn for the rest of your life. Imagine going from a Greyhound bus to a Denny's restaurant to a Holiday Inn for the rest of your life! The break from that routine is for the few hours you're onstage in a strange place in front of people you've never seen, during which time your job is to create joy, sadness, etc., with your emotions as the well from which you draw. Bad food, little sleep, constant temptation to drink, and, worst of all, there is the boredom. You can only write songs or practice your instrument so many hours a day. Then there's the fear of not being any good—"bombing"—stage fright. So with this type of patient, a doctor discovers the results of bad food, no sleep, no exercise, no sunlight, no vitamins, too many cigarettes, too much booze, almost constant boredom, and the stress of too much daily emotional outpouring. How do you advise this person or treat his particular problems? That's how you get these doctors that

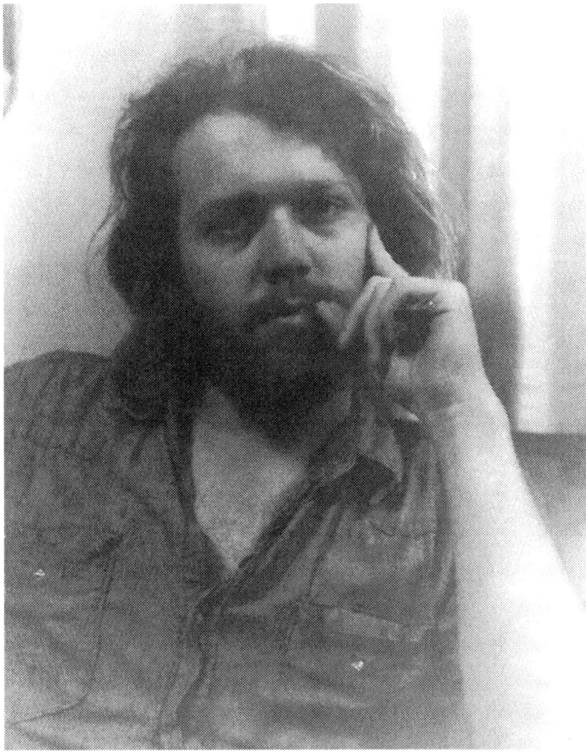

Gracey "getting and losing cancer."

will just go ahead and give him pills to sleep, wake up, create euphoria. Hank Williams and Elvis are prime examples of simple men who found a doctor who would give him anything he wanted, and the result was early death.

The doctor I saw in Austin was not a quack. He was kind and intelligent. He liked music and musicians, and he understood the kind of lives they led and tried to modify the worst aspects of it by telling them about nutrition and vitamins and sleep and the effects of stress and emotion and the lack of some kind of calm space that everyone must have. His office was in his house and he had a beard and wore blue jeans. He had a steer hide on the floor and a great stereo player playing his patients' records.

I says, "Doc, I have this sore on my tongue." (Since I had been a disc jockey and was a singer, my tongue was my second-most prized body part.) He looked at it and squeezed it a little and said, "Well, one of the symptoms of syphilis is a sore on the tongue." He took a blood sample and gave me a shot of penicillin and stuck a swab up into the front end of my most prized body part.

A few days later the tests showed that I did not have syphilis. He said maybe it was just a bad herpes sore and told me to put these little silver nitrate sticks on it every night. What they do is merely burn the tissue and cauterize the wound. So that didn't hurt anymore than putting a wood burning iron up to your tongue except that the sore itself had become terribly angry, with an evil sharp pain all its own.

Then I was sent to a dermatologist who said it was probably syphilis and took a blood test. Then he also said that if it wasn't syphilis, it might be cancer. This was the first time anyone had said that word. My reaction was one that I would come to experience many times in later months. I was angry. It made me mad that he would even bring up that subject. I immediately decided that he was an incompetent old fool and made up my mind that I was never coming back to his office again. What a ridiculous suggestion!

I went to another dermatologist who assured me that at my age, twenty-seven, cancer was a very remote possibility and that I probably had some type of obstinate infection that would be rooted out by antibiotics and treatment of the sore itself. He took a blood test and ruled out herpes. He gave me a week's worth of strong antibiotics and told me to return. In a week it looked a little better but not better enough. He told me to stick out my tongue, and before I knew it, he was squeezing on my tongue for what seemed like about six years until some stuff came out of it. I would have hit him but I was completely blinded by tears. He was gleeful and said, "What we have here is a necrotic infection going deep into the center of your tongue. More antibiotics and you'll be fine."

One week later, no improvement. He looked at it and said, "Son, this is bad. I'm scared. I'll be right back. We've got to do a biopsy." He walked out of the room leaving me with that kind of wrench in the gut that gets you when you hear that ominous tone come into someone's voice, especially a doctor's. He and the nurse came back in and did a biopsy. He gave me a prescription for some kind of painkiller and said he would check around with some of his doctor friends and see what needed to be done but that it would probably involve some radiation and a little surgery to remove the sore if indeed it proved to be malignant. He said, "Come back in a week." Well, I was going to be in Nashville in a week, but I said I would call and check on the biopsy results.

Here I experienced the first instance of another emotion I was going to get to know very well in the months ahead. Rather than the panic, I initially felt a sort of shock set in, a mixture of numbness, wonder, and curiosity, as if one could step outside of one's body and view it critically from ten feet away. I was immensely curious about this "cancer" that might be residing in my body. Then came a fear so monstrous that my mind just surrendered to it and lay down in front of it and was engulfed by it. At that point you and the fear become one, as if you are in it, as if in an ocean, floating, and you can just lie back in it and float in it because it is so big you don't even bother to try to fight it. You simply become it. In that way, you fool it. You are tactful and calm. People around you call it courage and admire you for it, but I think it was the only way I could cope with it, because I had no choice.

Bobby Earl had driven me to the doctor's and was in the car waiting for me when I came out. "The son of a bitch thinks it might be cancer," I said, eyes wide. "Oh, shit, Gracey! What did he do?" "He sliced off a piece of my tongue and sent it to the medical examiner for an autopsy or something. Fuck if I know! My tongue hurts like hell! I want to fill this scrip!" So we drove next door to pick up the pills and it was something called Demerol, which I had never heard of before. They were a hundred milligrams, and I hurt so badly that I took two of them just to be sure. By the time we got back to our basement office I felt like I was on a slow boat to China. I knew I had probably overdone it a bit when I slipped and fell out of the chair onto the floor and just lay there with a dumb grin. "Pill's strong, Gracey?" Bobby Earl asked. "Oh, boy," I says.

Demerol, as I came to find out, is a synthetic substitute for morphine. It is pure hospital-tested all-American "junk." Elvis loved it. At first I did, too, but after a few days of being junked out, it became tiresome and uninviting for me, so that's why I was never tempted to use it all the time.

Bobby Earl and I had been promoting Alvin's new single release on Puppet Records called "Nyquil Blues," a neo-'50s rocker about getting stoned on Nyquil, a cold medication that at the time contained chloroform and alcohol enough to get any self-respecting wino buzzed a couple of times. We had driven ahead of Alvin's bus all the way from Hilton Head to Texas wearing "Nyquil Blues" T-shirts, painting our tongues green, and handing out bottles to disc jockeys. Doing this, we had gotten enough airplay to put us at 99 on the *Billboard* Top 100 chart. When we called up Puppet Records and told them we'd made them a hit record and asked if they would be doing the final push it needed to get into the Top 40, they told us we should mind our own business.

So I flew to Nashville and checked in at the Hall of Fame Motor Inn, right across the street from the Country Music Hall of Fame. The mullets at the Puppet office were oh-so-glad to see me, especially since they loved people from Texas so much. The national director wanted to know how on earth the song had gotten on the charts with no promotion. "I guess you didn't hear that Bobby Earl and I have been buying cases of Nyquil and driving two thousand miles in one week and dying our goddamn tongues green and living on beer and Vienna sausages and visiting every *Billboard* reporting station between the Atlantic Ocean and the Mexican border with a quick stop off in St Louis?" I asked. "Well, no." I didn't realize you'd jumped the gun so badly. I guess now we'll have to step up our promotion on the record," the squirrely little guy with the thick round glasses said. "Well, I think I'll help you." I said, "Who's in that little empty office down the hall that I saw Little Junior One Hand using the phone in? (Little Junior had lost a hand in a pinball accident and was one of their top acts. He played slide guitar.) "Nobody's in there. You can use that phone if you'd like. Aren't there a lot of little stations in Texas you could call too?" "Why, yes, there are three hundred and fifty-one, to be exact." So first I called all of them for little chats about their wives and kids and dogs and Alvin. Then I called every major station in the country and Bill Mack and Charlie Douglas (who do the all night trucker shows on powerful stations in Dallas and New Orleans). I called WHN in New York, all the trade magazines, and *Rolling Stone*. And then I called my doctor.

He says, "Not too good, I'm afraid. The pathologist detects definite signs of cancerous cells, squamous cell carcinoma, it's called. I want a second biopsy to be done right away. This time we'll take a little bigger piece and get a better idea of the true nature of the thing." "Oh boy," I thought. "I'll be home next week so you can schedule the surgery then. Bye."

On a cloudy, cold, gray day, Nashville can be the most lonesome place on earth. I walked back to the Hall of Fame Motor Inn and went into the little lounge for a drink, or perhaps two. I had a couple of Jack Daniels and eavesdropped on conversations. Seemed like the bar was full of older guys in suits or call girls or younger girls trying pretty hard to get their hands in some old guy's pocket. The ambience was pretty much "gin and carpet." Of course, finding out I had cancer of the tongue might have influenced my perception of the place. I remember vividly the sense of tired, sick loneliness that got to me in that tacky room. Seems like even the walls were painted gray. My girlfriend and I were on the verge of splitting up, and she wasn't a particularly sensitive type anyway, so calling her to tell her the bad news wasn't such a hot idea. I don't think I called anybody. I just sat there and stared at the walls and felt horrible. Then I got a ten-dollar cab ride to the airport with Eddie, my favorite cabbie, and headed back to Austin.

I later discovered that MD Anderson in Houston is one of the most recognized cancer hospitals in the country. They know more about the treatment and diagnosis of cancer than most other doctors simply because it's all they do. They treat thousands of patients with every known type of cancer, and the knowledge gained from each operation is put to teaching and research uses. But I kept running into some sort of jealousy syndrome in Austin. Doctors who held my life in their hands would say, "Oh God! Don't go down there. They'll have half your head cut away before you can blink!" Or they would simply assert that there was nothing that MD Anderson could do that couldn't be done in Austin.

So, here I am, pathology report in hand, reporting that I have cancer and with a doctor who says he wants to "cut out the sore, just to be sure it's cancer." And if it is, he says, "We can probably remove it all during surgery." "How much of my tongue will you have to remove?" I asked, thinking of Barbary Coast pirates. "About a thimble's worth," he replies, holding up his finger and marking it at the first knuckle with his thumb. I grimaced. There is really no choice, and, besides, I think, as long as he gets the cancer out it's really no big deal.

So the following morning at 8:00 a.m. I go to the Bailey Square Surgery Center for a day surgery. Here I am with a bunch of little kids all having their tonsils removed. In my green robe and cute little paper slippers, I am terrified. I have never gotten over my childhood fear of anesthesia and operating rooms.

Back in recovery I really didn't feel too bad. I didn't notice the pain or some swelling in my tongue. The doctor came in and told me he had gotten all the cancer and everything would be okay in a few days, he was sure, so not to worry about a thing. I started having pain and asked for a shot and got one and passed out. When I awoke around 6:00 p.m., there was terrible swelling and a pain that felt like I had been kicked in the head by a mule. They gave me some codeine tablets and sent me home with my girlfriend, who took me back to her house.

By 10:00 p.m. that night my tongue had swollen hugely, and by 3:00 a.m. I woke up in a feverish sleep, realizing I was bleeding to death. We rushed to Brackenridge Hospital going about 140 miles an hour in my 1967 Cadillac. The doctor who was on call saw I was turning blue and bleeding profusely from the mouth but had no idea what he was confronted with. They called the surgeon who had performed the surgery earlier in the day, and he declined to come down, saying they could do just as good a job as he could. So I'm sitting there with a doctor whose saying he's "stumped," figuring, well, this is it. . . . I'm probably going to die. Then a surgeon shows up, puts a clamp here and there, takes out a big needle and some black thread and starts sewing me up. He gave me a shot of Demerol and left.

There was an old black gentleman who was complaining of breathing difficulty on the table next to me. I was lying there with my eyes closed trying to collect my wits when I overheard two doctors standing at the foot of my bed speaking in hushed tones. I caught a snatch of something that sounded like, "This guy doesn't realize it, but he really hasn't got long to go in this world." I'm thinking, "Oh no! Does he know something I don't know? Do I still have cancer?" One of your greatest fears as a cancer patient is that you have a terminal case and nobody is telling you. As it turned out, they were speaking of the poor guy next to me.

The quack who had performed the surgery and then refused to come sew me back up when I was bleeding to death became defensive and was clearly beginning to bend the truth about whether or not he had in fact removed all the cancer. I finally found my way to a head and neck doctor who was familiar with my radio show I had done at KOKE-FM. He quietly listened to my fear and confusion and finally said, "I think you are becoming entangled in a web of local advice. This contradiction is unnecessary. I think you should go to MD Anderson and get their opinion. They are the best people in the state on this subject."

So in early December my parents and I went down to MD Anderson. The Head and Neck Surgery department can be a terrifying place. Unlike most cancers that don't "show," this one can be quite disfiguring, people without noses or chins or eyeballs. As we waited for five hours, my terror increased. Finally an oncologist came in, nodded at my weary parents, and opened my mouth to have a look. I explained that I had had an "excisional biopsy" the week before and that the tests were inconclusive. The doctor became incensed. As he looked in my mouth he began to shout, "What the hell is an 'excisional biopsy,' and what is all this filthy black thread and why is this wound so infected?!" I felt he was mad at me, and I was close to tears. I had come to this great hospital in desperation, seeking help, and I was being ground under the menacing glare of a "great surgeon" and treated as if I were guilty of gross stupidity for allowing these things to happen. He disgustedly told me he couldn't see a thing until the swelling had gone down and these gross sutures had been removed. My father, torn with grief and fear for his son, calmly asked what the treatment might be. The doctor briskly stated that at least part of the tongue if not all would have to come out and then turned on his heels and strode out of the room without so much as goodbye.

I had made my living since I was fourteen with this tongue. I was a rock 'n' roll singer and a disc jockey in high school. My voice was a deep, rich baritone, and I had developed not only a career but also a personality, a character, around it. I had been a classical singer in opera choruses and choirs at the University of Texas. I gloried in the sound, the timbre, the inflections, the tricks I could make with my voice. I was a singer, on the verge of making records with one of America's greatest producers, who had promised me that once I was sufficiently groomed for the part, he would produce my records. He told me I had the ability to become a star. My voice and I were about to "make it." Now I was being told that at best I would be vocally handicapped and at worst, mute, if I survived. On the way out I told a nurse that I would rather die than let that bastard come near me again. I had told myself over and over during the early part of this ordeal that I'd rather be dead than lose my power of speech, and I meant it.

I was well into an identifiable stage that every cancer patient must endure. I was angry with the doctors because they were being unfeeling and insufficiently impressed, I thought, with the fact that my tongue meant more to me than to most people. I refused to believe that all this was really as bad as I was being told. I convinced myself that all I needed was a little bit of radiation and simple surgery and I would be okay. So in my rage and disbelief, compounded by this rather shabby treatment by the surgeon at MD Anderson, I resolved to seek every possible opinion. I frantically decided that somewhere in the country was a surgeon who wasn't ready to cut out my tongue between lunch and golf.

In the office of one surgeon I noticed a book on the desk. The surgeon was a kindly older gentleman, and I felt that I could trespass a little, so I picked up the book and started to look at it. It was called *Cancers of the Head and Neck* and had been published about ten years prior by the staff at MD Anderson. It was a textbook. I looked up cancers of the tongue and larynx, use of extensive tissue grafting to rebuild the floor of the mouth, radiation of the area, removal of the lymph system in all surrounding muscles in the chin and neck. There was nothing else, no options, arguments, or pleas of mercy. This is what statistics showed to be the most effective way of saving the life of a person with oral cancer. The older doctor came in with a younger earnest-looking doctor as I finished reading this succinct little wrap-up.

"Reading up on your case?" he asked with a smile. "Just checking it out," I replied. I could feel the sadness in the air. These men were unhappy about what they were about to have to tell me. My defiant outward show of courage was melting slowly. The younger doctor began to describe a radical surgery where a piece of tissue from my forehead would have to be removed to replace the tissue removed from the floor of my mouth. He kept talking, but by then I was far, far away. The room became as if underwater, and I heard his voice droning, and I kept hearing the words "tongue" and "removal." After he stopped talking, I begged them again if they were sure that radiation was not the answer. The older surgeon answered, "Our radiology team feels as if they cannot help you. I'm sorry."

I walked out into the sunshine. The feeling of unreality was becoming constant now in this waking dreamlike world. The gray cover of the surgical textbook, the slick white pages, the old-fashioned lettering that reminded me of our encyclopedias at home, black-and-white grainy photos of tumors and tongues and lips and jaws. But the sun kept shining, and it was almost Christmas, and I was sliding, sliding, all the time, backwards, downwards, into the maw at the other end of a mile of slippery fear and disease.

Cancer—the word itself has taken on primeval, disquieting shades of meaning that one only feels. It is the crab, the gnawing tentacled monster with too many legs and no brain to be told that inside of one's body is a disease that is growing and eating away at your flesh every minute of every day. I always picture a brown feces-like mass of cells that somehow grow. I remember the way the tumor felt when it was in my tongue. It was hard but not rock hard. Hard like a lump of scar tissue, hard and soft at the same time. Surgeons know the feel of tumor tissue very well. I was developing a violent dislike for surgeons and was convinced that they were sadistic and trigger happy and out of date in today's world of medical science, dinosaurs of the art of healing. In my fright I was sure that surgeons were just out to slice up one more victim needlessly.

I was a drowning man, and radiation was the log. Finally, a well-respected and experienced radiologist told us exactly what we didn't want to hear, that with radiation treatment only, my chances of survival were 25 to 40 percent at best. His last words were soft as he looked at my distraught parents' faces, "If this were my son, I would have the surgery."

We saw yet another surgeon in Dallas who came into his office on the day after Christmas especially to see me. He said my jawbone would have to be broken and wired back together and confirmed again that skin from my forehead would have to be moved to the floor of my mouth to replace the tissue that would have to be removed. We didn't even ask any questions or beg for a more lenient assessment. We thanked him and walked out into the crisp December day.

My parents rarely drink. My brother, Bill, the family psychologist by virtue of his degree, broke the stunned silence in the car by demanding that we stop at a 7-11 store to buy a coke. He and I went into the store, giddy with the "overwhelmingness" of it all, laughing and feeling like we'd taken a psychedelic drug. The world was not real. The people in the store were all grotesque, or hilarious, or sad-looking. We laughed insanely at everybody and everything in the store, then bought a six-pack of beer. Back in the car, Bill handed one to my father and then to my mother, saying he thought we all just needed a beer. My mother finally burst out laughing and said, "I think you're right." I had never seen my mother drink a beer. Our family's sense of humor has carried us through many a battle.

Finally, my doctor sent me to a doctor who sent me to a doctor who sent me back to MD Anderson, saying he thought he knew a surgeon there who had a sense of humor and was kind and that I would "get along with," Dr. Richard Jesse. I felt good about Dr. Jesse as soon as he walked into the room. He reached for one of those rubber things they use to palpate the inside of your mouth and dropped it. He either dropped or discarded a couple of them before he finally got grip on one and commenced to feeling around on my, by now healed, tongue.

He said he felt like there was still cancerous tissue in my tongue and offered several options. One of them, because he had spoken with my doctor and was aware that I wished to try to retain my speech if possible, was an option for minimal surgery, meaning he would stop as soon as he obtained a clean tissue biopsy, rather than continue to cut in order to maintain a safer margin, followed by heavier radiation to the tongue. Or I could have radiation alone.

My father asked Dr. Jesse if he would be willing to do the surgery himself. Jesse had hands that felt good while he was feeling around, and I decided to put him to the test. I said, "Hold on a minute. I ain't so sure I want you operating on me after the way I just saw you drop those three little rubber things before you could get one on your finger." I looked semi-serious. He just looked at me deadpan and said, "I was going to do you next Tuesday, but Tuesday is my drinking night, so I'll take care of you Wednesday morning . . . early. That was all I needed to know. I

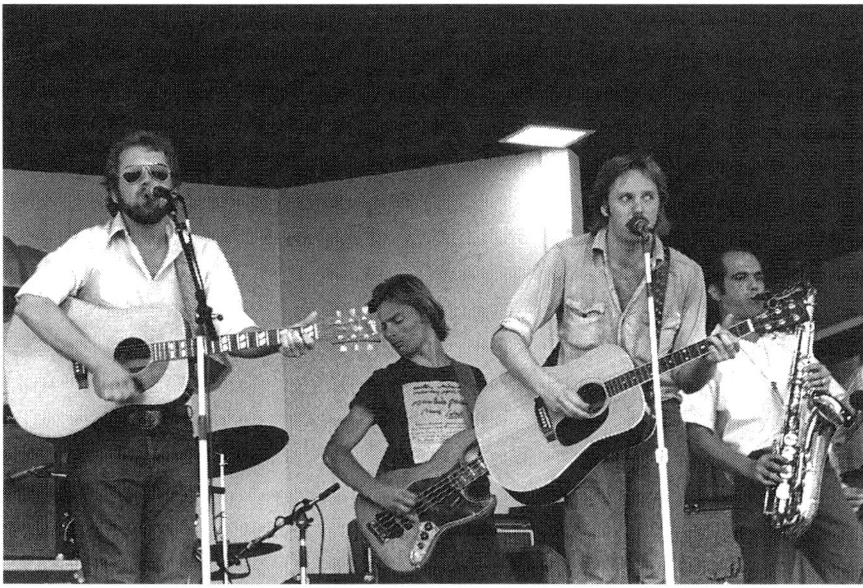

The Amazing Gracey Brothers.

realized that for the first time in this ordeal I felt true hope. The surgery was scheduled for the following Tuesday morning.

I went back to Austin. I had written a couple of songs that I had felt were good enough to record demos of. I realized that after the surgery there was the possibility that I might have relatively impaired speech, so I wanted to at least get myself on tape in case that happened. I was still playing a few shows with Alvin and his band, and they knew all the songs that Bill and I had done on the Eastern Seaboard tour. Bobby Earl and I booked time at Austin Recording Studios and asked the band to be there to back me up.

The session went remarkably well. Alvin arranged the songs, and we laid down basic rhythm tracks, using Rick Crow, Billy Nadeau (drums), and Alvin (rhythm guitar), and then we overdubbed Alvin on fiddles, Rick on electric guitar, Herb Steiner on steel and dobro, Roger Crabtree on harp. I did the vocals on "Deep in Love," a Ray Price–type twin fiddle shuffle, and overdubbed the main vocal, and Bill overdubbed the harmony vocal.

On "Him Again," sort of a Don Williams–inspired song, I played rhythm guitar and sang the vocal at the same time that the rhythm section did the basic track. It was considered to be a "work vocal," but as things turned out, it became the final vocal. My gut feeling that this would turn out to be the last time I sang turned out to be true. We finished the tracks on Sunday night and we mixed them down on Monday. I left for Houston Monday night to check in for the surgery the next morning.

One thing about my family is that we are close. My parents were there in a rented apartment across the street from the hospital. I was rapidly retreating into my childhood, back when I was a sickly kid and got a lot of attention from my parents. It was wonderful and also a little eerie, being twenty-eight years old and experiencing precisely the same set of emotions as when I had been seven and had to have surgery. We even ate tomato soup—Campbell's tomato soup—the staple of all sick kids in my family.

I checked into my room at the hospital and was told I could go eat with my family as long as I was back at 10:00 a.m. I went to Trader Vic's, near the famous Shamrock Hotel, and the only people there were my parents, my brother, my maternal grandparents, and my aunt and uncle. I began to be seized with terror. I sat next to my grandmother, who refuses to be daunted by fear, unhappiness, bad health, or unpleasant people. Her sense of humor is completely absurd, and she is one of the brainiest people I have ever known. Everything that comes out of her mouth is witty, sometimes delicately sarcastic, and in denial of the darker side of human existence. That helped assuage my growing panic. Damn if I know what I ate.

Jesse likes to operate early in the morning. They came for me at 6:00 a.m., and I was on the way to surgery at 7:00 a.m. I was first in line, full of morphine and scared witless. Then came the bright lights of the operating room, nurses in green, their calm chatter bouncing off tile walls, a cold sensation on my chest, a few quick strokes of a razor, another coldness on my forehead, a quick swipe of the razor there. Then I hear Jesse, and I open my eyes for the first time. "Ready, Gracey?" I nod. "Okay, I'm going to give you some sodium pentothal." Ten seconds and the world goes sweetly, quietly black.

The operation took four or five hours. When I came to Intensive Care I had never felt so miserable in my entire life. My tongue was already swollen terribly and was sticking out of my mouth. My mouth was packed with gauze, very dry, very painful. My neck was wrapped tightly in elastic bandages, and it burned along the incision line. I felt battered and beaten and shocked and sick and exhausted. I was breathing through a hole in my neck. I was dazed and confused. I started to call for help and realized I couldn't. A nurse came over and asked me how I was doing and handed me a pad and pencil. I wrote, "I feel terrible." She gave me a pain shot. I lost track of the hours and days. I began to wonder how long I had been there. I fixated on the clock above the nurses' station as a handle on reality.

I would experience a drowning sensation when fluid began to build up in my bronchial tubes. At one point I started to slide. My will to live was drained out of me. I was being covered in blankets of depression over losing my tongue, my voice, over having cancer, possibly dying, losing my ability to make a living. My lungs kept filling up and I didn't have the willpower to raise my hand and call for a nurse. I couldn't breathe any longer. I felt myself going black and sinking down, down, into a delicious warm blackness, with no more problems, no more pain, and no more need to prove that I could "handle it." I sank into a deep dark well that had a glorious light at the end of it, toward which I began to be drawn. I had the most delicious sense of going home.

Then I heard the sound of my name being called. It got a little louder. Then I realized that someone was shouting at me. Not only that, but they were shouting right in my face. I have never been too fond of having my face shouted in, especially in light of the newly found peace I was trying to slip off into. It made me so mad that I started backing up so I could tell the son of a bitch to get out of my face and let me die in peace! Then boom! I crash out into the green tile brightness and here's this guy screaming, "Joe! Are you listening to me?! Joe! Wake up and talk to me! Can you breathe yet?! Tell me right now if you can breathe yet! I'm not going to stop suctioning you until you tell me you can breathe!" Tears were coming out of my eyes and I was wracked with convulsive coughing. I calmed down and nodded that yes! I could damn sure breathe now! I was disgusted that my happy swim toward death had been interrupted by the man shouting in my face because it was extremely irritating in my floating euphoric state, but I'm glad he did.

I was moved to my private room, and Jesse came in to see me, followed by his retinue of interns and residents, and announced that the results of the lymph node biopsies had been negative, which meant clean, which was the most important thing of all. I stayed for ten days longer and then returned home to Austin with a little more than half my tongue intact and a short red scar under my chin.

I moved into a tiny little apartment next to Bill. I had a bed, a kitchen, and a bathroom. It cost a hundred dollars a month and was furnished. I had enough money to live on. I was independent, and it was a fine feeling.

The radiation treatments started, and after about three or four weeks, my skin began to look burned and I got to the point where I could barely eat because of the pain. When I reached the point where I couldn't eat, they would stop the radiation treatment for a couple of weeks. This went on from February to April. I looked weird going around all the time with red dye patches drawn on my face to delineate the areas that were to be zapped by the radiation. One night Bobby Earl decided to join in the fun and painted big patches on his face and we went barhopping. We got some good reactions from people.

It was during this time that I formed Joe Gracey Productions, Inc., with my grandfather, Cecil Morgan. He wanted to make sure I didn't starve to death, so he invested some money in me to get me started in the record business. I rented a set of offices across from the Crow Smith Productions office in the basement of the KOKE-FM building, borrowed a table from Tony down the hall, and set up a little Sony quarter-track machine in one room. I bought speakers, an amp, two fifteen-dollar microphones, and some wire, and I was in business. I generally began to gear up to become the man I had always wanted to be: producer, writer, thinker.

Sometimes it takes being led through the valley of the shadow before one realizes the meaning of what it is to be alive. I never had any trouble with the fun part of being alive—food, drink, etc.—but it really is more than that and I've known it all along. Maybe there's a compromise, if I can just let myself do the best for me and not ruin my life trying to prove something to myself that didn't need proving anyway. Life regained is in some ways better than life untroubled.

LETTER TO PEN PAL MARIAN IN MARCH 1978
PARTIAL LOSS OF SPEECH

My dearest Marian,

I'm sitting here listening to Jack Clement's album on a cassette. He came by the hospital today while on a promotional tour for his album, and I was overjoyed to see the silly old fucker walk in the door, truly wonderful surprise. I think he was surprised at how well I'm doing.

I thought I'd try to answer some of your questions. I may have said this in the other letter, but the tongue starts in the larynx and ends at the tip. It fills the floor of the mouth and forms the front of the throat. I have lost the part that goes from tip to back molar and most of the part that fills the floor of the left side of my mouth. All the right floor side is still there. So I have this odd, crater-like rolling and tumbling mouth and nothing even remotely resembling a tongue. I feel very confident that this time the surgery has fixed the problem. The nagging doubt still lingers.

However, I can still talk! I haven't yet figured out how, but I can still make sounds that people can figure out, and some of the words are almost perfect. I can still count on doing any of things I've been doing up to now, except the most blatant record promoting, which I hate anyway. After all the melodrama, I have returned with very reasonable speaking ability but markedly handicapped, but it will improve with time. I have no doubt. It is nothing short of a bloomin' miracle (which, of course, I believe in fully).

If I am to eat, I have got to figure out a relatively dignified way to get things from the front of my mouth to the front of my throat, something the tongue normally does. Looking up speculatively at the ceiling from time to time might do the trick, but after a while it would seem fairly eccentric to other people at the table. Poking it back there with a spoon might work. I could simply carry a little thing like they used to load cannons or muzzle loading rifles in the Civil War. I don't know. Oh yes, I can also wash things down with water after carefully chewing them. I imagine chewing will be a chore without a tongue to manipulate the food around. Dear. Dear. How disgusting that such a glorious thing should become a hassle and ultimately almost too much trouble to mess with! You wanna take bets I live on Nutrament?

I thought today with sadness about how I only got to record two songs before they got me. I've got other more primitive stuff but only two real-live studio quality tapes. Dear God. I wanted to sing. The main sadness is in knowing that something is irretrievably lost; same as funerals, graduation, dropping things in the lake. I remember Jack Clement once told me I was the best singer in Austin.

My speech will change my approach to the world. I won't know just how yet, but yes, my lifestyle has been dictated by ability to project myself through my voice and its sound. It's the first talent I harnessed to give myself status and self-image in school, way back in the fifth grade. In fact, my talking career can almost be viewed as my attempt to quit competing on the "hard, cold ground of thought" and shift to the glamorous territory of speech and drama and music and entertainment. In fact, as I write this I realize that I've been feeling guilty about the whole thing ever since, knowing full well that I have cheated myself by relying on my tongue to keep my brain from having to work. I know it's not that simple, but I also know that what I'm saying is true. Charm, glibness, blue eyes, sweet tongue, deep voice, all that shit, have carried me past the point where I wanted to "get off" and start being a man. It just won't be so easy now. I'm glad something has come along to put me in a position where it's "think, or else!"

Love,
Joe

ON NOVEMBER 23, 1978, in an article in his column for the *Austin American-Statesman* newspaper, Austin's beloved critic, Townsend Miller, wrote, "The 'Thanks Joe Gracey' benefit Thanksgiving night was an overwhelming success. The largest crowd in Armadillo World Headquarters history heard a fine program of music, ate some 400 turkey dinners, and contributed almost $10,000 to help pay Joe's medical

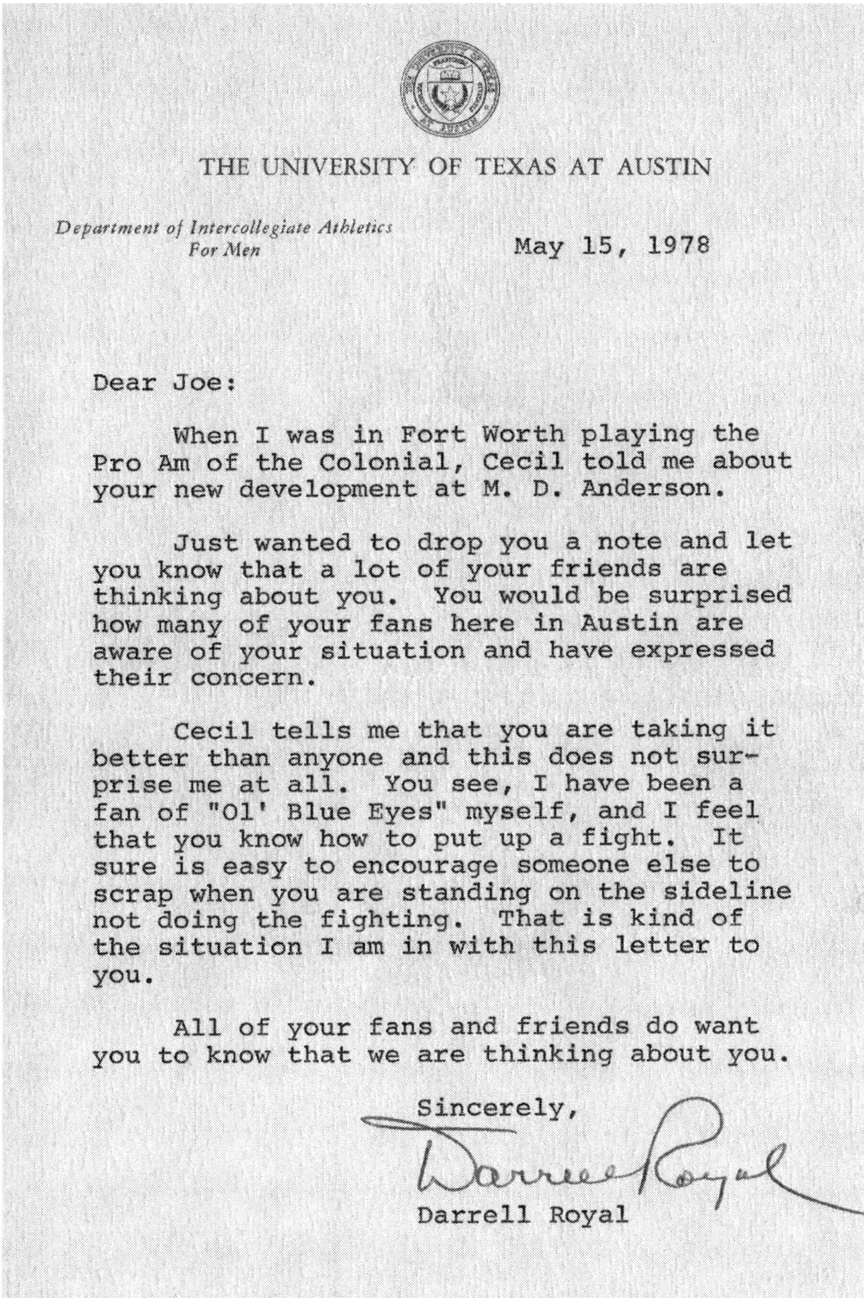

THE UNIVERSITY OF TEXAS AT AUSTIN

Department of Intercollegiate Athletics
For Men

May 15, 1978

Dear Joe:

When I was in Fort Worth playing the Pro Am of the Colonial, Cecil told me about your new development at M. D. Anderson.

Just wanted to drop you a note and let you know that a lot of your friends are thinking about you. You would be surprised how many of your fans here in Austin are aware of your situation and have expressed their concern.

Cecil tells me that you are taking it better than anyone and this does not surprise me at all. You see, I have been a fan of "Ol' Blue Eyes" myself, and I feel that you know how to put up a fight. It sure is easy to encourage someone else to scrap when you are standing on the sideline not doing the fighting. That is kind of the situation I am in with this letter to you.

All of your fans and friends do want you to know that we are thinking about you.

Sincerely,

Darrell Royal

Darrell Royal

University of Texas Coach Darrell Royal letter to Gracey.

Gracey,

well here i am home and just heard the bad news. what can i say?what x can you you say?(bad joke #1) we all send our best(the band) and just to let you know things are as hectic and fucked up as can be. But the real thing is that it keeps on going almost like it don't even need people or so itseems. As of rite now Floyd has left the band and we're having the other cats Danny and Link play the thing and get on with the business of making music and money. If we ever get out of this inceesssant touring thing i mite be able to set back and see what it is that all our(meaning you me the band speedy alvin et al) collective ramblings babblings and ixx gross neglect of our own selves have done in the broader scope of american musical and cultural life.Sounds heavy don't it well i hope we have been just that,heavy. Sometimes when we give of ourselves to another person or thing we give away the best part and wind up short changing ourselves, the one who needs it the most.You certainly know that and my poor body is beginning to feel the worst after all these years of misuse. Anywho we've had a ball and burned the candle from the middle out so.... maybe we're gettin what we asked for idont know. Me and you are a lot alike joe and the things that happen to you usually happen to me and vica versa in a lot of ways. what i mean is that in you i see a lot of me and sometimes it helps me to see what i look like and what i act like from another angle.Don't worry Joe we arn't that much alike it's just we have similar goals and attitudes about music life and all that and we're both performers of the highest order because life is our stage if we are denied that release on stage.It's not music or history or any of that jazz that is the ultimate stimlant,it is our love for communication and attention that is being fed and txxxx tongue or no tongue you'll find a way to satisfy that part of you.Hell I've had to come to the realization that i wasn't a great singer and that i was gonna have to communicate this thing some other way which i ain't got figured out xtxx at all. Anyway Remember; if ther is anything i can do name it(besides learnin to type) I feel like your brother and miss you a lot you son of a bitch and for gods sake or anyones for that matter get well and stay in touch.

I guess you'll be in Ft Worth for a while so i'll catch up with you there.

Adios amigo drop me a line if you get a chance

Power to the Proper People

Ray

Ray Benson (Asleep at the Wheel) letter to Gracey.

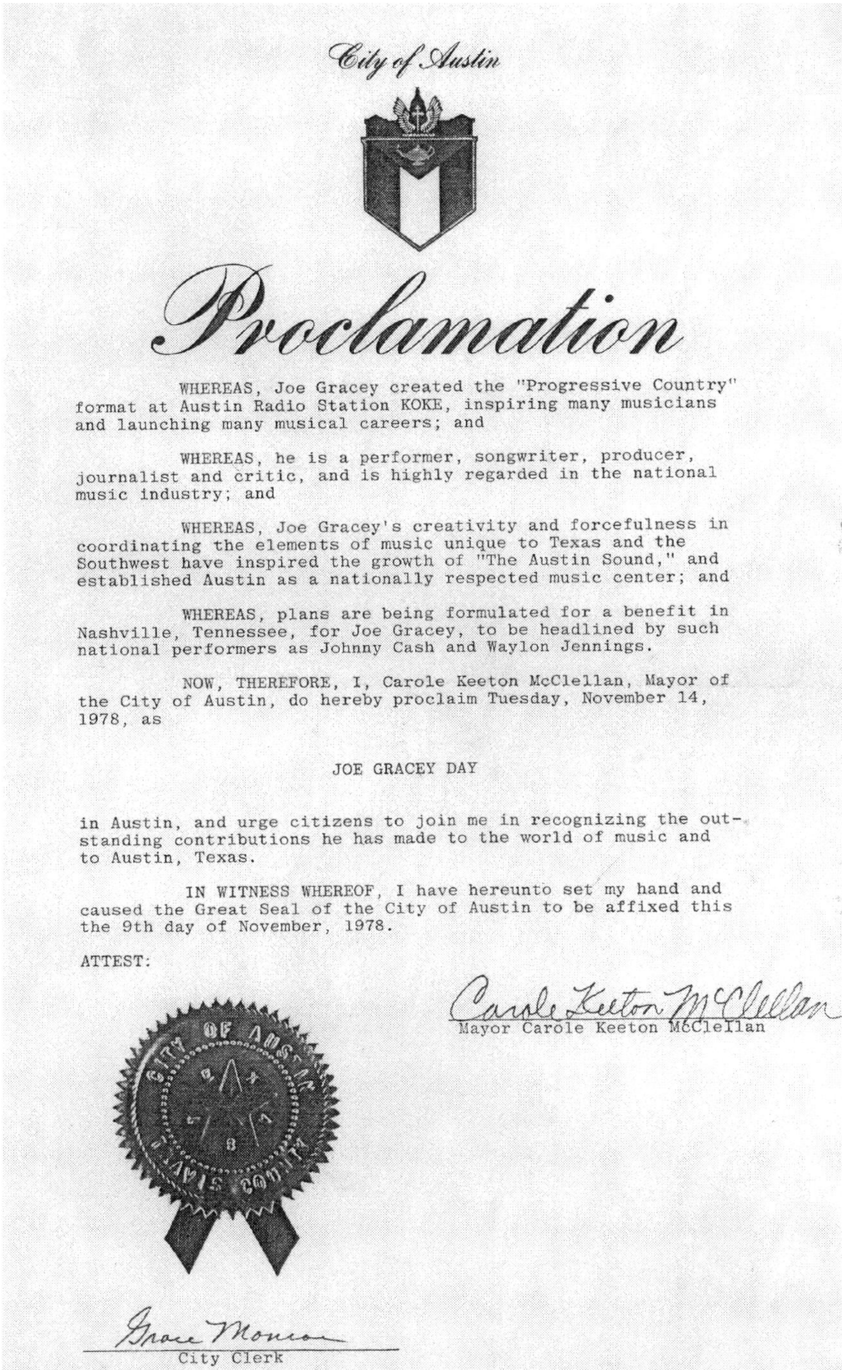

City of Austin

Proclamation

WHEREAS, Joe Gracey created the "Progressive Country" format at Austin Radio Station KOKE, inspiring many musicians and launching many musical careers; and

WHEREAS, he is a performer, songwriter, producer, journalist and critic, and is highly regarded in the national music industry; and

WHEREAS, Joe Gracey's creativity and forcefulness in coordinating the elements of music unique to Texas and the Southwest have inspired the growth of "The Austin Sound," and established Austin as a nationally respected music center; and

WHEREAS, plans are being formulated for a benefit in Nashville, Tennessee, for Joe Gracey, to be headlined by such national performers as Johnny Cash and Waylon Jennings.

NOW, THEREFORE, I, Carole Keeton McClellan, Mayor of the City of Austin, do hereby proclaim Tuesday, November 14, 1978, as

JOE GRACEY DAY

in Austin, and urge citizens to join me in recognizing the outstanding contributions he has made to the world of music and to Austin, Texas.

IN WITNESS WHEREOF, I have hereunto set my hand and caused the Great Seal of the City of Austin to be affixed this the 9th day of November, 1978.

ATTEST:

Carole Keeton McClellan
Mayor Carole Keeton McClellan

City Clerk

Proclamation issued by Austin Mayor Carole Keeton McClellan declaring Tuesday, November 14, 1978, Joe Gracey Day.

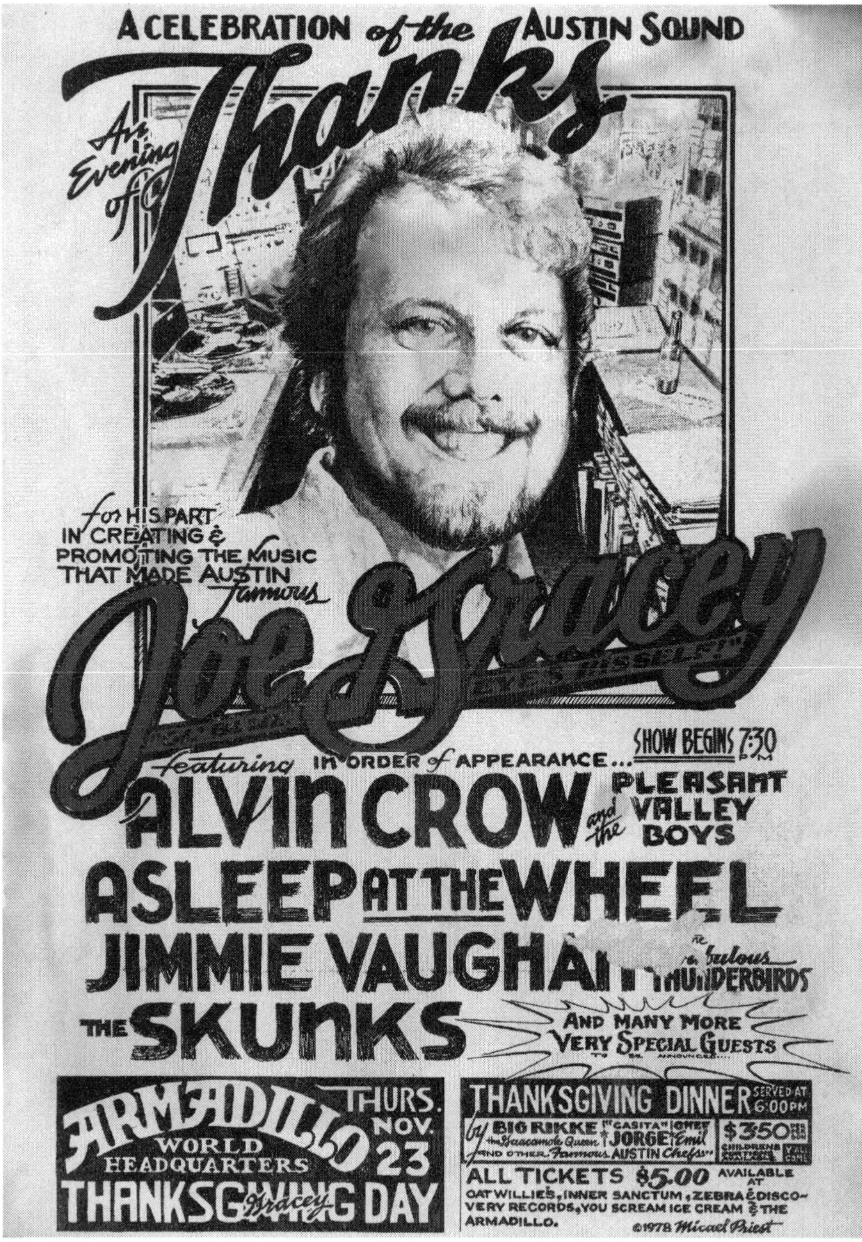
A CELEBRATION of the AUSTIN SOUND
An Evening of Thanks
for HIS PART IN CREATING & PROMOTING THE MUSIC THAT MADE AUSTIN famous
Joe Gracey
featuring IN ORDER of APPEARANCE...
SHOW BEGINS 7:30 PM
ALVIN CROW and the PLEASANT VALLEY BOYS
ASLEEP AT THE WHEEL
JIMMIE VAUGHAN the Fabulous THUNDERBIRDS
THE SKUNKS
AND MANY MORE VERY SPECIAL GUESTS
ARMADILLO WORLD HEADQUARTERS
THURS. NOV. 23
THANKSGIVING DAY
THANKSGIVING DINNER SERVED AT 6:00PM
ALL TICKETS $5.00 AVAILABLE AT
OAT WILLIE'S, INNER SANCTUM, ZEBRA & DISCOVERY RECORDS, YOU SCREAM ICE CREAM & THE ARMADILLO.
©1978 Micael Priest

Thanks Joe Gracey Day, Armadillo World Headquarters poster.

expenses. Doug Sahm on the same night passed the hat at Manhattan's Texican musical hangout, the Lone Star Café, and raised some $500 to push the night's total to more than 10 grand."

FROM A LETTER TO MARIAN REGARDING THE SUCCESS OF THE "THANKS JOE GRACEY" BENEFIT

My benefit was a howling success. Ten thousand dollars in the bank, show was perfect, and the audience was the biggest one Armadillo has ever had for anything! Everything came together in perfect harmony, PR, tickets, 400 turkey dinners, great music. They even sold autographed posters and T-shirts. I got a couple of standing ovations with cheers and have now mixed a tape recording of the whole thing. Ego is now satisfied!

LETTER TO MARIAN IN AUGUST 1979 ENTIRE LOSS OF SPEECH

Dear "Marina,"

Well, I got your card and it was exciting to receive a postal card from such an exotic place. I wished immediately that I could have gone with you. I think you deserved the trip more than most.

My fucking health . . . I went back with terrible pains in my head and went under a general anesthesia for a short biopsy. Cancer had spread to a small area in the floor of my mouth where my tongue used to be. This meant that the floor of my mouth tissue had to go, along with what was left of the base of my tongue, which extends to the top of the larynx. You guessed it. In order that I might be able to swallow without the liquid running into my lungs through my larynx, it had to go. No more golden throat . . . the cords had to go!

I had been in awful pain (from the tumor squeezing some nerves) and so unable to speak anyway from the encroaching stiffness in my mouth. So the prospects of never speaking again didn't seem so bad after all. I have been essentially hamstrung in that department for so long anyway that I just said, "Get it over with." I have experienced a few frustrating incidents without any speech at all, but for the most part I haven't minded. Trying to break up with my most recent girlfriend was hell with nothing but a writing pad, if you can imagine that . . . "I don't love you anymore" . . . then her screaming for ten minutes. She's still living in my fucking apartment pretending I never wrote it!

The surgery was eight hours long and rather interesting. They rerouted my trachea to a little hole between my collarbones, creating a permanent breathing hole, like a fucking dolphin. No air now passes through either my mouth or nose . . . forever.

At this point I would imagine that I am through with this whole mess, since such a massive amount of tissue was removed from my neck, surrounding such a tiny little tumor. The biopsy on the lymph nodes on the left side of my neck was okay, so no spread had taken place. Now if I can just get my drunken girlfriend to get out of my apartment (in the old Terrace Apts., which Willie bought and rents out to derelicts like me), my life will be a wonder of peace and happiness.

Love,

Joe

A SENSE OF HUMOR REGARDING LOSS OF SPEECH

Here I am a thirty-year-old man going around writing to people on a child's toy. It makes for great situations in places where people don't know me. Most people start shouting at me, thinking I'm deaf. I usually just play along because it's easier than trying to tell them any different. In fact, I think I'm getting a little hard of hearing from being yelled at by people. One time I drove up to a drive-in window at a bank and I was trying to mouth the word pen to the guy in the cage. He said, "I can't hear you, sir." So I wrote a message on my pad that said, "That's because I can't talk."

When they see the Magic Slate, people think I'm being cute, or the worst is when they say something like "Oh, I see you have laryngitis"—which I can understand, but which always makes me want to say something like, "Yeah, a permanent case, you bozo!" But that's really just *my* problem. I try not to take out my frustration on people, because nobody is ever intentionally cruel. In fact, most people go out of their way to be nice.

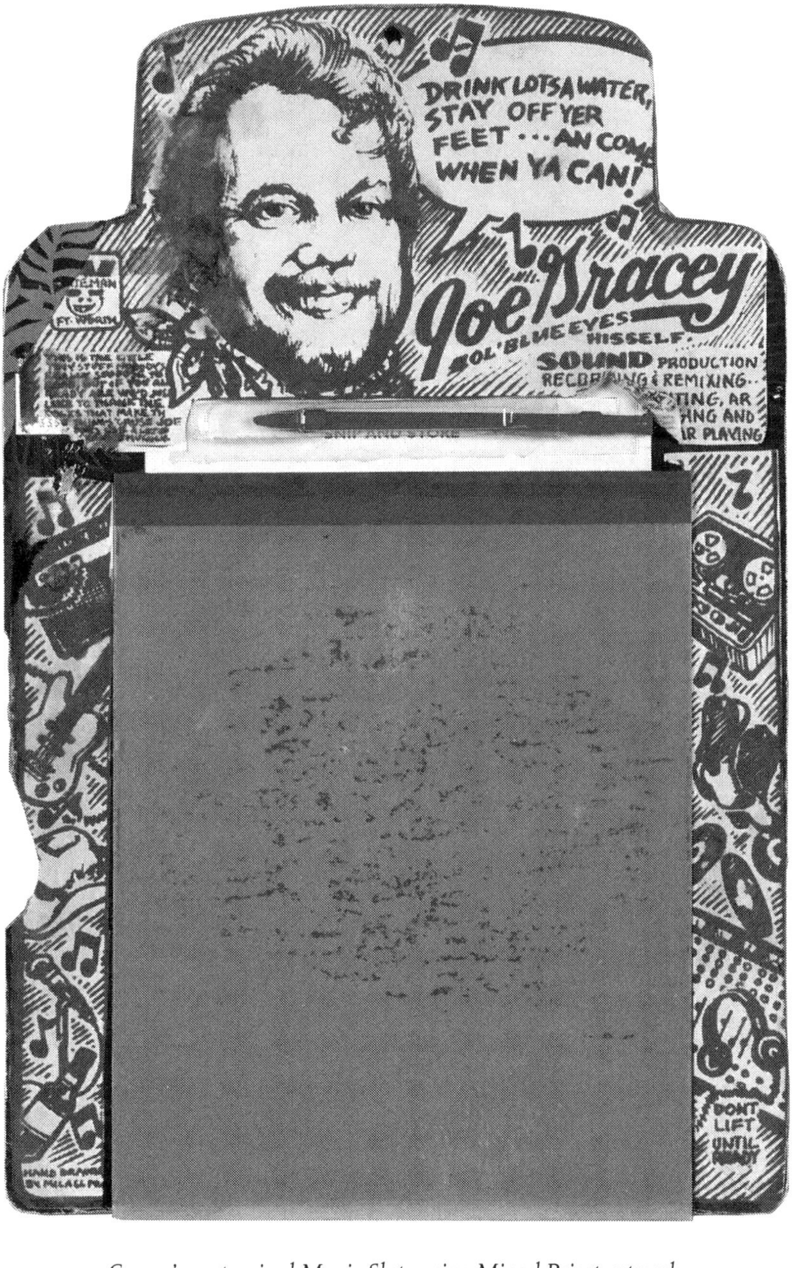
DRINK LOTSA WATER,
STAY OFF YER
FEET ... AN COM
WHEN YA CAN!
Joe Gracey
OL' BLUE EYES
HISSELF
SOUND PRODUCTION

Gracey's customized Magic Slate using Micael Priest artwork.

The sun melts my Magic Slates, so summer is a trying time for me. I usually go through about one a month in winter and about twenty-five a week in summer. I'm the manufacturer's best customer. I'm gonna ask them if they'll do a Joe Gracey model!

One time I met Johnny Winter on his bus outside of the Armadillo. I shook his hand and then just stood there, since he was blind and I couldn't talk . . . for fuck's sake!

Wanna know why I know all about Huntsville Prison? I was there because of a little minor mishap with a woman at the Department of Public Safety, where I went to renew my driver's license, a matter of mere formality here in the Republic of Texas, since anybody who can move even one muscle can drive, regardless of how drunk/insane/blind/senile/deaf/bedridden they may be. My grandfather, bless his soul, was still driving a giant Cadillac at eighty-five years old, when he couldn't tell a stop sign from a rhinoceros, and his idea of driving on the freeway was to go forty-five in the fast lane with ten miles of murderous traffic stacked up behind him, oblivious. Anyway, I stood in line with all of "The Infirmities" for an hour and finally made it up to the little hole, behind which was an enormous woman who looked like something out of a movie titled "Enormously Fat Trailer Park People." She began to question me, and I answered her on my ridiculous child's Magic Slate (which you may or may not have in your area of the world but which is a popular toy here), which I am forced to use to communicate because of an unfortunate smoking accident in 1978 in which they ripped out half my head, mainly the speaking half, but I looked cool smoking, so it was, of course, worth it. I wrote my name, etc., and showed it to her, and she began to make signs to me as if I were deaf, which is all too common in my ironic little life, and as always, I hastened to assure her in my laborious hand that "I can hear" (mainly because I couldn't read sign language . . . if it meant getting the last drop of tequila in the world). Being polite, that's all it was. She rose up, all quivering three hundred fifty pounds of her, and yelled, "I know that, you asshole; if you are going to act like that you can just go back to the end of the line!" This confused me, since if she knew I wasn't deaf then why was she signing incomprehensible things at me? And why was I being an asshole to tell her this humble, simple fact? I am proud to not be deaf, merely horribly mutilated, and I should be able to state this, seems to me. I became mildly enraged, took out my grandfather's gun, and shot her through the center of her third eye exactly once, stilling her expertly, like the old deer slayer that I am. I was satisfied with this. We all were.

LAST NIGHT I DREAMED

Last night I dreamed that some asshole took away my Magic Slate and tore it up and said, "Stop using that crutch and start talking," whereupon I did. I have dreams like that all the time, in one form or another. This feeling that I am dreaming is with me at all times; it is just another of my routines. At times I realize I am full of bitterness and anger at my condition. Do you know the feeling of dreaming that something terrible is happening, then realizing that it is only a dream? I realize something terrible is happening, then I know it is only my life. Of course, I am glad to be alive, and I have no expectation of ever being sick again, but there are times when I feel this is a horrible thing I am forced to deal with. Oh God! If I could only sing again! I go through my days in a controlled fury. My happiness at being alive is balanced by my anger at my inability to command.

KIMMIE RHODES—LIFE'S OTHER PLANS

John Lennon sang to us, "Life is what happens to you while you're busy making other plans." Oh, how true this statement became for Joe Gracey. On the very day he was diagnosed, he quit smoking cigarettes immediately, realizing that he had been "a fool . . . to think cancer was a thing that happened to other people," and he always swore he never experienced the withdrawals that make quitting so difficult. He would for the rest of his life breathe through a stoma at the base of his neck and never again utter an audible word. He learned to use a primitive version of American Sign Language, which he used to speak to the immediate family who found the time to learn it, but, of course, most people were unable to communicate with him in that way.

Having been an eloquent speaker with a strong Texan drawl and a great vocabulary, he also always felt that the language was too limiting, so he opted for a child's toy called the "Magic Slate," which enabled him to express himself in roughly a 5 x 7–inch space on a piece of plastic film that could be lifted and erased due to a black wax coating that lay beneath the plastic film, using a red plastic stylus that was kept in a special slot just above the writing area. It was a very charming little pain in the ass. He was creative and would reinvent his Magic Slates by covering the cartoon artwork with his own designs, which humorously reflected whatever his artistic adventure might be at that particular time.

The well-known phrase from Shakespeare's *Hamlet,* "Brevity is the soul of wit," became his mantra. He was already long on wit but very short on brevity, and for the next thirty years, the writer who had shown such extraordinary talent that even his grade-school teachers had encouraged him (by way of letters sent home to his mother) to become a professional writer, would be learning how to express himself quickly in eight-to-ten-word phrases. It was a lifelong frustration for him that most people, no matter how well meaning, would just not be able to stay with more than two to three lifts of the magic film. Until computers and the Internet came along to free him from that reality, the brilliantly gregarious, chatty personality with the deep, rich voice, who had daily enjoyed having the faithful Austin listeners of whatever musings were uttered off the top of his head between spins, was forever silenced.

Thanks to his indomitable spirit, determination, tenacity, and courage, he found a way to carry on by taking the counsel of his beloved mentor, Jack Clement, who had also been a fan and regular guest of Gracey's show on KOKE-FM. Cowboy advised him that since he would no longer be able to sing, he should turn to record producing because he knew exactly how a great record was supposed to sound. Gracey's loving grandfather, Cecil Morgan Sr., literally the cotton-picking son of a dirt farmer from Pendleton, Texas, and a visionary who had elevated himself to the status of successful Fort Worth lawyer and oil speculator, understood what it was like to "start from scratch." Cecil made a business arrangement to support his grandson by injecting a thousand bucks per month into a company they formed, Joe Gracey Productions, Inc.

The Best of Electric Graceyland, a collection of music recorded at Electric Graceyland Studios in Austin, Texas, 1978–1980, includes the song "Contrabandistas," cowritten with Bobby Earl Smith. It was ironically the last recording made by Gracey, and you can hear in his vocal that a good part of his tongue had already been surgically removed. Although it was written as the soundtrack for a film in which the main characters are smuggling marijuana from Mexico, the lyrics profoundly foreshadow the philosophy Gracey would have to continue to embrace for the rest of his life while bravely enduring a humility he would never truly and openly acknowledge as a handicap.

— CONTRABANDISTAS —

Texans and Mexicans been fussin' and fightin'
Been loving and dying for years
Contrabandistas drinking tequila
Drink up, we have nothing to fear

I'd rather be flying and risking my dying
I've no fear of flying, been flying for years
I'm flying under the radar and thunder
I'm leaving down yonder and I'm going home

JOE GRACEY—ONE DAY ON THE BEACH

One time I took a little rented Piper Cherokee down to Padre Island to an old WWII landing strip on a part of the island you can't get to by car, only by airplane, so we flew down there with another couple and had this vast gulf beach all to ourselves all day. We also had a bunch of hashish brownies. Sunscreen hadn't been invented in 1973. I am fair-skinned, and I sunburn fairly badly after about thirteen seconds on a beach, so after a whole afternoon of it, I was just beginning to realize that I had made a terrible, terrible mistake.

My second mistake was in forgetting that hash brownies take a long time to come on, and when they do, it is like being on an up elevator with no floor in sight. By the time we had to get back in the plane, the pilot (me) was: a) redder than any boiled lobster and getting worse by the minute, and b) so stoned that the very idea of going up into the air seemed ridiculous, since we all know that big metal objects do not fly.

I got redder and sicker and "stoneder" all the way back to Austin, which seemed to take six days. I somehow managed to land the plane intact while I wondered who was flying the damn thing using my hands. I laid in bed in wet sheets for three days waiting for my skin to shed and my brain to inch back to within shouting distance of its former self.

I think that was my next-to-last pyschedelic excursion, except for the occasional time when Willie will hand you a joint that he has cleverly inserted mushroom powder into, and twenty minutes later you think, "Uh oh, something feels very '70s-ish around here."

6

JACKALOPES

KIMMIE RHODES AND JOE GRACEY

KIMMIE RHODES

ONE AFTERNOON in December of 1979, I walked through the door of Electric Graceyland in Austin, Texas, at the invitation of a new acquaintance, T. J. McFarland, to meet the Jackalope Brothers, Joe Gracey, and Bobby Earl Smith. I was there to record some songs, the melodies of which I had composed in collaboration with a lyricist named Kim Banks, who had introduced me to T.J., or "Tiny," as we called him in those days.

All the "bells and whistles" of my intuition went off the second I laid eyes on Joe Gracey and shook the elegant hand he politely offered. There was something on an unseen level that unnerved me when I looked him in his deep blue and remarkably expressive eyes. I had inherited a family trait from the side of my Yugoslavian grandfather, Mijo Grbavace, which we all refer to as "The Shining." I have these painfully vivid dreams that to the exact physics, temperature, and even lighting capture snippets of time in frames that I later find myself having to pass through in the future. It's a sort of a déjà-vu-to-the-tenth-power experience. I had it explained to me once by someone who said it was a frequency thing that certain people are attuned to, like dogs to a dog whistle. Who knows?

Trying to ignore the fact that I had recently seen this very face in a true-to-life dream from which I had awakened in a cold sweat and in tears, I quickly scanned him and assessed him to be an extremely hip and soulful cat (who for some reason seemed exhausted far and beyond the hangover, which he soon admitted to be experiencing). He was skinny and unhealthy-looking, and his hair was still uncombed from the night before. He was wearing jeans, cowboy boots, and a T-shirt that looked like it had been washed too many times and had never stopped shrinking. By all accounts he appeared to be a "bad boy" with a really sweet heart, just the kind I like. Then he picked up a child's toy, a Magic Slate like the one that I had played with when I was a kid. Instead of talking, he wrote something in Texan-speak, like, "Hidy, glad yer here." I'd guess I'd been told that he had lost his voice to cancer recently, and I couldn't help but notice that he had extensive scarring on his neck just under his chin and was wearing a chain with a blood and mucous stained pad over a hole in his neck. It was curious how he seemed to have adapted to it all with what was clearly a keen sense of humor and overall sense of being "cool."

There was just a lot to take in with this guy, and, as he wrote a few words and then lifted the film and then wrote a few more words and lifted the film, something—like some kind of odd "knowing"—started dragging me under. I hung on every word, every letter, in fact, and was overly fascinated by the way his writing looked etched into the wax beneath the plastic film.

It's hard to explain, but I'll try. It was like it didn't matter what he was saying so much as how he was saying it, like I was meant to be inexplicably engaged with every word he wrote for some strange reason. Never mind the dream. . . . I instantly felt a bond with him, like I'd known him for many, many years, like he was someone closer than a mother or a father or a brother. I'd never experienced that feeling before upon meeting anyone. It was peculiar. I have no way of knowing for certain, of course, about reincarnation, but I can say that if I were to meet him in a next life, introduced as strangers, the way I felt that day is probably exactly how I would feel again. It was like there was a lifetime of deep, meaningful history between us.

Meanwhile, since I had just entered the studio and about ten people were standing around making introductions, I was forced to come out from my shell of inner thoughts and feelings and participate. There was this other fella there, Bobby Earl Smith: polite, confident, energetic; he appeared to be this Joe Gracey guy's sidekick, or "partner," as he was introduced. He was really quick-witted and seemed to have an unusual knack for being jovial and dead serious at the same time. If I'd had to compare them to cartoon characters, Gracey was like Bugs Bunny and Bobby Earl was like Daffy Duck. They had this slapstick vibe about them that I could tell had been purposefully honed to an art for years. Together they were stunning, and maybe it made me feel a little bit like Minnie Mouse. Time would prove that my reckoning at first impressions was off, because, in fact, it turned out that I was to be Bugs; Bobby Earl, Daffy; and Gracey, W. C Fields. Everything else about my instincts, however, was dead-on that day. I'll never know why I seemed to know what everyone else in the room didn't, and mostly it made me toggle between wondering whether I was losing my mind or if some sort of miracle was at play.

Gracey didn't pick up on any of this nonsense. I think maybe I fell in love with him that day, but it was hard to tell because I was married (albeit unhappily), and my joy was directed toward the excitement of being there for the first recording session of my first songs. After the introductions were over, I was shown into a small room across the hall that had blankets and empty egg cartons attached to the walls. I met "the boys" who would become my band for the next several years: Johnny X Reed (a guitar player with an infectious laugh and sense of humor) and Ron Howard (a soft-spoken fellow who had intense dark eyes and played the piano a little bit like Floyd Cramer). T.J. manned the drums, and I sang. As soon as we started playing, it was like the music conjured up this magic that had the power to dim lights and that descended and permeated every molecule of oxygen in the windowless room.

The day passed as we'd record a song however many times it took to get through it without anyone screwing up and then go back across the

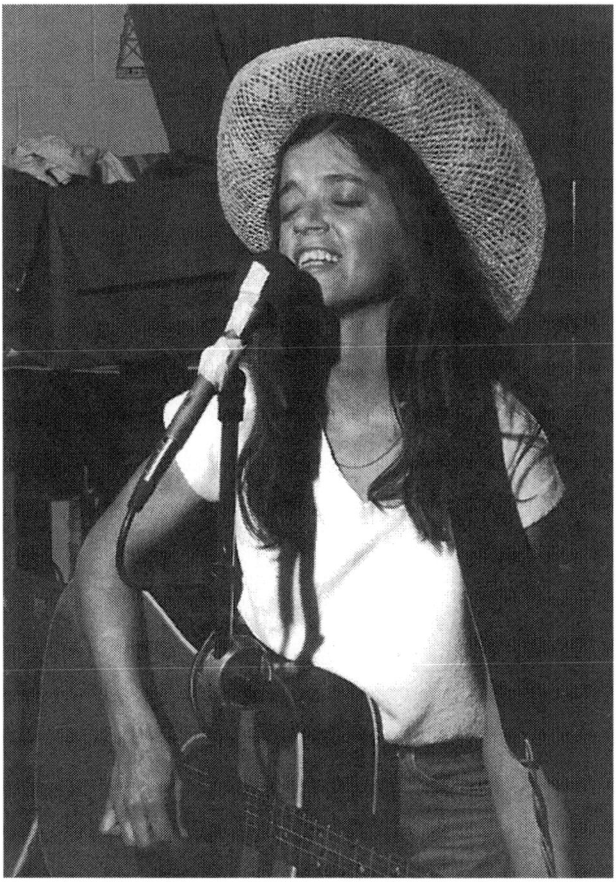

Kimmie at Electric Graceyland, 1979.

hall and listen to the playback. At one point I wandered into the adjoining office to catch a moment to myself, and my mind drifted back to the face in the dream that had definitely been this interesting person who was now sitting in the other room recording my voice. As I pondered what it might mean, I felt dizzy, like the earth was moving under my feet; I blamed it on the jumbled squealing sound of the rewinding reel-to-reel tape.

I ended the day feeling grateful and elated, as though for at least one afternoon I'd been wondrously transported to the place where I had really belonged all my life. Then I went on back home to where my reality was still taking place.

Gracey married just a few weeks after I'd met him. In a very primitive attempt at artist development, the week before his wedding, Gracey and T.J. drove through a bad snowstorm up to my farm, set up a four-track recorder in my living room, and started teaching me Gracey's songs. T.J. coached me to breathe in the right places, hold my notes longer on the ends of phrase, and things like that. Their dedication to music and passion and excitement for working with me as their new artist was exactly what I needed. It was like the whole world was sparkly and new and belonged to me for the first time in my life.

A week or so later, I was thrilled when I went to my mailbox and found a letter from Gracey saying he loved the way I sang his songs and was looking forward to helping me with my career any way he could. I decided the dream was a bizarre fluke of some sort and didn't mean anything. I was happy that he had at least fallen in love with my voice.

So, we started to have fun making music, and I learned to ignore anything I thought I might have felt otherwise, although every time I was away from Gracey, I missed him terribly. I wondered where he was in the world without me and hoped he would survive cancer and wondered if he was thinking of me, too. Then every time I was finally back in the room with him, I felt a very big love, like an angel or something was looking on. Being with him made me feel like the world was safe and right and like I was finally where I was supposed to be and doing exactly what I was meant to be doing, even if I wasn't doing anything besides sitting in a bar watching him write things on his Magic Slate.

I stayed at T.J.'s house a few times and slept on his couch when I'd drive my little junker of a yellow Volkswagen to Austin from Sunset to record demos and learn new songs. He was like a big brother to me, and that whole new world was made possible because he had heard me singing and believed in me and introduced me to Gracey and Bobby Earl. T.J. gave me a life.

Then a terrible thing happened just about a little over a year after I'd met him. T.J. was arrested for cocaine possession and sentenced to a couple of years in a "white collar" prison in Big Springs, Texas. On May 15, 1981, I wrote a letter to the parole board pleading for his release, which resulted in my being listed as a security risk and being barred from visiting him.

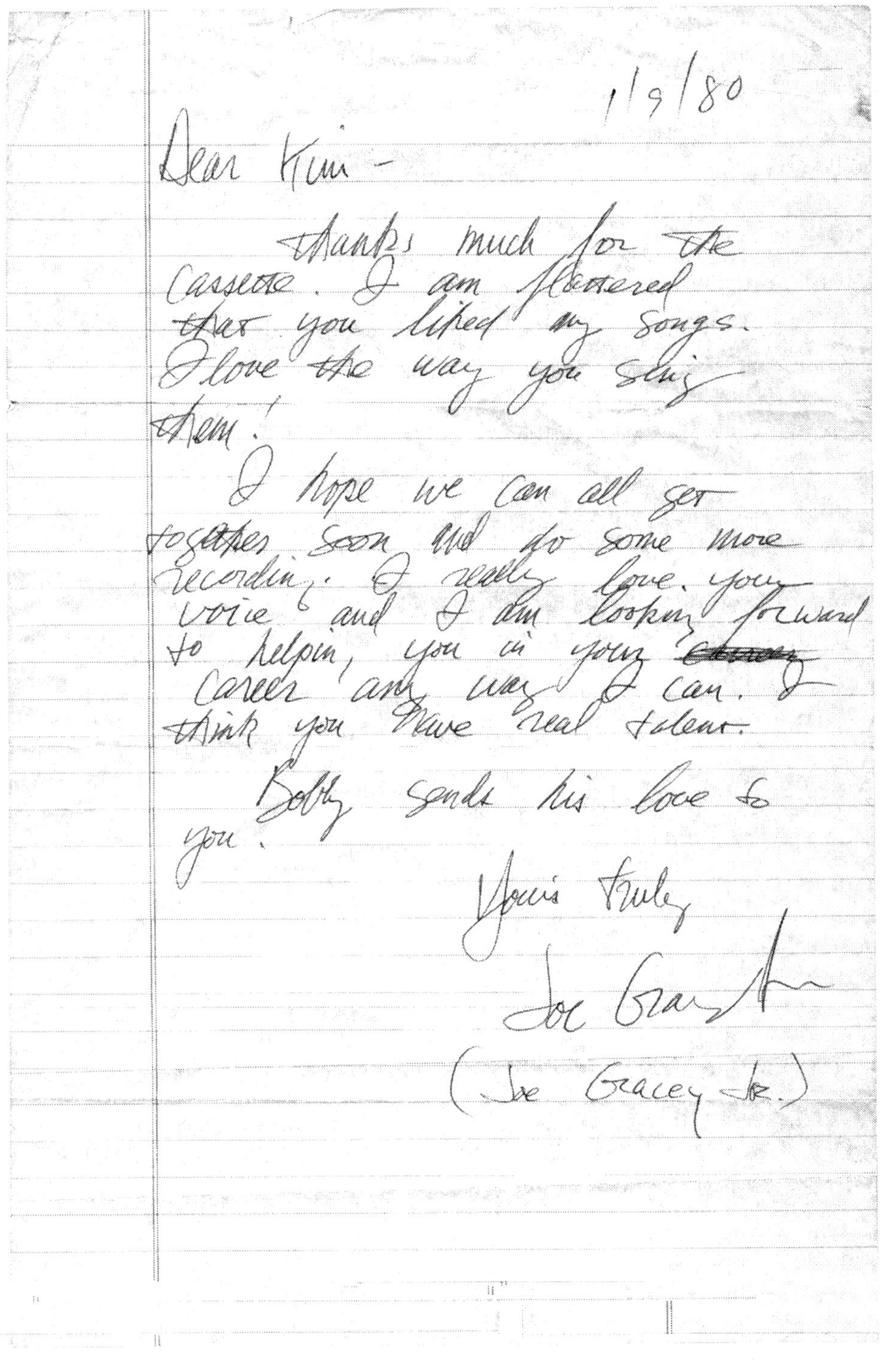

1/9/80

Dear Kim -

thanks much for the cassette. I am flattered that you liked my songs. I love the way you sing them!

I hope we can all get together soon and do some more recording. I really love your voice and I am looking forward to helping you in your ~~[illegible]~~ career any way I can. I think you have real talent.

Bobby sends his love to you.

Yours truly

Joe Gracey

(Joe Gracey Jr.)

Gracey's letter to Kimmie.

LETTER TO THE PAROLE BOARD

Dear Sirs,

I am a country singer-songwriter from Texas. Since December of 1979 I have been writing and selecting material, arranging rehearsing, and making demo recordings for my first album, which will be recorded, hopefully by the end of this month. This has been a long uphill climb for me. Many times I might have abandoned this project if not for the help and encouragement of T. J. McFarland. It takes a person with a unique ability and patience to seek out artists like myself, encourage their efforts, and finally produce a product and present it to radio markets.

I hope soon to complete these past two hard years of work spent preparing to make my first album. It means the world to me. T.J. is one of those rare persons that the public has to thank for taking music from the private rooms of musicians and off the scribbled pages of writers and composers into the hearts of the people.

Still his letters come regularly to me saying, "Keep working, be confident, keep taking lessons, keep practicing, keep singing. I believe in you, kid." This is a fine, Christian man who, like all of us, finds himself in a life that offers first the test and then the lesson. He has made his mistakes, but he has learned his lesson.

He is unique and vital to my own and many other people's careers. Please consider his release at the earliest possible date. Thank you so much for your time.

Sincerely,
Kimmie Rhodes

KIMMIE RHODES

I had become good friends with Bobby Earl, and we wrote each other letters weekly and started sending each other song lyrics. After T.J. went to jail I started staying with Bobby Earl and his wife, Judy, and their two young songs, Jon Marc and Eric. I went off into a couple of years of denying what I knew in my heart was true. I had accidentally and totally unacceptably fallen in love with someone who was unavailable, and I was a married mother of two young boys. But still, I was over the moon with excitement at the prospects of making my first record and loved being with like-minded artists.

Although things were rather grave in my relationship with my husband, I carried on and tried to make another go of it, better able to dodge the daily emotional punches with newly found inspiration and happiness. I felt like he liked "the idea of me" but had never really approved of who I was. He was unreasonably jealous, though openly unfaithful. I felt like he didn't really want me and yet he didn't want anyone else to have me. It was bizarre, and it was beginning to take a toll on the kids.

Then the plot thickened. Joe Gracey pulled out all of his songs for me to record, and, after everyone else had left the session, he and I spent many hours alone together working on my vocals, which really helped me find my voice. He would pick up a guitar and play notes that he suggested I try on harmony overdubs and things like that. It was touching to have him play for me on guitar what he couldn't sing. I loved his courage. We were both still committed to being loyal spouses to our significant others, but being an infamous rogue, he did make some "pear-shaped" suggestions—as he liked to call them—quoting his hero, W. C. Fields. I was flattered but resisted what would be considered casual infidelity because I didn't want to ruin what had become a great working relationship by having sex with my producer, and I wasn't the kind of person who would cheat with or on a married man. So we focused on the music, which had also stolen my heart and was, in fact, really both of our priority and greatest passion at the time.

At some point it became hard to tell where the love for the music stopped and where the love for each other began, because it was all becoming so intermingled. Being a singer and reveling in the joy of hearing and controlling my voice, I felt his sadness that he could no longer sing. He had at least found a surrogate voice in me, and we became each other's muse. The more I empathized with his struggle, the more it gave me purpose beyond my own goals; I was honored that fate had landed me in such a place with such a man who was so creatively reinventing himself. And besides, it was really fun.

I think one reason that life with the Jackalope Brothers felt so natural was because I had been raised hanging around with my dad and his buddies in bars, privy to their grand business schemes and singing songs I'd learned for them. I fit right in. They liked having me around and nicknamed me "Kupcake." I joined the Jackalope Brothers band, and we played around town in the clubs for songwriters: the Armadillo Beer Garden, the Alamo Hotel, the Tavern, and Emmajoe's.

Finally, after recording lots of demos, we got the funds to record two songs at Lone Star, a recording studio where Gracey had started working as an engineer. And that's where I met the legendary steel guitar player Jimmy Day.

The single was really good, and Bobby Earl was a fantastic promo guy. We recorded Gracey's songs "You'll Take Care of You" and "No Next Time," a honky-tonk shuffle that Bobby Earl and I sang as a duet. It was the one that all the disc jockeys picked to play because it was up-tempo and rockin'. Armed with our new single, we'd jump in the car and take these regional road trips that were a real blast! We would stock up on Fritos and cans of Beanie Weenies and Pearl beer and head off in some general direction with a sketchy idea of where we were headed, looking for radio towers. *The Loretta Lynn Story,* in which Sissy Spacek had done such a prodigious portrayal, had just come out, and it was strange to be viewed as a sort of Loretta character. The shoe did kind of fit, although I was from a totally different generation that had been hip in a completely different way. I even had the accent to live with!

I remember the first time we took my record to a disc jockey who said he'd put it on after the commercial. We ran out and jumped in the car, and I got to hear myself on the airwaves for the first time with all that radio station compression and everything, sounding like a real recording star! Bobby Earl and Gracey looked at me so proudly, like big brothers, while I soaked it all in, beaming with gratitude, amazement, and pure innocent glee. They had sacrificed so much and worked so hard by that point. That my joy was their reward was humbling.

Daily, Bobby Earl would hand me a list of stations that had played the record. As soon as I had called to thank them and done interviews or station IDs for them (usually they were really surprised and put me

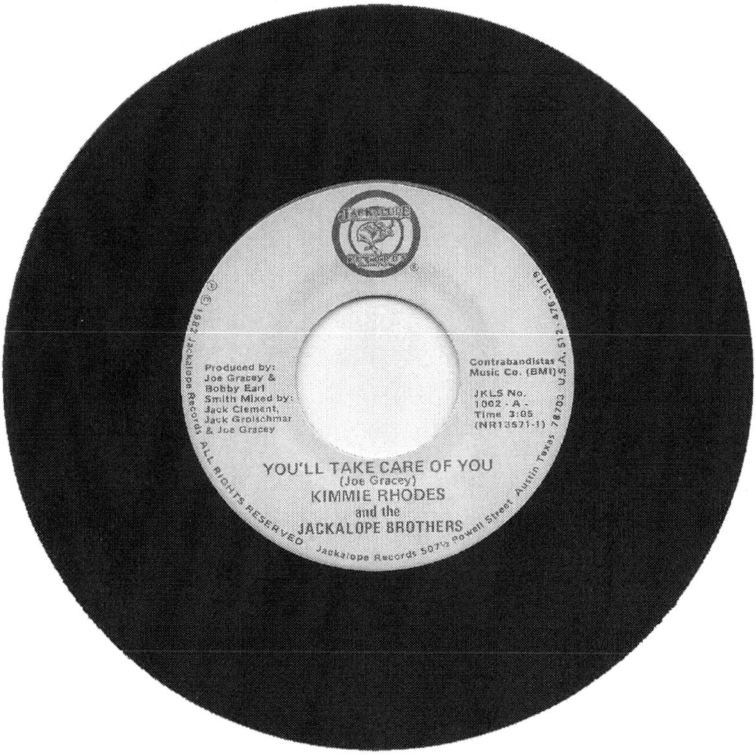

Kimmie's first 45 single.

straight on the air live), they would add it to their rotation. Then I would call and thank them for adding it to the rotation and they'd ramp it up even more. We got a regional hit that way.

We were diligent and dedicated, and we were doing our job and giving ourselves wholeheartedly to our goals, but we still romped and played like kids who were getting away with something. It was just so damn wonderful to be doing what we loved. One day we headed for KELG, this cool AM station in Elgin, Texas, that was in a double-wide trailer next to a big ol' antenna. There was a plowed field behind the station, so Gracey decided to start doing donuts in it. We were bumping and bouncing along through the furrows, whooping, hollering, and laughing hysterically, like teenagers. After we stopped, we looked up and saw Tom Hale, the disc jockey, standing in the open back door, taking it all in. So Gracey headed for the station, and as we approached the building, Bobby Earl rolled down his window and sailed the 45 to Tom, who caught it and went in and put it on. I think that memory best describes the wild abandon of who we were and how we wanted to live as fellow Jackalopes on a mission from God!

JOE GRACEY—LETTER TO HIS PEN PAL, MARIAN

Dear Marian,

We just did a session on Kimmie Rhodes, the girl from Sunset, Texas, who is like a replay of the Loretta Lynn story. Kimmie, of course, is "our new fair-haired boy" at Jackalope Records. We expect her to be a big star and make us all rich.

We used the best musicians in town and bought a brand-new box of tape and went for the most commercial sound we could get, while still retaining our concept. I finally decided to use studio cats instead of us trying for the next five years to get a usable take. It came out really well. I view it as my best production job to date. I engineered it and wrote one of the songs, a great maudlin waltz tune about a man who comes back to his small hometown without his wife and laments that he's finally realized "You'll Take Care of You." I played it for Cowboy Jack, and it is the first thing of mine that he has liked, which is a huge milestone for me. After all the years I've known him, and as old as I am, and after all the things I've been through, I still had to psych myself up to mention to him that I had "a tape that I'd like him to hear sometime," and I swear that as I said it, my heart was pounding in my chest a hundred beats per minute. He said, "You got a copy of it anywhere?" And I bounded up the stairs and grabbed it off the machine and breathlessly threw it on his tape recorder in record time. As I played it for him it seemed that my whole life was focused into this tiny room and this moment—my song—my singer—my studio (it might as well be)—my choice of session musicians—my engineering—my mix. And the crusty old fart liked it, played it over and over, said it "didn't sound like

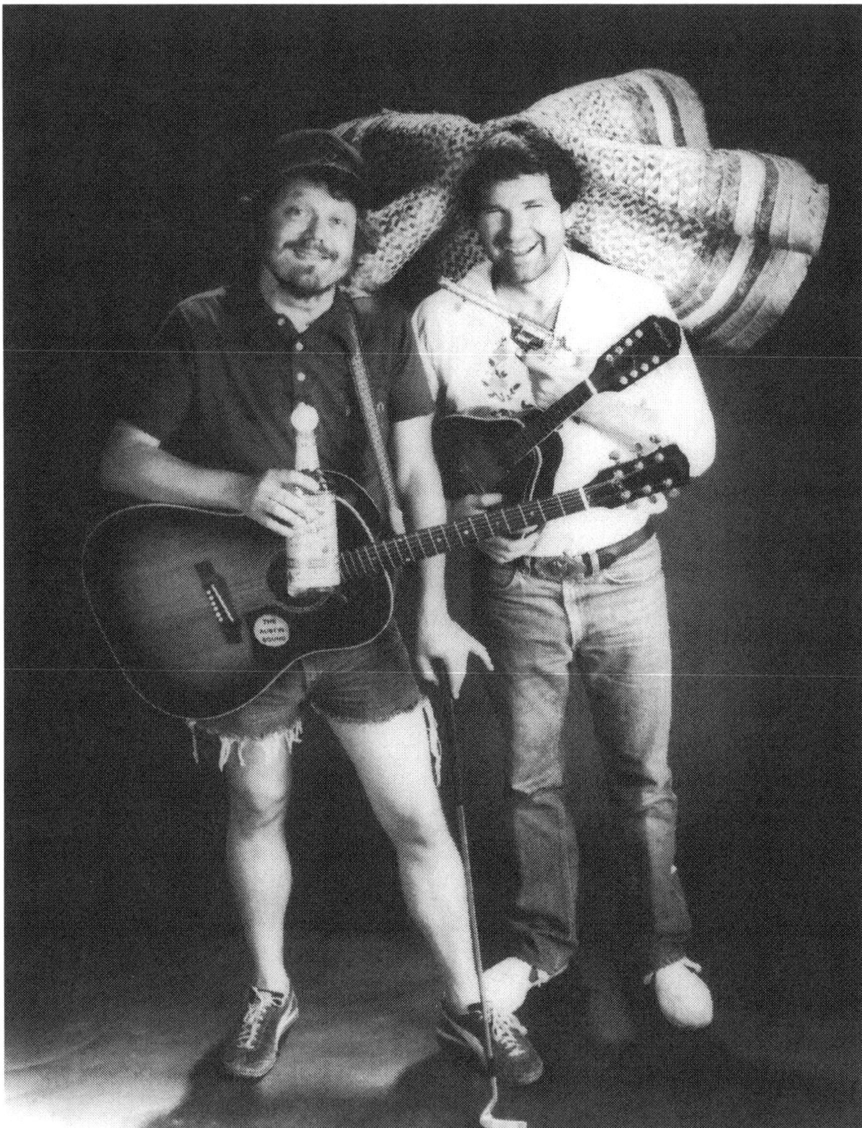

The Jackalope Brothers.

Nashville" and said Kimmie had "an innocent quality." Why would it matter to me what he thought? Why would my heart race as if it were my first kiss? (Why was my first kiss such a disaster?)

It's her first 45 single and should be out soon. Kimmie is growing artistically, and we'll all be ready for the big time by fall.

I went out to Willie's with Ray Benson to play golf and ran into Darrell Royal, and he looked at me with a deadpan expression and said, Oh! Joe! I didn't recognize you without your voice."

We've been playing more live gigs in the local commie folk club here. We are the bastion of magic, John Reed, Ron Howard, Me, Kimmie, and Bobby Earl.

Love,

Joe

KIMMIE RHODES

We got kicked out of the basement of KOKE-FM because of our incessant partying and carrying on and because someone threw up in the bathroom we shared with the incompatible tenants down the hall, a company that manufactured dentures. The putrid smell of their burning materials mingled with the disgusting smell of the Graceyland trash cans, filled with beer cans and cigarette butts, in such a way that it's hard to imagine how a little vomit could make such a big difference, but apparently it did. So we bummed around homeless for a while.

Bobby Earl started ragging Lana, Willie Nelson's mightily soulful and lovely daughter, thus nicknamed the "Princess of Redneck Rock," to let us come out to the studio and record. One day the call came, and we grabbed a six-pack of Shiner Bock and went to check out the exclusive Pedernales Studio, located just outside of Austin, in the country and which belonged to Willie, who was at the top of his game by then. Bobby Arnold, the assistant engineer (who later became a very dear friend after forgiving my son for taking a joyride in his car), and Larry Greenhill, the engineer, showed us around. Lana showed up, too, at

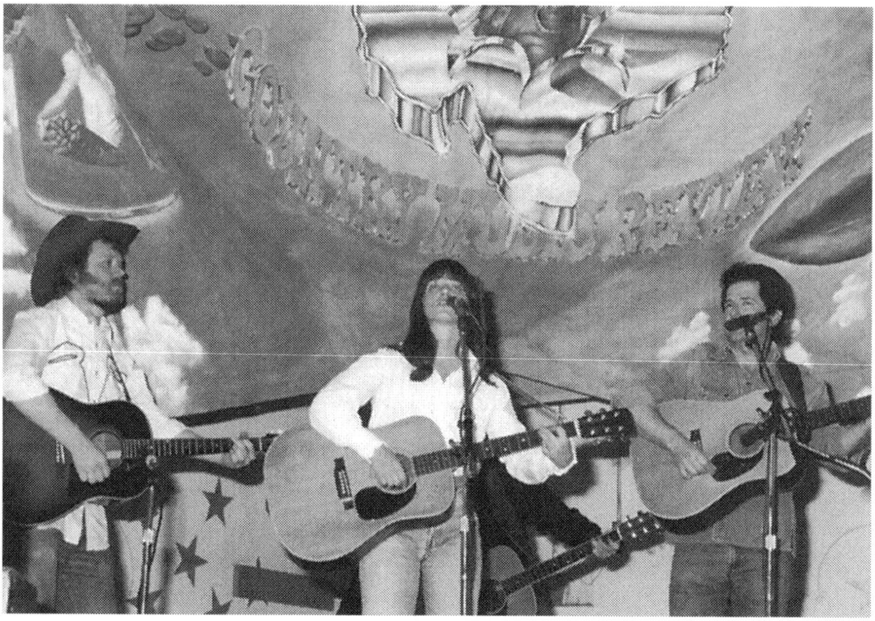

Kimmie Rhodes and the Jackalope Brothers at the Armadillo Christmas Bazaar.

some point. We were all standing around joking about how God was our distributor because we didn't have a record deal. Lana disappeared but came back around just as we had gotten in the car to leave and asked, "Have you seen Daddy?" Bobby Earl said no, so she took us out to the golf course where Willie was hanging with his buddies. Just as we were walking up, Willie made a perfect drive that landed right on the green and then turned his attention to us.

He honed in on me immediately with his deep black eyes and went straight to it, firing three questions at me in rapid succession. First, "How long have you been singing?" I answered, "Since I was six years old." Second, "Do you write?" I replied, "Yes, we all do, and Gracey's my favorite writer." And finally, "Who is your distributor?" I balked at the question, not wanting to blaspheme in my conversation with Willie, and Lana said, "Tell him." So Bobby Earl answered, "God." We all laughed, and somehow his dark eyes turned even a shade deeper, and he said, "Well, why don't you come out here and make a record?" I said, "Okay!" He asked, "When?" Bobby Earl jumped in: "Next week." Willie pitched it to Lana, who said that she figured that the studio would be available in three weeks, so it was confirmed that we would return to record my first album, *Kimmie Rhodes and the Jackalope Brothers.*

It was so surreal to have everything turn around so fast like that; it took a while to sink in. I remember asking the guys on the way back to town why Willie had repeated, "Why don't you come out here and make a record?" three times right in a row. Bobby Earl said, "He didn't. That was just the question reverberating around in your brain." Then I had to go back to town and go to a laundromat; it just felt so weird to be standing there folding clothes, trying to figure out what had just happened and what it all ultimately meant. We had been recording on a four-track reel-to-reel at Electric Graceyland, and the session to record the 45 at Lone Star Studios had been a big deal, but this was a bona fide miracle, and Willie was the angel.

JOE GRACEY—LETTER TO MARIAN ABOUT BEING INVITED BY WILLIE TO RECORD AT HIS STUDIO

Dear Marian,

We've suddenly had the most amazing luck. We went out to see Willie Nelson's new studio on the Pedernales River and to talk to his daughter Lana about maybe helping us someway. So we went out there and she listened to our tapes of Kimmie Rhodes and liked them and then disappeared for two hours, leaving us sitting in the studio playing our tapes to ourselves. So we got tired of sitting around and got up to leave, and as we were getting in my car, Lana drives up and says, "Did y'all get a chance to see Daddy yet? He's around here somewhere, and I know he'd like to say hello." So we follow her out to the golf course. (He bought a fucking country club and he keeps the golf course for him and his buddies to play on and turned the clubhouse into the studio.)

Willie is out on hole five and he sunk a long putt just as we drove up, which I was glad of. We say hello all around and my mouth starts going dry. I mean Willie has gotten so fucking big these days I'm actually a little in awe of him now—he's become a little bit like Midas. He gives us that big, weird smile, and Lana says, "Daddy, Joe and Bobby Earl are producing Kimmie and they have some real nice things on tape and a record out that is real good (meaning the 45 single of "You'll Take Care of You.")

Willie says, "Do you write?" And Kimmie says, "Yeah, we all write, and Joe is my favorite songwriter," which I thought was pretty cool of her to say to him. He says, "How long you been singing?" She says, "All my life." He says to Bobby Earl, "Who's your distributor on the record?" And Earl says, "God." Which was the perfect cosmic cowboy response and got a big laugh. So Willie says, "Well, why don't you come out here and cut a record?" We all just started bobbing our heads like a bunch of chickens in a circle. He says, "When do you want to start?" Earl says, "Next week." He turns to Lana and says, "Book them whenever the studio is open."

What that all means is that he has now become a major financial backer in our next album project. At his rates he's given us about a twenty-five-grand recording budget. Then Saturday I went back out to play golf because he'd invited me to play anytime I wanted. He asked me if I had set up the time yet and I said yes, and then out of the blue he said, "Do you have everything you need?," which meant do you need any money. I was so completely flustered by the directness of the question that I could only scrawl "yes" on my slate, which is completely untrue since we need about six thousand more dollars to pay the band.

So all of the sudden we've been capitulated into the position of being able to cut a true big-time album master. We don't have to watch the clock or worry about using up tape too fast. I don't have to produce, engineer, and play guitar all at the same time. The equipment is the best on earth. I feel like somebody cut a hole in the top of my skull and let the sky fall in.

I avoided going to see Willie for years on the theory that, until I was ready, I didn't want to waste the chance. What a sweet old outlaw! The session is now twelve days away, and I can't sleep a wink. Songs go through my head all night. All the new material is delicious and exciting and rare.

Have fun in Outer Mongolia and tell them I said, "Come when ya can."

Love,

Joe

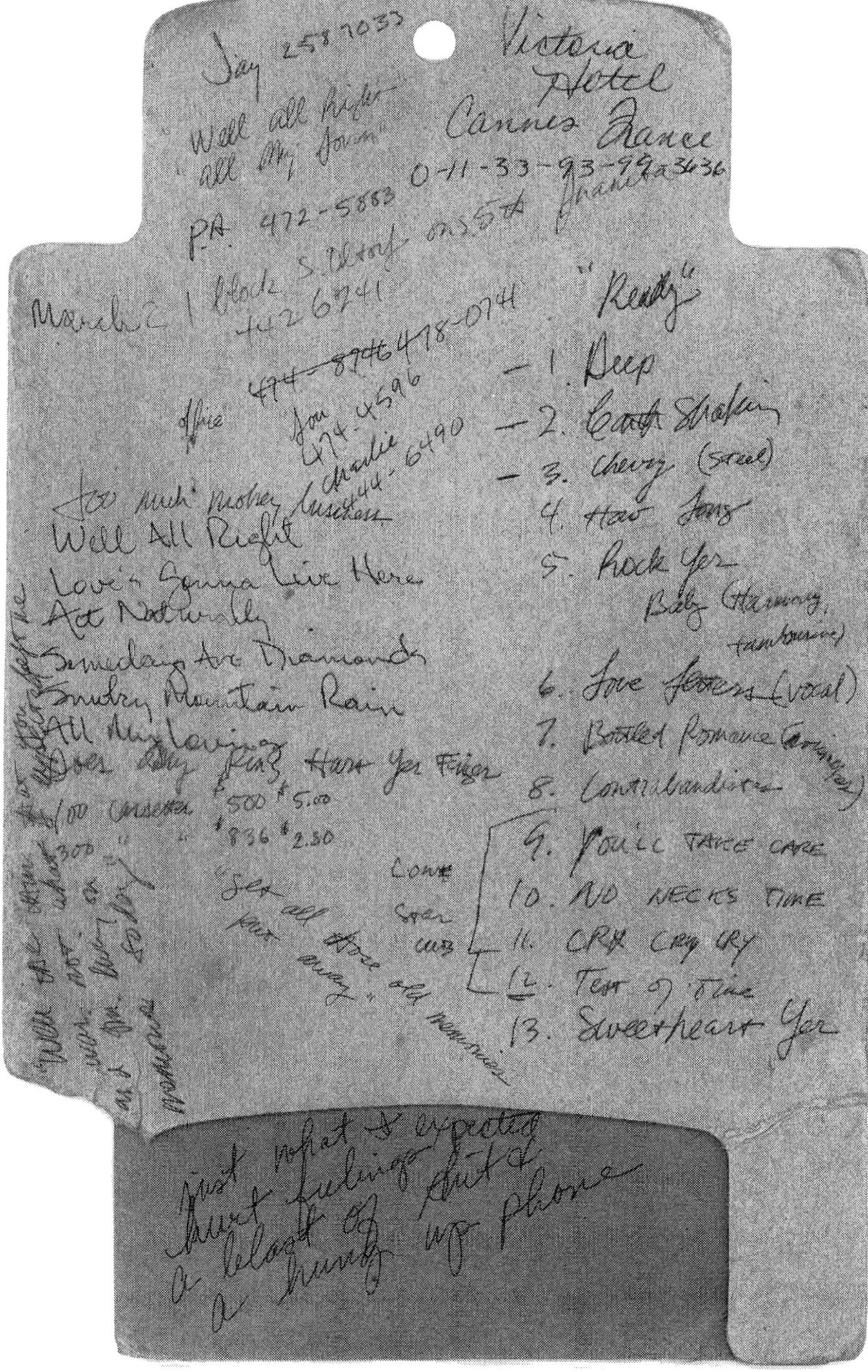

Gracey, Kimmie, and Bobby Earl production notes written on the back of a Magic Slate.

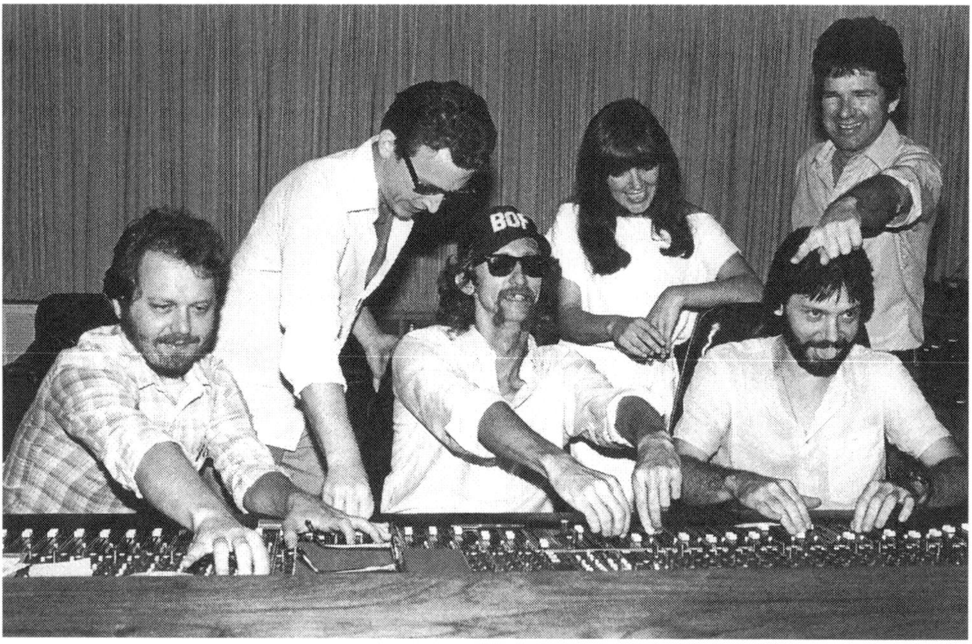

Jackalopes recording at Pedernales Studio, 1982. Left to right: Joe Gracey, Johnny X Reed, Bobby Arnold, Kimmie Rhodes, Larry Greenhill, Bobby Earl Smith. Photo by Scott Newton.

JOE GRACEY—LETTER TO MARIAN, MARCH 6, 1983
FALLING IN LOVE WITH KIMMIE

Dear Marian,

Thanks for your "critic's-eye view." What's interesting about your comments concerning the slow songs is that Bobby Earl and I have been complacently assuming that they are her forte until last week or so when we woke up to how good the fast ones are. She likes to sing the slow ones. I should have guessed when all the radio stations picked the fast side of the single to play last summer.

I don't know if I wrote you about any of our promotional swings on behalf of the single I sent you, but that is part of the game I really enjoy. Bobby and Kimmie and I would take off in my car (I always drive every mile. I must be compulsive about it. I love to drive.) and wheeling through ten or fifteen little towns on all the back roads between here and Corpus Christi one time, then up toward Lubbock the next.

We roar into some one-horse sleepy Texas place and stride into the station with our fantastic-looking promo kits and wow 'em and then go jump in the car, hearing the record played on every station as we pull out of town. Then we pull out the map and look to find the next town in the general direction of where we're headed and tune that station in, memorize the DJ's name, and descend on him next. By doing it that way we garnered thirty to forty stations playing it and had a great time, too. Bobby Earl and I have been on the road together so many times in that manner that we have it down and it's always fun.

Last summer on our trip through Mexican South Texas to the Corpus Christi beach stations was when I finally gave in to my overpowering, unnerving love for Kimmie. After trying to keep it at bay for two years and denying it and turning away from it and burying it, I fell to my knees before it and surrendered. On the road down through all the old historical revolutionary towns (Goliad, Gonzales, Victoria, the places where the meat of the war was), things were all business and all seemed reasonable and I thought I had my life under control.

After we went to the stations, we drove over to Port Aransas to the beach cafés and ate shrimp and drank Cuba libres and some beer and then went down to the billion-year-old Gulf of Mexico, with its brown-sand beaches and roaring breakers and a hundred miles of ocean, just on the other side of which is Spain. I feel the presence of the galleons every time without fail when I go there.

Bobby and Kimmie went down to the water and took off their shoes and socks and started playing, and I leaned on the hood of my car with my mirrored shades on, feeling the blinding sun behind me and watching these two people I love. I thought about how glad I was to be alive . . . and there . . . and slightly drunk, and how I loved Texas and how I loved Mexico, and how somehow my marriage was starting to take Texas and Mexico away from me, some insidious anxiety that my wife had about going ahead and being alive was beginning to take my essence and my at-oneness with this country, which is my heart and soul, and I looked at this amazing gutsy little Texas girl in front of me and I caved in.

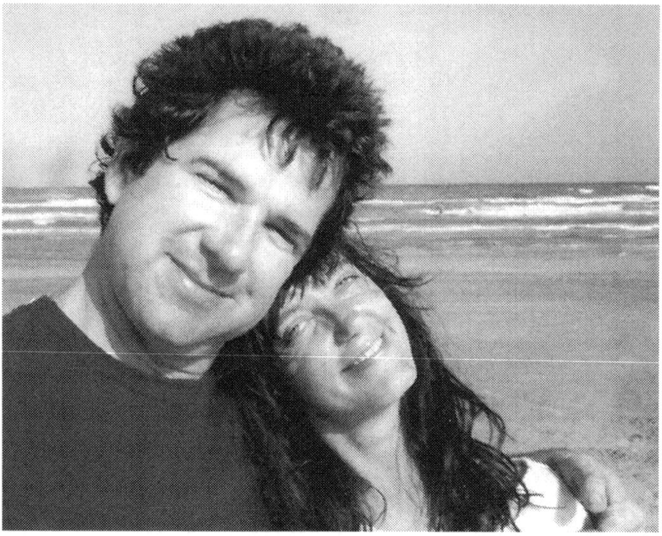

Bobby Earl and Kimmie on the Corpus Christi beach.
Photo by Joe Gracey.

I went down to the water, and as I came up, Bobby Earl started on a long walk down the beach and I took her in my arms. Time stood still. The sun got brighter and brighter and the waves roared in our ears and I could feel her wet Levi's and her girl's body against me, and we were there like that for a thousand years, two huge figures in a huge empty landscape, nothing but us and the ocean and the sun and our pure patient love.

So now I'm living in the Willie Oaks, the old motel Texas Opry Hall apartments complex owned by Mr. Nelson. Now, I've got a bed and a frying pan and a coffeemaker and an icebox full of soothing substances (flour tortillas, hot sauce, brown speckled farm eggs, real butter, bacon, homemade pinto beans, cheese, expensive baloney, foot-long loaves of dark German-style bread, milk, beer, wine, and vodka (in the freezer). I've armored myself with great food.

On the walls I've placed the photo of my grandfather Gracey with a group of cowboys herding his cows to the railhead in Fort Worth, a photo of the mansion built by my great grandfather, Lafayette K. Miller, up on the hill overlooking the football stadium until it was torn down by LBJ to build a monument to himself, and a marvelous painting done by Kimmie, which reminds me of summers at my grandparents' house in West Texas, and the Texas flag, a quilt on my bed made by my marvelous great grandmother, Lucy DeLoach Davenport, who loved to tell me stories about coming to Texas from Alabama after the war by way of Mobile to Galveston and then by wagon all the way up into Indian country on the far reaches of the Brazos River. She was a powerful cooker of fried chicken and mashed potatoes and brown gravy and black-eyed, by God, peas and pumpkin and chess pies, and a pretty fair hand at sneaking off to dip snuff. She told me about my great-great-uncle Overton Davenport (whom I uncannily resemble), who left Georgia to cross the great desert in 1849 to go to California. I have his

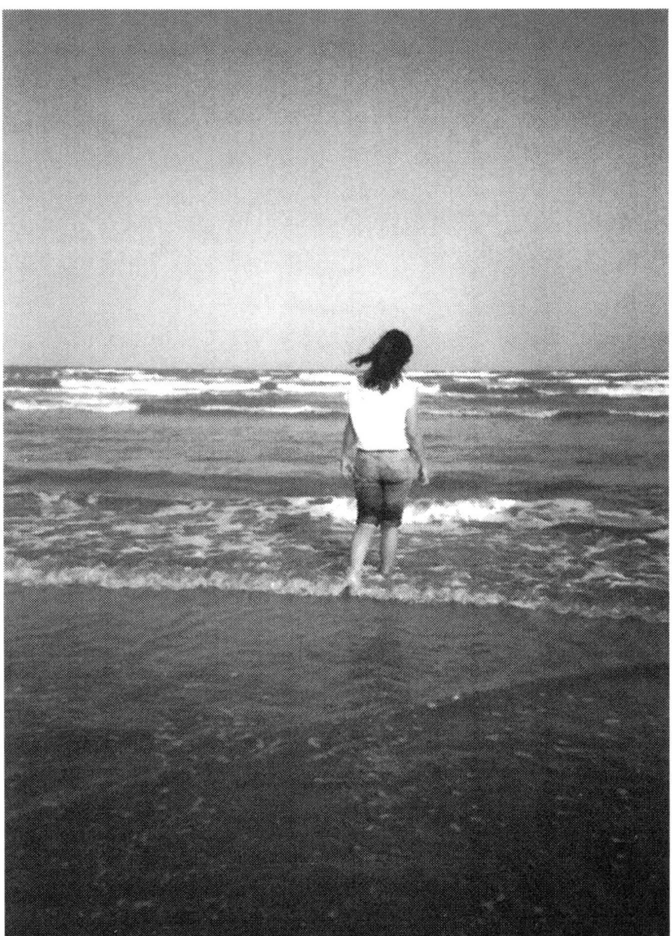

Kimmie on the Corpus Christi beach. Photo by Joe Gracey.

letters written to home. He later got a Yankee mini-ball to the tongue during the Civil War. He once shot a man out the window of the church during the service for trying to make off with his horse. Got the son-of-a-bitch, too!

I know my ex feels betrayed and flayed for reasons she probably doesn't understand, but, on the other hand, her behavior has been fairly bizarre, and to quote John Lennon, she has kept me apart from the things that I love: past relationships with friends, family, travel, food. I have just recently decided what it is exactly that I want out of life. I am rather focused these days, and I'm impatient to get on with living my life the way I envision it. I suppose it's also possible that at the time I met Linda, I was reeling from the pain and horror of my all-too-recent cancer experience and my judgment was severely out of whack. In any case, there you have it. I am relieved to be here, in this chair, in this apartment, writing you this letter.

We are receiving letters every day from radio stations in England that are playing and loving our records. We will take England by storm. Tokyo needs us. My vision has never failed, and I can see all of this clearly. Kimmie will be to international music what Ricky Skaggs is to American radio right now. She has star quality. We shot a video of her at Clement's place, and she is a natural actress with tremendous camera sense and presence. Some people look bloated and unhappy on camera. She looks normal and warm and glad to be there.

Right now at this moment Bobby Earl Smith is singing "Dry Creek Inn" on the air in Wales, the Celtic enclave of my ancestors who fled from the Saxons. Ah, it is balm to my soul to contemplate it! Kimmie Rhodes, on BBC London, capturing the hearts of the Texas-loving English crazies!

Soon as the mixing is done, you will have Kimmie's new album, and I think you will be surprised at the improvement, with the addition of Kenny Malone on percussion. The Tex-Mex songs now sound completed, and "Rock Your Baby" has a nice coffee-percolator kind of New Orleans feel, and "Sweetheart You're a Lot Like Texas" has a Bob Wills sort of snare sound to it. After doing rough mixes in Nashville, I learned to my disgust that Willie's engineer is better than I am, so I return to my role as producer when I go out there, and merely look officious and nod sagely. Learning never stops, does it? Just like all these damn computers. I realize I have no choice, but all my lazy bones cry out in pain at having to learn a new way to think.

Hope I see you soon. You will find a happier man here than you did before. Next time you'll also find a home open to you, with all the gracious hospitality that Texas stands for.

Love,

Joe

KIMMIE RHODES

The day finally came when it was time to go record a full album at Willie's, and we were ready. We had rehearsed a bunch of the best songs that we had chosen from all the songs we had written. I met Johnny Gimble in the kitchen before the session. He was such a gentleman and encouraged me in such a beautiful way. Looking at it through my eyes, he talked to me like he was just as excited about my session as I was, as if it were his first, too. It really put me at ease because he was the big man that day in my eyes.

Then we all moved into the pristine studio with white carpet, wooden walls, and recording booths, and the band set up their instruments. The engineers, Larry and Bobby, loaded the giant reel of tape onto the twenty-four-track machine. I was about to cut the first track at a big-deal session at this incredible state-of-the-art studio that belonged to the biggest regional superstar, at his own invitation! I put my lyric sheets on the stand, got my chair and mic situated just right, and ran to the bathroom while the band put the finishing touches on their tuning. I said a little prayer of thanks while I was taking a pee, washed my hands, and excitedly headed for the door. It wouldn't unlock. I tried and tried and couldn't get it to unlock! A lot of time passed, and I wondered what they must have been thinking in the studio since I hadn't returned. Finally, someone realized that I must be locked in the bathroom because the door had taken to doing that of late. It was a big guffaw for everybody and actually a perfect way to start the session because I had become sort of the goofball of the bunch, being the youngest and the only girl. I admittedly had this Gracie Allen knack for sticking my foot in my mouth and saying air-headed things. Gracie would say, "Say 'Goodnight, Gracie.'" And I'd say, "Goodnight, Gracie." I laughed along with everybody at myself and decided it was a good, rather than bad, omen because we all went in laughing.

Despite our best efforts, the more we made music, the more deeply in love Gracey and I fell, until it finally became impossible to ignore. A jealous mind is a guilty conscience, so my husband just couldn't believe that I was ever faithful to him, although I always had been, not as much for his sake but for my own sense of dignity. Gracey's wife, who was a really nice person, had her own life and was not able to participate musically, although to her credit, she had made an attempt. I had tried hard to be friends with her, but it was forced, and she was understandably unkind to me.

They always say that after a life-threatening trauma, you should wait a while before making big life-changing decisions. Gracey hadn't done that and had gotten in over his head. Our spouses just didn't have much in common with us, and we quickly grew apart from them. Of course, it was frustrating for them to watch the two of us working so happily together. The more we worked, the madder they got, so the worse they treated us, the more we turned to each other to be loved.

One day Gracey and I were at the new Jackalope Records office, and both of our spouses phoned within mere minutes of each other to give us our respective daily abusive verbal thrashings and to inform us that they had better things to do and wouldn't be around over the weekend. After fielding those calls, we looked across the desk at each other, and he said, "Want to go see George Jones?" We drove out to this overdone "modern" honky-tonk on the outskirts of town and waited, along with the rest of the punters, for a long time, hoping for "no-show Jones" to show, which he finally did. Ol' George was great, but he was so coked up that he could barely keep his clothes on, and that's no exaggeration. He did a few songs and started having so much fun that he announced, "We're gonna be here until three or four o'clock in the morning," to which the grateful audience cheered gleefully. Then he did one more song and left, so we did, too.

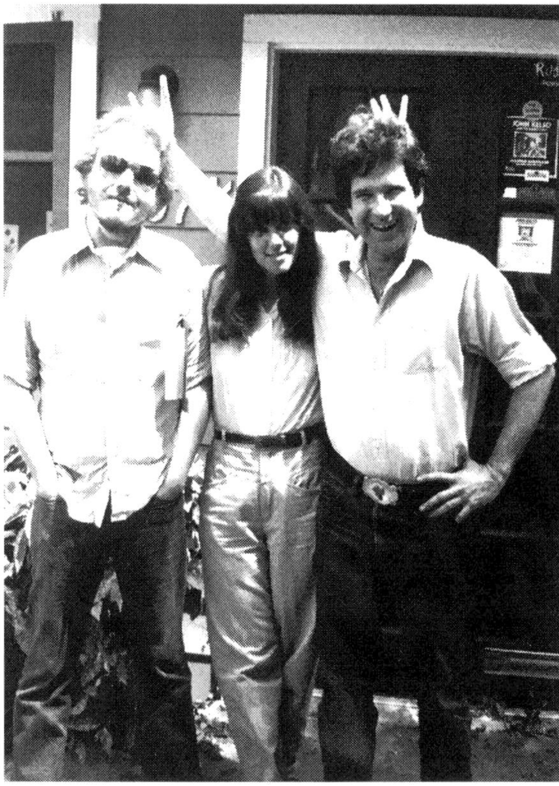

Jackalopes at the Powell Street office, Austin, Texas.

The record was finally finished, mixed, and mastered, and Gracey and I went to Nashville to turn it in to the pressing plant. We hadn't given a lot of thought to a cover but, of course, had to have one before we could turn it in, so I took some pictures that I had, one that had been taken at my first real photo shoot by Butch Hancock, and one that Gracey and Bobby Earl had gotten drunk and had taken one afternoon in Austin of the two of them together with all these ridiculous props. For the cover we used a drawing done by Micael Priest (of Armadillo poster fame) that had already been used on the release before mine for *The Best of Electric Graceyland* of a girl riding a jackalope. It was almost prophetic how it was so perfect, so we didn't mind using it again, and besides, it was what we had. I spent all of thirty minutes designing the layout on a table upstairs in Cowboy's studio. We jumped in the car and made it to the pressing plant just minutes before they closed for the day.

We'd been running back and forth to Nashville with Bobby Earl, but this time it was just Gracey and I, and we were so in love that we could hardly stand it. We turned the record in and went to Brown's Diner, the dive where all the hit songwriters and artists, like the Everly Brothers, would go to hang out every afternoon and drink. It was Valentine's Day, and we celebrated for hours, and finally Gracey blindsided me by suddenly proposing to me! The trouble was that we were still both married to other people, though basically separated by then.

While we waited for our divorces to become final, Gracey and I and my two sons, Jeremie and Gabriel, moved into an Austin apartment complex off of Congress Avenue that I honestly don't think I ever knew the name of because we all called it "Willie's Arms." Lots of the musicians in town lived there on the cheap. Just a stone's throw away was the Opry House, which was run by Tim O'Connor and his partner, Willie. To those of us who had been beating the pavement on Nashville's Music Row, trying to get a deal so we could record, it was like the beatnik antithesis. We had this weird bathroom that was fitted with industrial fixtures, so it had a commode that seemed like it might suck everything in the tiny space away when you flushed it. You were inclined to sort of stand back and brace yourself first. We called it "Mr. Bathroom." Outside Mr. Bathroom's window was the view of a rather crooked, smallish, green street sign that read "Music Row." We thought that was hilarious because it wasn't a street at all but more of an alleyway that led to the rehearsal complex everybody used. So our Music Row was filled with trash cans and winos!

Across the street were two hotels that were brothels (which later became top-end chic places to stay after the renovation of South Congress that turned it into "SoCo"). The boys would walk down Congress to school every morning, and the sweet little whores who worked there would wave at them and say, "Hi Honey! Have a nice day!"

It was a one-room apartment except for a tiny side area/entrance outside Mr. Bathroom with a dressing table. Gracey and I trekked on over to Academy Surplus and bought a foam mattress and put it under the dressing table, and that was what we called "the boys' bedroom." Gracey and I slept on the double bed that was in the living-room/bedroom/kitchen area, next to the fridge. It didn't matter that the bed was so small because we held each other so tightly when we slept that we'd have taken up about the same area in an ultra-king-sized bed.

The boys, though still very young, seemed to be having a lot fun discovering the joys of "city life," after having been raised in the country up until then. They liked having a celebrity stepdad and were impressed that everybody in town seemed to know Gracey everywhere we went. There was the unavoidable pain of being put through the ordeal of a divorce and the awkwardness of having a new adult show up in their lives, but we all did our best to rise to the occasion, and everybody handled it pretty well. Looking back, I marvel sometimes at how oblivious I was as a parent, and I know I could have done better, but given my upbringing, I still had a lot to learn and was still a kid myself in a lot of ways, but we had a lot of love and a sense of humor, and life was really fun and interesting, so we all got through it okay.

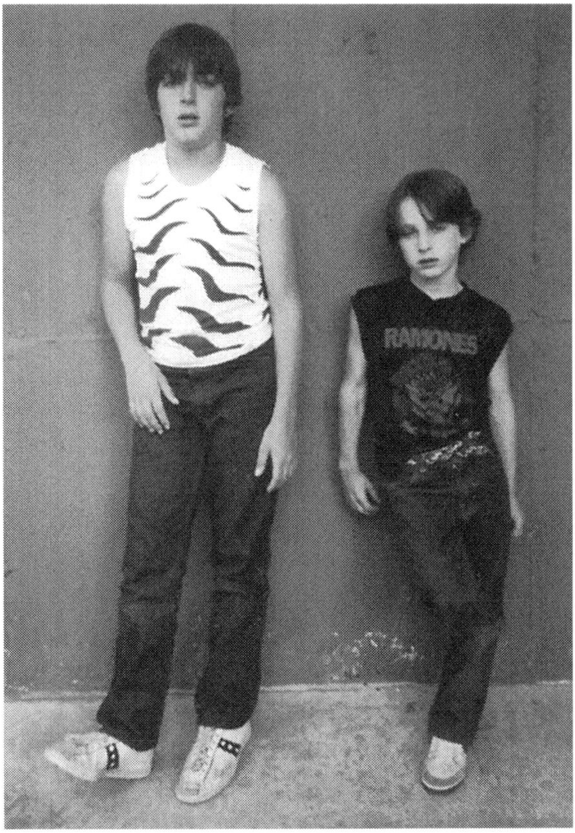

Punk kids. Left to right: Jeremie and Gabriel Rhodes.

Gracey only owned a cast-iron skillet and a couple of beer glasses stolen from the Continental Club (which was just down the street) when we moved in, and I'd left everything I owned at the farm because I hadn't been able to bring myself to officially leave there yet. (In fact, for a while I continued to hold down a part-time job at a greenhouse there and commuted between Austin and Sunset.) Within a week I'd managed to save up enough "value points" at the nearby grocery store to get a free set of dinner plates. I cooked everything we ate in the cast-iron skillet and bought a small saucepan so we could boil potatoes.

I was working as a florist as my day gig, so I would bring home a plant or two every day to plant in the tiny flowerbed outside the door. There was this crazy old woman named Eleanor living next door who would sneak over and steal my plants every night, and I finally caught her when I spied them planted in paper cups on her windowsill. She just would not stop absconding with my flowers, so I finally abandoned gardening. T.J. lived across the parking lot from us. It caused big excitement in the neighborhood one day, when Ray Charles knocked on his door, thinking he was at Willie's apartment, which was next door to T.J.'s.

We soon married "properly" (a quiet church wedding, family only, in a little wood-framed Baptist church in Sunset) and moved to a larger place in the complex, where Gracey and I had an actual bedroom and the boys moved into the kitchen/dining room/living room area. "Daddy Pop" even came down from Fort Worth to visit and had dinner with us one night. I made a homemade blackberry pie with vanilla ice cream, which he loved. We had nothing really, but we were so in love that we thought we had everything. We were very, very happy.

We finally got a great deal on a big two-story house in Clarksville, the area near downtown Austin where all the slaves had settled and built clapboard houses after they had been freed, which had been taken over in the '70s by the hippies because the rent was cheap and it was in the heart of town. We paid a mere three hundred bucks a month for a kitchen, dining room, living room, two bedrooms, and a bathroom upstairs. It also had a big wooden deck out the back door that overlooked a nice little backyard. I had real flowerbeds at last! Joe King Carrasco, Charlotte Herzele, and an actor friend, Brady Coleman, were neighbors. It was a very hip street to live on. Joe King paid the boys five dollars to walk his dogs daily while he was on the road, and he'd come over and hang out. I fed him homemade biscuits, and we all acted like we were domestically normal. He liked my paintings so I gave him an oil painting I did of some sunflowers. I saw him years later and he told me that he still had it and was waiting for me to get famous so he could sell it for a lot of money! I wonder if he still has it.

Gracey was doing some engineering and producing, working with the Supernatural Family Band and others and was also doing some mundane work, recording radio ads to help pay the bills. The Jackalopes had disbanded by that time. Bobby Earl, having a family to feed, had decided to make use of the law degree he had worked so hard to get. The *Kimmie Rhodes and the Jackalope Brothers* LP was finally out, and we marveled, as reviews from all over the world—Germany, Austria, Switzerland, and even Japan, but especially the UK—came trickling in weekly.

I had quit my job as a florist, and, having decided to try my hand at acting, was taking acting lessons at a really soulful little actors' co-op in town, where we all taught classes to scratch out a living, and we swapped lessons with each other. We also all volunteered to answer the phone one afternoon per week and helped each other recruit "students" for our classes, the lesson plans for which we all just basically "made up out of thin air." Everyone convinced me that since I knew how to record, use a microphone, and wasn't afraid to sing in front of an audience, I should teach a class called "Singing for Actors." This brought in as much money as my full-time job as a florist had, but it was more fun, and, besides, I had become pregnant, and this reduced my workload considerably.

Gracey soon began working as the sound engineer for Butch Hancock at his television studio, Dixie's Bar and Bus Stop. It was an amazingly ambitious enterprise where the multitalented songwriter had designed and built a great little room with a stage and was running all the local acts through every single night of the week. I would cook dinner for the boys and get them settled in for the night and then run downtown to the studio and take Gracey dinner and see what was going on. The Jackalope Brothers' nickname for me, Kupcake, had stuck, but Gracey had shortened it to call me "Kup." I called him "Blue," short for "Ol' Blue Eyes," which had been his radio moniker at KOKE.

Every day I would swing by the grocery store and pick up the most ridiculously decorated cupcake available to add to a magnificent lineup we had going across the back of the recording desk. Gracey was really proud of his cupcake collection. I moved my afternoon actors singing class there. It was a really great scene to be part of and really suited our lifestyle and dreams at the time.

I had accumulated enough of my original oil paintings to have my first art exhibit at a restaurant on the east side, Nadine's, where all the local actors and old-school writers still hung out, so I could go there and eat tacos and "get seen" in and among my own creations and feel like all my hard work was paying off, and like I hadn't been just living a pipe dream after all. I even sold a couple of paintings, which for me was yet another dream come true. It was absolutely magnificent to be deeply in love and surrounded by actors and musicians and artists every single day, people who not only encouraged me but also truly appreciated my efforts. For me it was like a modern-day Renaissance, where Austin was Florence and the Texas Capitol building was the Duomo.

Our daughter, Jole Morgan Goodnight Gracey, was born on Mexican Mother's Day, May 10. All the family and friends came to see her and hold her. Everyone had to wear these yellow sterilized robes. It was fun to watch everyone all dressed in paper hospital garb passing the baby around the room. Jeremie and Gabriel were there, of course, to welcome their new sister. They were starving for something to eat, so we ordered a pizza. When the pizza deliveryman came in, he said that he was a gypsy and was obliged to have to touch the baby's forehead and give her a blessing or it would be bad luck. I agreed, on the condition that he first wash his hands. We took Jole home from the hospital and placed her in a little crib at the foot of our bed. Everyone delighted that rather than sucking her thumb, she had been born sucking her two middle fingers, which made it look like she was giving the "Hook 'em, Horns" hand gesture of the Texas Longhorns football team, which we all worshiped.

On my first official outing with Jole, to the downtown post office, a bum on the street came up to me as I was getting out of the car with her in my arms. He said the same thing that the pizza man had said and insisted on touching her head and giving her a gypsy blessing. So she was twice blessed in her first few weeks of life.

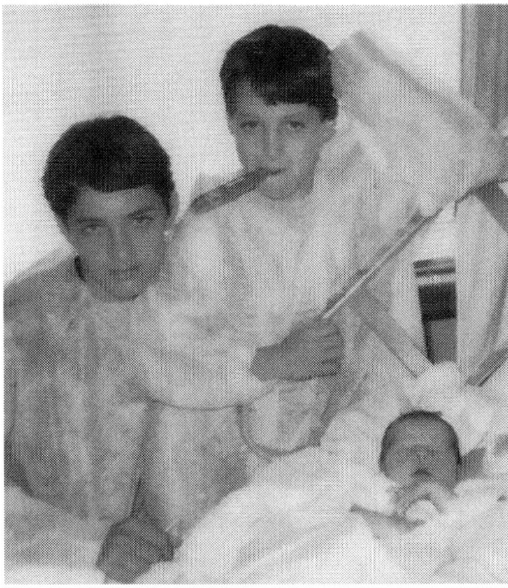

Jeremie, Gabriel, and Jole on the day she was born.

Oddly, I woke up one day missing being a florist, which was good because the actors' co-op had disbanded, and although I had done a few auditions, the whole acting scene in town just wasn't burgeoning; most of the serious actors had run off to Los Angeles to seek their fame and fortune. Gracey still had part-time work at Lone Star Studios, but we needed cash. I went back to work part time at a flower shop, and Gracey loved keeping Jole in the daytime while I was working. He wrote a lot on his old typewriter, shopped for food, and developed a real interest in cooking. He would shop at Whole Foods, the hippie store down the street, every day and study cookbooks. He began cooking really fabulous meals every night and began to cultivate a taste for fine red wine. He even borrowed a small winepress, bought some wine grapes, and gave winemaking a try.

All this time the *Kimmie Rhodes and the Jackalope Brothers* album just kept finding its way around the world and getting good reviews, due mostly in part to the continued efforts of Susan Jarrett, who had a small regional business called Austin Record Distributors and was good at getting the music out to indie labels in Europe, where there was a real buzz about Texas music at the time.

JOE GRACEY—LETTER TO MARIAN ABOUT MARRIAGE AND KIDS

Dear Marian,

I was just sitting here reading about Texas cooking, and I heard my youngest stepson, Gabriel, counting up to fifty so he could go look for his brother and their friend in an entirely too-noisy game of hide-n-go-seek. Them boys are fine, courteous, respectful, intelligent, and sensitive, but, of course, I and their mother spend about 50 percent of the time trying to raise them up to be decent human beings.

You see, the doctrine of Original Sin was thought up by a parent, since it is obvious that a kid has no natural sense of morality or decency, so if a kid grows up to be a nice person, it is entirely the result of some poor parent who bribed them, seethed at them, grounded them, lectured, yelled, begged, denied, praised extravagantly, listened to, lied to, shielded, altered, babied, spoiled, laughed at/with/about, cajoled, argued with, and laid down the—by God—law, too. You would be amazed at how awesome the yawning abyss of their ignorance is . . . at least I was, anyway.

But I love these kids, and we get along just fine, which is more than some stepparents get. The young one is still malleable and has developed a kind of hero-worship for me, akin to a crush, that is touching and sweet. He comes and sits close to me or in my lap and in one of those innocent gestures that only kids can offer. The older one is admirably already his father's son. His loyalty is engrained but he likes me and we have more of a brotherly relationship, which is fine, too. I always wished I had a big brother to help me through the crisis of adolescence.

Me and my perfect mate are going to try to time our baby so that it will be born next spring. That means we'll be working on that pretty soon. At the typing of that sentence my balls contracted in a reflex of pleasure and fear. Now I realize what all this love and marriage business is really about. It really helps if the person you pick to love and marry is a nice, intelligent, steady, competent type. It makes things run ever so much more smoothly.

We've moved into a swell old house in the quasi-Clarksville section. I feel like I've come full circle, having lived here in a previous marriage and loved it in 1970. This is the Austin everybody idealizes and fights to preserve. We're near great little neighborhood shops that combine to give you a sense of belonging to the place. The house is an old frame story and a half with a fireplace and dining room and a bedroom for the kids and everything!

I feel full of life today. My ho-hum job as a recording engineer is proceeding in the proper manner; I'm very good at it and I gave myself a raise to fifteen dollars an hour, so I don't feel so put upon when I have to do mundane recording work. I work in groups of a few days then I'm off for a few, so it doesn't normally interfere with my dreaming. And, of course, it is a perfect trade for a producer to keep up. Kimmie works at the flower place so we have enough to pay the bills and eat out at will and buy crazy food to take home and play with.

Now Austin has this new "Whole Foods" store, which is like a cross between those old hippie natural food stores and a gourmet market. My ongoing interest in food and cooking makes these places a natural for me, and we spend a considerable hunk of our money there. I got me one of those old drum barbeque deals, and I have been investigating the wonders of smoked meats, or, you could say, "burnt meats." You see, the real secret of barbeque has nothing to do with direct heat or sauces or herbs. The real item consists of a piece of meat that has been cooked as far away from the fire as possible so that the smoke and overall heat of the unit does all the cooking.

You go out upon arising and build a fire of mesquite wood (which regrettably has become trendy with the cursed gourmets), and when it is mere coals, you stick the salt and peppered meat in the far end of the drum, under the chimney so that the draft carries the heat and smoke over the meat. You then drink beer and stoke the fire gingerly as the day wears on, and by nightfall, you have "burned meat." Or, if you prefer to actually eat the meat, you remove it from the pit about a half hour before I normally do, thus preserving some of the juices and texture. Otherwise, you bring it in and drive nails with it. Oh, it is grand!

I also have become a wine expert; I've been checking out books about wine, a subject that I have assumed was impervious to, these many years, which I find has some basic tenets, which, if grasped, can at least cause the beast to yield slightly to assaults by redneck Texans. I've been trying my hand at Beaujolais, which are great amateurs' wines, and next, I intend to work on some Cabernets and see if I can discern any of the "chocolate with a hint of cherries" I keep reading about.

I am recovering from a terrible hangover. Stan (the studio owner) and I went to a Texas football game in great weather yesterday and drank some bourbon in our cokes, then repaired to the Hole in the Wall and decided to have a few shots of tequila, then bought a couple of beers on the way home and opened a bottle of New Beaujolais 1983 crop and drank most of that, then watched my W. C. Fields movie on the rented VCR machine while drinking a couple of Pearl beers as a nightcap. As Fields would say, "I feel as though the Russian army had been marching across my tongue in their stocking feet last night."

As I was making breakfast, around 2:30 p.m. today, Gabriel came home with his new recorder (a flute-like instrument) and proceeded to play "Three Blind Mice" about four hundred times in the kitchen with me at high volume and unsteady timbre. It was a very "Fieldsian" scene, what with me with a throbbing headache and all.

You are in for a huge surprise. You have no idea what rotten little bastards kids are. So, anyhow, congratulations on your pregnancy!

We're still plugging away at Kimmie's LP, with most of it mixed now. We've been cutting some music for a movie soundtrack. We used Johnny Gimble and Jimmy Day, so that was fun. I played rhythm guitar and amazed myself at how good I'm getting. Bobby Earl is opening his law office and trying to make some money at his true profession, which is handing out great advice.

Let us know when your kid is born, etc. Love y'all.

Joe

JOE GRACEY—LETTER TO MARIAN ABOUT HIS DAUGHTER BEING BORN

Dear Marian and Reid,

How are you? I'm writing, not typing this, because Jole Morgan Goodnight Gracey(!) is asleep in her little "play prison," sucking two fingers with the two outside fingers up in a "Hook 'em, Horns" sign!

She was born May 10 around 7:47 p.m. after two hours of labor and no anesthesia and no problems. I was taking photos of her yelling her little head off. She has big blue eyes like her mama's and big ears like her daddy's and hair of some intermediate light-brown-red hue.

Her brothers are crazy about her and spoil her to death. Kimmie is very happy to have a little girl to dress up and be on her side. I'm ecstatic to have a kid and especially a girl who will grow up thinking I'm worthwhile instead of worthless, like boys do. Also I think it's important that Kimmie gets to train up a girl to be like Mama.

Love,

Joe

7

WE MUST BELIEVE IN MAGIC

KIMMIE RHODES AND JOE GRACEY

JOE GRACEY—"MAGIC"

I THINK WE HAVE STOPPED admitting openly that we believe in magic, but we still do the things that we always have—pray, engage in superstitious rituals, go to psychics, read horoscopes in newspapers, and put horseshoes over doors and Christmas trees in our houses. We just deny that any of this is magic, unless we don't care if people think we are crazy.

My mentor, Jack Clement, began his career as the engineer/producer at Sun Records and wrote great songs like "Miller's Cave" and "I Know One" and "The One on the Right Is on the Left." He produced Johnny Cash and Jerry Lee Lewis and Charley Pride and Don Williams and Waylon Jennings and is the most brilliant rhythm guitar player on earth. Every morning in his sun-filled office in his studio/playhouse, he takes down his old Gibson J-200 guitar, the one he played on a million hit records, and starts to strum that beat that you've heard on records like

"Ring of Fire" and "Bob Wills Is Still the King," and people filter in there and pick up guitars and mandolins and start playing counter-rhythms to his beat. After about fifteen minutes, it settles in and takes on life, and you can play it all day if you want to. It is magic, called down from someplace where the groove resides. Some people like Jack can call down the groove any time they want to. It is an act of invocation.

One day I walked into Jack's office, over at the Cowboy Arms Hotel and Recording Spa, and his mentor, Sam Phillips, who had owned the Sun label and Studios, had just come in from giving a speech at Vanderbilt. He was still pretty wound up from his speech, and I sat down and proceeded to listen to the two of them for the next six to eight hours. Hooch was produced, the afternoon wore on, and I got the full Sam Phillips treatment coupled with the Cowboy retorts . . . pretty amazing day in my life. I remember watching the sun sinking through the trees in the backyard, thinking, "Am I dreaming this?" When we broke up, I ran back to my hotel room and scribbled every word of it down while I could still remember. I sure hope I can find it someday.

Sam is a man of strong opinions, many of them dead-solid-on. You can imagine what he thinks of the current state of things in American music. The funniest part of the day was listening to him and Jack arguing over why and how Sam fired Jack. Suddenly it was if they were transformed into the same two people they were at Sun; Jack was still pissed off, and Sam was still trying to tell him why he had to fire his ass. Jack says his proudest accomplishment at Sun was building a bathroom off the control room so he didn't have to go through the studio to piss.

Later we recorded a record at Sun, and that piled on more magic because Jack showed us his bathroom. He says Jesus was the greatest general contractor the world has ever known and that he thinks that would be the ideal career. I figure Jesus could probably play rhythm guitar better than Jack and probably build a better bathroom . . . but he's the only one who could!

Jack still has his big Gibson J-200 guitar from the Sun days, and it sounds otherworldly. I try to play it every chance I get, and it always sounds just like it did on all those great, great, great records. Praise Sam Phillips and Jack Clement for midwifing rock 'n' roll! (Think "Ring of Fire.")

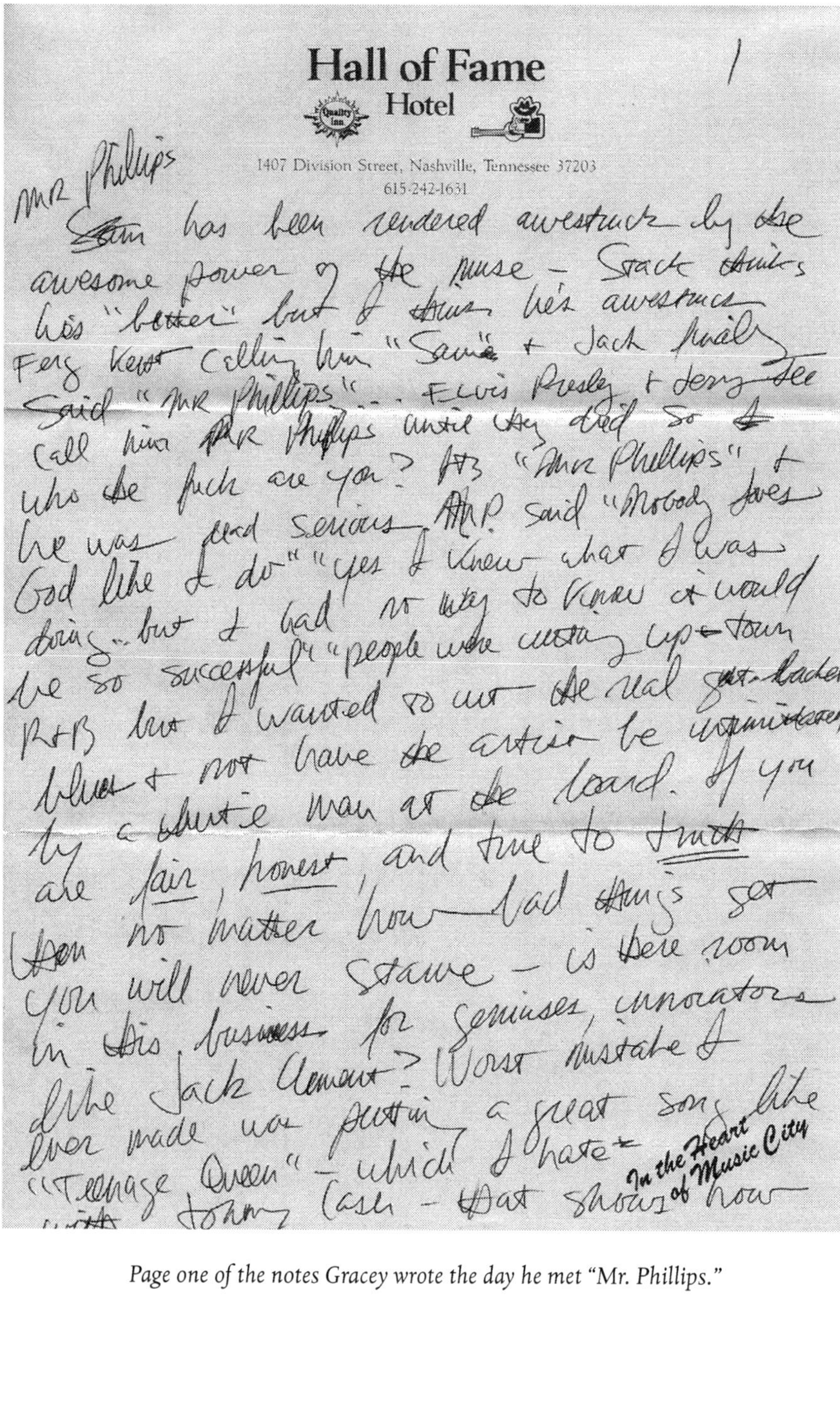
Hall of Fame
Hotel

1407 Division Street, Nashville, Tennessee 37203
615-242-1631

1

Mr Phillips
Sam has been rendered awestruck by the
awesome power of the muse – Stack thinks
his "better" but I think he's awestruck
Ferg kept calling him "Sam" + Jack finally
said "Mr Phillips"... Elvis Presley + Jerry Lee
call him Mr Phillips until they died so I
who the fuck are you? It's "Mr Phillips" +
he was dead serious. Mr P. said "Nobody loves
God like I do" "yes I knew what I was
doing.. but I had no way to know it would
be so successful" "people were cutting up-town
R+B but I wanted to cut the real gut-bucket
blues + not have the artist be intimidated
by a white man at the board. If you
are fair, honest, and true to truth
then no matter how bad things get
you will never starve – is there room
in this business for geniuses, innovators
like Jack Clement? Worst mistake I
ever made was putting a great song like
"Teenage Queen" – which I hate –
with Johnny Cash – that shows how

In the Heart of Music City

Page one of the notes Gracey wrote the day he met "Mr. Phillips."

KIMMIE RHODES

As if by magic, we were living a life in which it seemed like almost everything we wanted came true, and pretty quickly, like all we had to do was settle our intent and know that stars out there somewhere would begin lining up to make things happen. Yes, we worked hard, but this was not the kind of success that's forced. There was a definite "groove" to the way things were going. We weren't really in control so much as obliged to be creatively "ready" and rise to the occasion when opportunity knocked. Things just happened. So it became easy to trust what was meant to be and accept what was not meant to be.

It was before computers and the Internet and smartphones, back when business was conducted via landline and FedEx and, later, fax machine. Nobody had a website, and we still snail-mailed press kits and contracts if we weren't able to hand-deliver them. Part of the fun of it was sowing the seeds and then having that period of waiting to see what "came up." The world was turning our way, so the idea that the phone would ring and something good would happen became a reliable philosophy for living.

We still weren't out of the woods yet, where Gracey's loss of speech was concerned. He was a dreamer but a hardworking and ambitious one, with a work ethic forged by being the son and grandson of successful trial lawyers, so he felt plenty of frustration in those days at not being able to speak on the phone and get things done. Remember, this was the guy who, by the time he enrolled in the University of Texas, had already been a disc jockey for several years and was writing a music column for the *Austin American-Statesman*. He stayed busy.

He wrote a lot of letters, which, for most people, was becoming a lost art. He enjoyed the "intelligence factor" of communicating in that way. He had an antique cast-iron typewriter that he called his "old dinosaur." He always had a stack of yellow legal pads, which were his medium of choice if a typewriter wasn't available. He kept a stack of envelopes and a roll of stamps on his desk and mailed letters daily. He was a list maker.

He seemed to take his loss of speech in stride during the few years following the final surgery that took his voice completely. He was astoundingly steady, patient, and calm, but then frustrations would build up inside him. When he would have a meltdown, it was almost always over some incident that involved an inability to communicate by phone. He would ask me to help him make a call, and, prior to me dialing the number, he would, in a very clear and premeditated way, explain exactly what he wished to be said. It was touching how openly humble and grateful he would be for my help every time. Now, this wasn't solely to make important business calls; he also had to deal with the usual bill that needed to be straightened out or the booking of a hotel or car or flight for travel. He spent a lot of time running errands because he had to physically drive to places to have a discussion using his Magic Slate. He couldn't just pick up the phone, ask questions, and get answers, a convenience most people in the world take for granted. He learned to have phone conversations with people who knew him by tapping on the receiver with a pen: one for "no," two for "yes," three for "maybe" or "I don't know." So you had to be good at asking only yes-or-no questions. I soon got to where I could talk to him for hours. If you made a mistake and posed the question incorrectly, he would start banging on the phone and make the wheezing sound that he produced when he was chuckling. A hard laugh was signified by slapping on his thighs and wheezing louder . . . laughter, another thing we all take for granted, the singular expressiveness of our very own laugh.

The first time I saw Gracey kick a trash can across the room in anger, I thought to myself, "Oh, no, this guy might be trouble." But in time I realized that that was not the case. In fact, sometimes it seemed like he had the patience of Job—too much, in fact. Time revealed that his anxiety over not being able to speak would take on a pattern that ran its course about once every eighteen months. He would finally explode, as I've said, usually triggered by a problem involving a phone call. Then he would become incredibly sad.

At this point we would have a late-night "heart to heart," which usually began with a laundry list of things that had been driving him crazy and a discussion about how we might make adjustments to reduce the frustration. This talk naturally progressed to the deeper issue of how he was "getting on," in terms of adjusting to not speaking. He was also beginning to show signs of depression, inherited from his father and his father's father, so, as with all depression, it was difficult to tell where the burdens of everyday living stopped and the chemical aspects of the condition began. In the early days there seemed to be more anger than sadness, but eventually we reached a new plateau. One night we talked for a long time, and he began to realize that somewhere in his psyche he had still held forth hope that he would speak again someday, like when you wake from a bad dream or finally heal from an injury. As time passed he began to comprehend that this, unlike most problems, was not going to disappear . . . ever.

He always quoted these words of wisdom from his father, like a mantra of cool, calm collectedness: "The lawyer who loses his temper loses the case." Gracey would use his hands in many expressive ways, but when he wanted to quiet a situation in order to discuss a solution to a problem, he would gesture with both hands, palms down, look you square in the eye, drop both hands about six inches, as if tamping the chaos down, point to his head to gesture, "Let's think about this." Then, adjusting his poise, he would take his Magic Slate in hand, as if wielding a sword, and calmly write and erase, write and erase, phrases in eight to ten words maximum, because of the space limitations, and write his way to the core of the matter. He avoided law school because it wasn't his heart's desire, but he would have made a fine attorney.

It was truly inspiring to watch him go forward in the days that followed these episodes. He was so very fortunate to have had strong role models in his life. His dad had been a war hero, who, although sometimes withdrawn, had suffered any burden of trauma handed him with grace and dignity, and balanced the world strapped to his back with a poignant sense of humor. It was as if, once Gracey survived the cancer that threatened his life, he made a conscious decision to "grow up" (and his grandfather had judiciously come to the rescue with funding for a production company). So he adopted the wearable parts of the strong respectable men who raised him and added them to his own nonconformist ways in order to somewhat domesticate a lifestyle that would never be normal. He took account of what he still had (like a sense of taste, although having lost his tongue) and used it to rebuild his life. He read books and took on hobbies, like winemaking and cooking (which would later become a passion and then a sideline career).

If the magic had stopped right then and there, I could have easily lived out my days on earth, with Gracey and my three children, my art and music, and all the new friends, just having fun and believing that I was the luckiest person. I felt happier than I had ever been and woke up every day feeling like my life had purpose. But as it turned out, the magic was just beginning.

One day we were recording at Pedernales Studio, and I walked over to the big plate-glass picture window and pointed out a secluded spot down the hill. I told Gracey, "If we built a house down there, we would be able to see if the kids have burned the house down while we're at work." He laughed and agreed, so with the expertise of Randy, a realtor who was a grade-school friend of Gracey's, we bought a lot from Willie in the Hill Country on Lake Travis. We built a classic Texas country-style clapboard house with a tin roof and a covered front porch so we could sit outside and watch the sun go down. We painted the house blue. We had just celebrated Jole's first birthday the month before we moved into our new home in June of 1986. Everything was perfect. Now we were not only conveniently near the studio, but we fit right in to the thriving artistic community that Willie had surrounded himself with, located near both the western town, Luck, Texas, where he had filmed his movie *Red Headed Stranger*, and his golf course, Pedernales Cut and Putt.

I remember one day in July. I was soaking in a bubble bath, listening to a live broadcast of Willie's Fourth of July Farm Aid picnic, which was taking place near our new neighborhood, and thinking about Willie and how natural it seemed that he would be the one out raising money to help family farms survive. It had only been a few years since I had been one of those family farmers that hadn't made it. I began to ponder that time.

When I was still living in Sunset, Texas, we had started dryland truck farming (meaning vegetables with no irrigation), the first year of what had turned out to be a seven-year drought. We had switched to commercial growing in a greenhouse, but soon after, Walmart moved into our community and sold plants cheaper than we could grow them. By the time we went broke, I had already started coming to Austin to record, and, anyway, my heart just wasn't into farming anymore.

My mind drifted back to the morning when I had been at the farmhouse alone, except for my two young boys. Two men from the bank showed up at my door to repossess the tractor and whatever could be salvaged in greenhouses and equipment. I was twenty-six years old at the time. They were really kind, and I felt bad about not being able to pay the debt, so I was just as apologetic to them as they were to me. However, I was greatly relieved that the worry was finally over and said, "Hey, it's okay, really. I'm sorry we couldn't make the payments anymore but here, let me help you." That's when I learned that "being under" is a lot easier than "going under."

I was snapped back to the present time by the voice of Kris Kristofferson, who was being interviewed just before he was to go onstage, saying something about waiting for Rita Coolidge before he could go on and joking about how he'd spent a lot of time in his years with her, "waiting for Rita Coolidge." I started daydreaming, imagining how fun it would be to play on that stage to Willie's fans, and before I knew it, I was clicking my "ruby slippers" together again, wishing that we would be invited to play it someday.

Not long after that I was driving down the road and heard "Uncloudy Day" come on the radio and thought, "Wow, wouldn't it be fun to be able to sing that with Willie onstage someday?"

Jimmy Day asked me to join his band the Texas Tunesmiths, which I happily accepted. Gracey also joined to play rhythm guitar. This was how we met David Zettner. When Willie had left Ray Price's Cherokee Cowboys to form his own band, Zettner had become Willie's bass player for a while, until he was drafted to go to Vietnam. Zettner had escaped with an honorable discharge and was living on the Pedernales River, just down the road from our place. He was one of those people who could do about a million things really well, and we connected

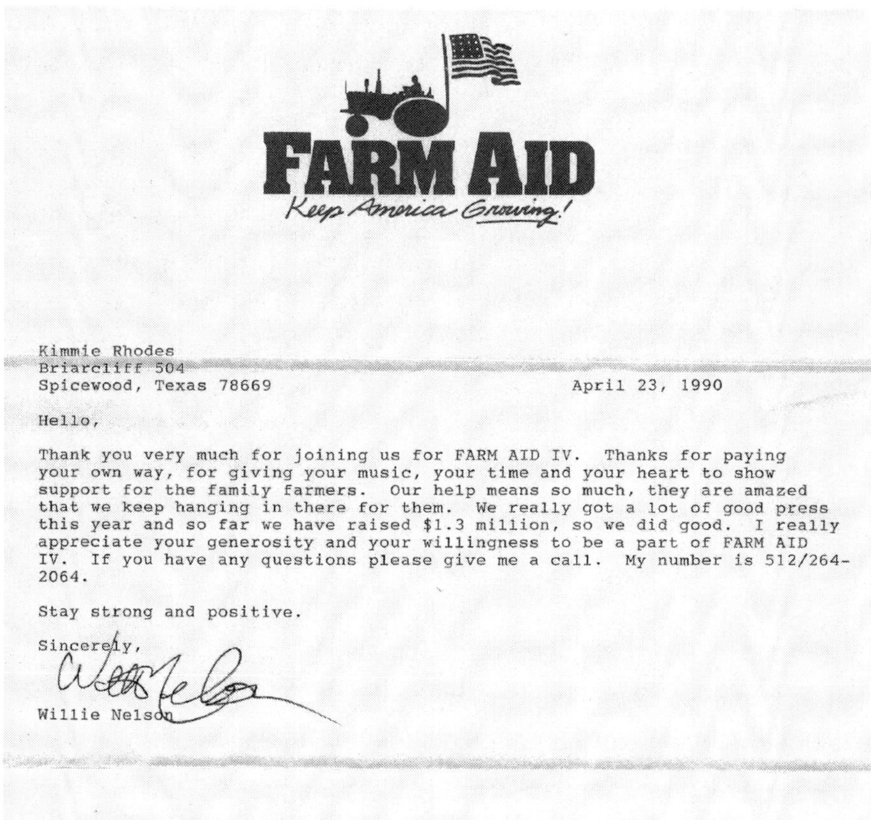

FARM AID

Keep America Growing!

Kimmie Rhodes
Briarcliff 504
Spicewood, Texas 78669

April 23, 1990

Hello,

Thank you very much for joining us for FARM AID IV. Thanks for paying your own way, for giving your music, your time and your heart to show support for the family farmers. Our help means so much, they are amazed that we keep hanging in there for them. We really got a lot of good press this year and so far we have raised $1.3 million, so we did good. I really appreciate your generosity and your willingness to be a part of FARM AID IV. If you have any questions please give me a call. My number is 512/264-2064.

Stay strong and positive.

Sincerely,

Willie Nelson

Farm Aid thank-you letter sent to Kimmie from Willie.

immediately because we shared a love not just for music but also for painting. He was an extraordinary artist and had painted all the murals at the studio, in addition to painting Willie's bus and designing the *Tougher Than Leather* album cover.

Jimmy was a Ray Price and Willie band veteran, too, and he had also played with just about every country act that ever came out of Nashville. When asked about it, he would say that it was easier to list the acts he hadn't played with than ones he had. He'd grown up in Louisiana with the pianist Floyd Cramer ("Last Date"), who said he developed his distinctive style while trying to play chords like a steel guitar on piano. Gracey and I absolutely devoured the "war stories" from the road that passed around the room when all these guys would get going backstage on breaks.

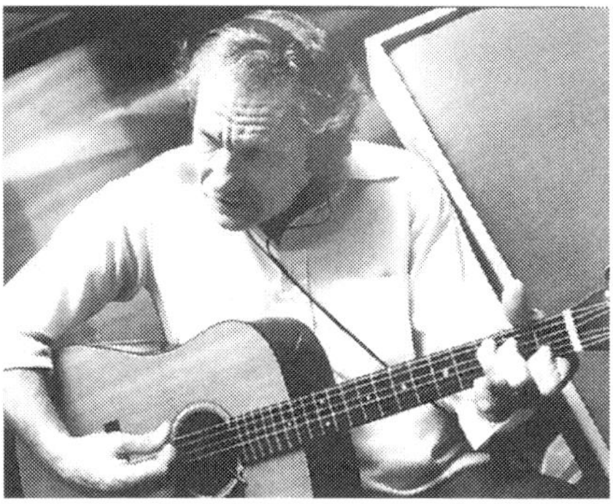

David Zettner at Lone Star Studios, Austin, Texas. Photo by Butch Hancock.

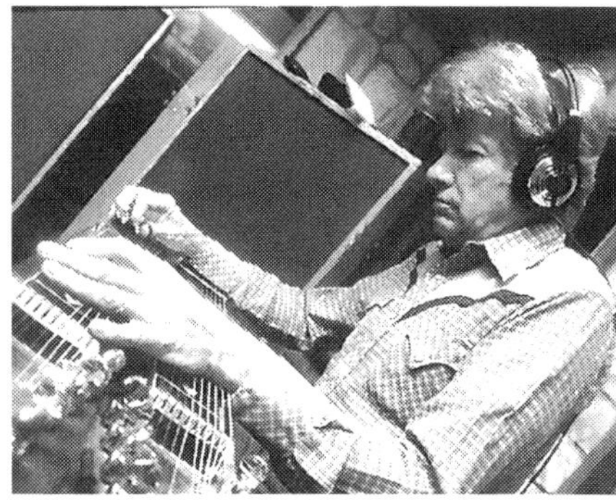

Jimmy Day at Lone Star Studios, Austin, Texas. Photo by Butch Hancock.

Jimmy was the maestro of the steel guitar, and I got a major crash course in classic country music by playing dance halls with him. One of the highlights of those days and, actually, a highlight of my career, was getting to open the show for the Texas Playboys (post–Bob Wills incarnation) in San Marcos, Texas. It was the penultimate show before they were to permanently disband, and I had a ringside seat. After we finished our set, I sat on the steps leading up to the stage and watched and learned "how it was done" by the masters of western swing. They played the old-time favorite "Faded Love" three times in a ninety-minute set that day. Someone would call it and count it off and they'd just play it again!

There were two shows going on, really: the one for the audience, which was as professionally played as could ever be done by any band of any genre, and the show they put on for each other onstage. They cracked dirty jokes, switched instruments with each other, and zinged hilarious "asides" and one-liners at each other, off mic and on. During the short intermission, they took turns at the merchandise table, like a tag team making sure that at least two of them were there at all times to visit with fans and sign autographs. I don't recall ever having seen a happier audience! I was particularly infatuated with Smokey Dacus, the drummer, because he played the drums like they were pots and pans and with an incredible sense of humor. All the jazz music I had been exposed to watching cartoons as a kid came flooding back to me, and I remembered how my dad would entertain me by banging on the pots and pans with wooden spoons while singing the words to an old blues song, "Get out in that kitchen and rattle them pots and pans."

I was as inspired as a girl could be by all this, and Gracey was having a ball getting to play jazzy rhythm chords on his treasured acoustic Gibson. I began to gain confidence and experience and turned a corner as a songwriter. I signed a deal with a British label, Heartland Records, during this time, and a swing tune I wrote called "Man in the Moon" became the title track of the first album released. Gracey produced the track, and Jimmy Day played extraordinary steel guitar on it, gracing it with a signature intro and outro. It was an instant hit and led to a successful tour in England, where I headlined the Wembley Country Music Festival in London with a band assembled by guitarist singer-songwriter Wes McGhee, who had recently recorded an album with Gracey and me in Austin called *Landing Lights.*

It was the first time I'd played for an audience this size, about twenty thousand people in a large arena. We were well rehearsed and the band was smokin' hot; we made absolutely no mistakes and killed it! But I was used to rowdy dance halls and had zero experience at playing for a polite British crowd, so I left the stage crushed, thinking we had failed completely. To make matters worse, the guys from the label were there in the wings screaming, "You went down a bomb!" I hung my head in shame and said, "I'm sorry. I know. I'm really sorry." And they said, "NO! You're getting an encore!" Where I come from, the word "bomb" means you "bombed"—you could not have done worse. But in England "going down a bomb" translates to "You've destroyed them!" Wow! Was I ever relieved! We played the encore, and afterward, it was a real eye-opener to step outside the elevator on the way to sign autographs and be rushed by a bunch of fans who acted like they were desperate to meet me. I had just never experienced anything like that before. (Mind you, it had only been a few years since I had been living on a dryland farm picking squash and going bankrupt.)

We followed that show with a bizarre tour of Europe that was like a roller-coaster ride that swooped along somewhere between the big-time arenas and small-time theaters in the middle of nowhere, where nobody showed and my name was spelled wrong on the marquee. They had started putting "Kimmie Rhodes and Her Band" on the posters, so we decided that was the name of the band: Her Band.

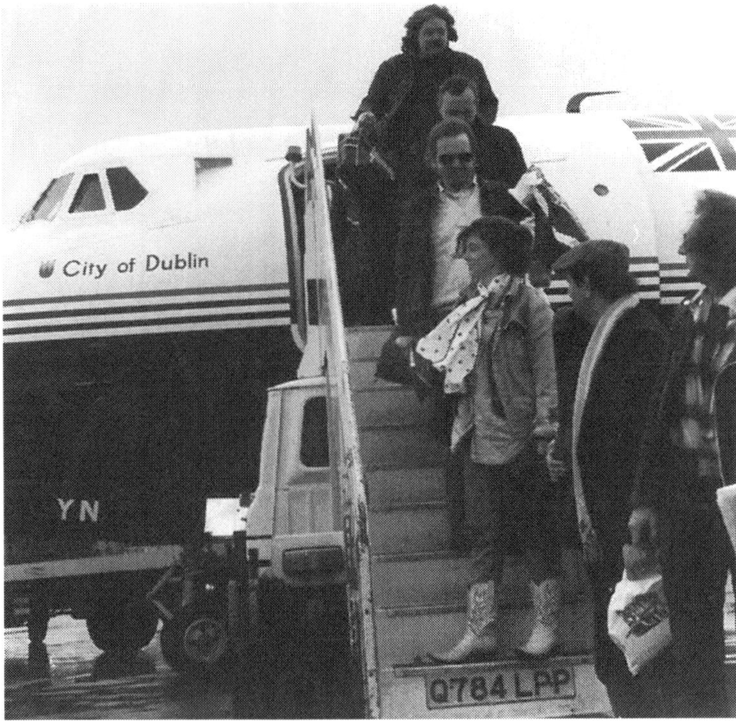

Kimmie and "Her Band" arriving in Dublin, Ireland.

A memorable gig on that tour was in a gorgeous area in a town on the border of Switzerland and Italy. The town was called Locarno/Ascona because half of the town was in Switzerland and the other half was in Italy. The accommodation for the band was in this ancient castle that in contemporary times had been taken over by a weird ballet dance company that did this avant-garde performance piece they had created in the puppet theater across the street, which was where our show was to be that night. As we all passed through the arched doorway of the castle, a strange chill passed through every fiber of my being, all the way to the bone. I exclaimed, "Wow! It's freezing in here!" and then I realized that everyone was standing around looking at me like I was crazy because it was actually a pretty warm day. The band spread out, and Gracey and I were escorted to the very top floor to a room with a domed ceiling that had been painted with strange Day-Glo-colored psychedelic images. Our room shared a large bathroom with the room behind a locked door that was located in the old original tower.

I went into the bathroom to get ready for the show and started to put on my makeup. It was dark and cold in the room, and I had a very eerie perception that someone was not just watching me but was actually following me around. When I leaned over the sink to get closer to the mirror so I could put on my eyeliner, I had a very distinct feeling that someone was standing just behind me, leaning in with me, curiously observing my technique. It really freaked me out because I'd never really encountered anything invisible that was this vivid before, and it was beginning to dawn on me that the place was definitely haunted, so I hurriedly finished getting ready and left the room as quickly as possible.

We went downstairs to meet the band and walk across to the theater. It was the first time in weeks the guys had had an opportunity not to have to share a room with someone, but in no time at all they had all moved down to this cavernous room with peeling paint on the walls, filled with twin beds that had a black grand piano in the corner, and decided to all sleep there!

We played a really good show that night to a sold-out audience, except for one small glitch at the end when they were thunderously stomping their feet and clapping their hands, yelling for a second encore, making it impossible for our drummer, Maurice, to count a waltz. But he somehow did, and we ended on "Waltz Across Texas," because it was the last one in our repertoire that the band knew.

We then returned to the castle elated, collapsed into our beds, and passed out. I was awakened around 3:00 a.m. by a big, cracking sound, like a skeleton key makes when unlocking a heavy door. I thought to myself, "How odd that the gardener lady who lived in the cottage outside and was the caretaker, would come into the castle in the middle of the night and enter through the tower room. I looked over at Gracey, who was asleep in the twin bed that was pushed next to mine. He was obviously dreaming wildly because he was making noises like laughing or gasping or something. I closed my eyes to drift back to sleep and then I felt it . . . again—the same undeniable presence from before, standing beside the bed next to me. It was so strong a feeling that I opened my eyes, sure to see someone standing there, looking at me. Yet, while I still very much felt it, I could see no one.

I somehow knew the ghost was a woman. She moved to the foot of the bed, stood for a while, and then walked across the room. I heard the woven grass seat creak, as if she were sitting in the rocking chair by the window. I was petrified but grew extremely exhausted, as this went on for a couple of hours. Whoever she was, this lonely ghost was clearly expecting my full attention because anytime I began to fall back asleep, she quickly moved next to the bed and made her presence known by bending close to my face. Finally, I thought, "Look, whatever you want and whoever you are, I'm too tired to stay awake anymore. I'm not afraid of you, and I'm going to sleep now. Good night." I closed my eyes, whereupon the ghost grabbed the end of my bed and violently jerked it! It was insane! And it went on and on like this until daylight finally started to creep through the blinds of the open window. I jumped out of bed, threw my clothes on, and announced, "I'm out of here!" Everybody laughed at me, especially Wes McGhee, who was on the tour as guitarist. The promoter laughed, too, and confirmed that all the bands that had stayed in the castle reported hauntings, some even seeing people dancing around the room. He said most assuredly it was the spirit of the woman with the dance troupe who was merely craving the company of a fellow artist.

When we returned the next year to play that theater, I had agreed to come on the condition that I would not be staying in the castle. So they put us in the cottage down below the castle. We returned from the show, and as soon as we switched on the lights, they immediately went out. I said, "That's it! Call the promoter and tell him I'm moving to a hotel!" While we were waiting for the promoter to come, Wes said, "I saw an altar niche on the street around the corner. I'll run down there and nick a candle." He returned with a taper candle and stuck it in a beer bottle in the center of the table, and as soon as he held the flame of his cigarette lighter to the wick, the lights came on. The promoter arrived and explained that it was too late and there was nowhere to go, so since I hadn't really been having any of the feelings of being haunted like I had from the year before, I agreed and climbed into Gracey's twin bed with him just to be on the safe side. Wes went to his room, and he would never say exactly what happened during the night, but this time he was the one who was ready to get going quickly the next morning! I sympathized and even carried his guitar to the van for him. Gabriel, who was also on this tour, had been given a room above the puppet theater. When he awoke and opened his curtains, he discovered that his room overlooked a graveyard. He reported that he'd had the feeling when he was taking a bath that someone was standing beside the tub wanting to push him down and hold him underwater until he drowned. That was our last visit to the castle in Locarno.

One of the greatest places in England where we played was a pub called the Weavers Arms, where people who were massive fans were packed, standing room only, like sardines. Those shows put a lot less pressure on me than the big shows, so I could let my hair down, tell jokes, and tease the hecklers in the audience. It became sort of an impromptu comedy act on those nights, so I finally got to use the improvisation techniques I'd learned back in acting classes after all.

It was also on one of these nights that I met a fan named Barry Dixon. I was leaving the sound check, and he met me on the street outside the London venue with a bouquet of flowers. Barry gets a mention because he caught on to the fact that I had a passion for flowers, so every single tour I have ever done in England for the several decades that followed, he has, without fail, come to a show and brought me flowers. Like the lyrics of one of my favorite Tom Waits songs: "I remember the showers but no one puts flowers on a flower's grave." Ironically, it's one of life's

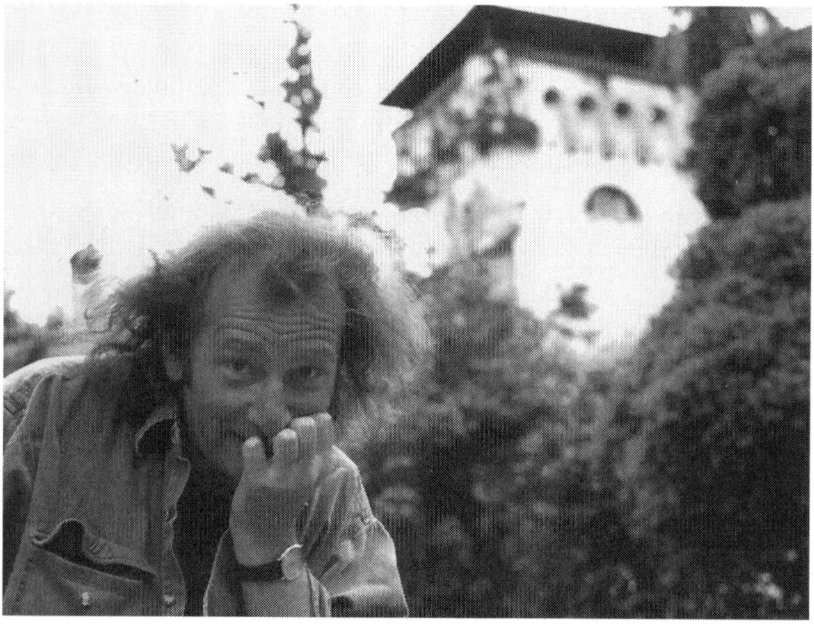

Wes McGhee at the haunted castle, Locarno, Switzerland.

mysteries that nobody gives flowers to a florist, although it's the thing we love the most.

We learned that shows could be characterized as feast or famine. Some nights were diamonds, and some nights were, well, . . . not diamonds. But "that's show biz!" Luckily, we also learned that those times could mostly be avoided if you have a good promoter and don't get booked into the wrong venue. Butch Hancock always said, "No matter where you go, there you are." If even a handful of people decide to see your show, get dressed, park the car, buy a ticket, and honor you by showing up, those people are every bit as deserving as an audience of eighty thousand. I'm grateful for the days I played with Jimmy, even when had some pretty low attendance. He always explained it away by saying they were "good rehearsals."

One time I was hanging out with Willie while he was being interviewed, and the reporter asked him a question. "If you could write your own epitaph, what would it say?" Willie really thought about it before answering, "I'd like it to say 'He did a great show. He gave people their money's worth.'" The reporter then asked him, "What is your favorite recording of one of your songs?" Again, Willie really thought about it and gave the honest answer, "I really like the way the singer Patsy Cline sang my song 'Crazy.'" I just thought to myself, "How cool is it to be able to answer that question like that?" I think it's that attitude that made him not just famous but a superstar. People love to be loved and appreciated. Thelonious Monk famously said, "Everyone is a genius at being themselves." Willie is truly an artist who seriously paid his dues and became a genius at being himself.

JOE GRACEY—"WEGETARIAN PROMOTERS"

We have had this kind of thing happen to us more than once, and one time it was a long-ass way from home, and we had put a bunch of rooms on our credit card and laid out a bunch of bread on gas and per diems, and the guy kept saying, "I'll have it, don't worry," and finally he just stiffed us. If we hadn't gotten half up front we'd have really eaten it, because this dill weed couldn't get his shit together. This was when I learned that you: a) get half in front and see if the check cashes before you leave town, and b) get the bread, in cash, in your hand on the day you arrive, and if it ain't there, c) get back in the van and keep going. It is the only way to protect your ass from scammers and well-meaning-but-unfortunate losers.

My God, one time it happened to us in Switzerland in a little town, and the promoter was a nice little guy who rode up on a bike and told us he was a "wegetarian." We started setting up for the show, and it soon became apparent that a crowd was not drawing; in fact, there were about fifteen of his friends there. We said, "Look, pal, nobody is here and you are about to get soaked, and you obviously can't possibly pay us the dough, so we'll let you off the hook, call off the dogs, and go home and have a night off, 'cause we're tired anyway." No, he insisted that we play anyway and he'd pay us what he promised. Warily, we finally agreed and played to the little bitty crowd, and when it ended, we went to collect our money, which he said he didn't have! It boggles the mind to contemplate, even to this day! About four of us relatively large and very angry, very road-weary, very drunk men, stinking of meat and hooch, gathered around him and pointed out that we had offered to go home, etc., etc., and that he would either pay with money or pay with delicate body parts, which would be ceremoniously ripped from him one by one. We made him get on his bicycle and we got in the van and followed him all over town going 20 mph as he went around borrowing the money from people. I got to be damn near delirious in the van, as we puttered around this village behind this guy on a yellow bike, getting twenty here and forty here. Man, the shit people will pull on a band is just amazing. People just don't realize how tired and nuts and don't-give-a-shit you are after six weeks in a van.

JOE GRACEY—MERVIN CONN TOUR WITH JERRY LEE

When we were on a big package tour of Europe one time with Jerry Lee and about ten other acts, he cleaned out his room's minibar, ordered boxes of Cuban cigars from room service, and then summoned the

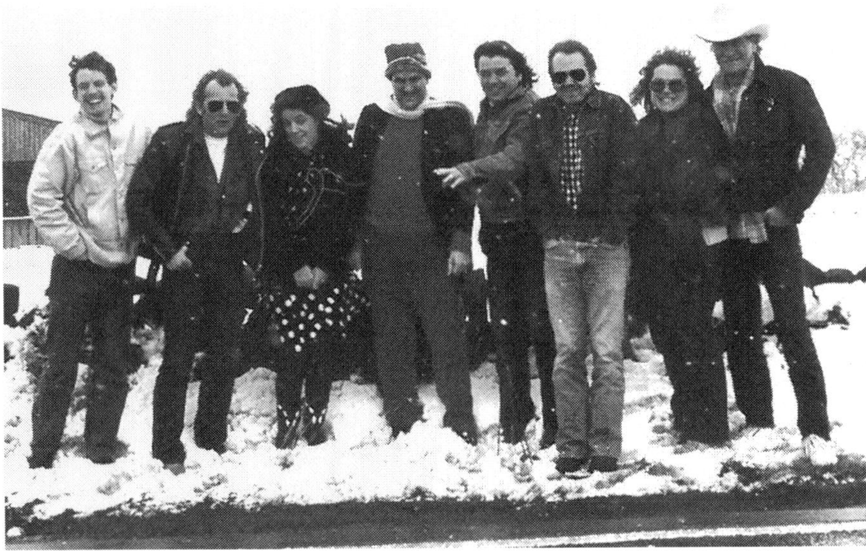

Kimmie and "Her Band" on tour in a blizzard.
Photo by Maurice McElroy.

promoter to his room at some ungodly hour and threw shit around the room, demanding that he get special travel arrangements because we were all having to board a train from Stuttgart to Lucerne at like 6:00 a.m., and he didn't dig it. He finally just said, "The hell with it," and went home. The problem was that nobody, including his band, knew he had left, so they had to go on and play a whole set of his stuff with one guy pretending to be him. I don't think the audience ever even caught on to the fact that he never showed up. It was a pretty bad deal.

Man, you should have seen all of us milling around the breakfast buffet at 5:00 a.m., waiting for the buses to take us to the trains. I have never seen a sorrier-looking group of pale, bleary-eyed, hungover, wasted human beings. Three hours of sleep and a body wracked with German beer toxins is not a pretty sight. When they told me the "Killer" refused this treatment, I understood completely. My God, I bet he looks bad at five o'clock in the morning. I was just thankful that none of us had to see that. It was bad enough seeing David Allan Coe. I never actually saw the Killer on that tour; he was in the final stages of one of his downward spirals and never showed his face outside his room.

KIMMIE RHODES

On the way home from one of our pilgrimages to Nashville to visit Cowboy Jack, we passed through Memphis to stop off at the legendary Sun Studios, which had just reopened. Cowboy had been bragging about hanging out with his new buddy, Bono, and the band U2 to help out with the making of the movie *Rattle and Hum*, which they had been shooting there. Just as we walked through the door, a tour was beginning, so we thought, "Well, why not?" So we played along as the tour guide told all the tourists who had gathered all about the days when Elvis, Johnny Cash, and Carl Perkins et al. had recorded there. All these pictures from the old days were hanging on the walls, and it really was all vibed-out and cool in there. Gracey started wandering around clapping his hands in different areas of the room to check the acoustics before the tour had even ended, and the guide, who was winding up his spiel said, "Does anyone have any questions?" To Gracey's surprise, I raised my hand and said, "Yes. What are your rates?"

Once we were back in Texas, we talked to the owners of the label I was with, Heartland Records, who were house. To their credit, it didn't take much hustling to convince them to fund a recording session at Sun. In fact, they liked the idea so much that they started begging me not to change my mind! I finally got the courage (and money) to quit the last "real job" I ever had, working at a folk art gallery, and we were back at Sun Studios within three weeks with a band assembled, partly from Texas and partly from Memphis and Nashville, to record all the new songs I'd been writing. David "Fergie" Ferguson came along to fill Cowboy's shoes from the olden days, as engineer, which made Cowboy free to play rhythm guitar and sing along. Believe me, with "The Cow" in the room, the bar was definitely raised. Johnny X Reed, guitarist for the Jackalopes, was there, as was Wes McGhee (guitar), Dale Dennis (bass), and Joey Miskulin, who was Cowboy's current resident genius and played keyboards and accordion.

We arrived the night before the sessions and set up the studio so we would be ready to go the next morning. Then we all sat out on the backsteps as the sun was going down. It was one of those extraordinary "golden hour" evenings. Because he knew how excited we were to be there, Cowboy started strolling down memory lane, telling stories, and we soaked it up. He was really sweet to entertain us in that way and add to the experience. Besides, anyone who ever knew him can attest to the fact that Cowboy loved to hold court. He said that back in the old days, when directions were given to get to the studio, they'd say, "Just look for the tiny building with all the Cadillacs parked out front." Then he pointed to a long building next door that ran far past the studio to the end of the big parking lot and said, "There's why Sun didn't make it. That's where they kept all the returns." There are two things that can kill indie labels. One is getting the returns of records that didn't sell, and the other is not being paid by the distributor. Sometimes they get this thing going where they collect the money from your sales but use it to pay people they owe farther back in the pipeline, figuring they'll catch up. But if they can't keep up with that game, they eventually go under and take a lot of small labels with them.

I had a song to record with Joe Ely as a duet, "Just One Love," that I had literally written on the way to his house to play it for him before I left for Memphis. It's crazy, looking back now, to think that I would decide to write the song on the way to his house, which was only about forty-five minutes away!

Once we were in Memphis, at Sun Studios, Joe flew in from Austin to record it with me. After we had cut the first take, we were all standing around in the tiny control room listening back and trying to decide if it was "the one" or not. This went on for a while, and I finally said, "Well if it's 'the one,' why are we all standing around trying to figure out if it is or not?" Cowboy's head jerked in my direction, and he grinned and said, "She's right. Let's go do another one." We went back into the studio and did another take, and when we came back in to listen, Cowboy grabbed me and started dancing all over the tiny room! (He had, after all, been an Arthur Murray dance instructor and even still carried his business card from those days and enjoyed whipping it out and showing it to people from time to time.) It was truly joyous. Ironically, not

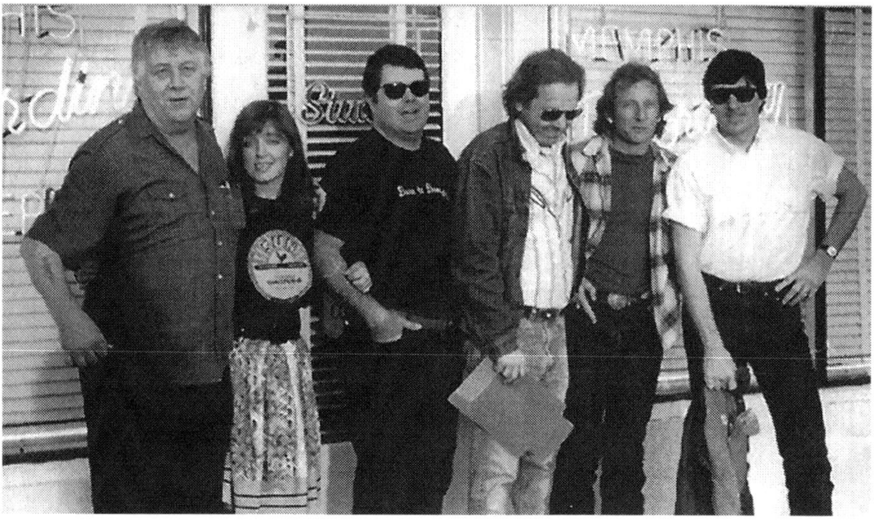

Kimmie with the band at Sun Studios, Memphis, Tennessee. Left to right: Cowboy Jack Clement, Kimmie Rhodes, Dale "Cowboy Dick" Dennis, Joe Gracey, Wes McGhee, Wes Starr.

long after that, I was in Nashville at the office of some record executive who had just rejected me as a viable artist. He made the remark that "if Jack Clement danced to your song, legend had it that you had a hit." I didn't even bother to tell him. I figured he wouldn't believe me anyway.

When we got back to Austin, we cut a few tracks at Lone Star Studios to complete the album. Jesse "Guitar" Taylor was there and blew us all away with his intro to a blues tune I'd written called "Trying for My Heart." As an added bonus, Chris O'Connell and Maryann Price arranged and sang killer backing vocals on it.

Also that day, we recorded a song I had written titled "I Just Drove By," which would eventually open many doors for me. I had been pulling the song out and rewriting it for seven years. Each time I'd had a go at it, I had ended up with a pretty good song, but I knew every time in my heart that it just wasn't finished. Like a painter knows when to stop painting a picture, I had an instinct about the song. One day, just after Gracey's grandfather, our beloved Daddy Pop (who was like the only grandfather I'd ever really had too), had died, the family had gathered at the house to sort through and decide what to do with all of Daddy Pop's worldly belongings. I was new to the Gracey family but had asked for what I always ask for when someone dies, their Christmas ornaments and their Bible, because those things have a patina that feels so time-worn, loved, and vibrant with history and important milestones and memories. I also asked for the antique hand-carved rocking chair that he always sat in when we would visit him.

As I rocked in my "new" old rocking chair, I observed my new family and the kind way they shared with each other. I laughed along at the ironic jokes and silliness . . . appreciating that unique sense of humor that had gotten them through a lot of very hard times. I drifted off into myself and soon felt distant somehow, as if I were seeing something they weren't realizing at the moment because they were so immersed in the tasks at hand. I looked around the room at the objects that had been placed individually where they were, each with a purpose, one day at a time, year after year, by either Daddy Pop or the one-of-a-kind grandmother I'd never gotten to meet, Gladys, or "Mom," as they all called her.

It was like the whole house shimmered with stillness yet teemed with life at the same time. I felt a deep sadness in knowing that within a few hours, like a company striking the theater after the finale, all these players would be leaving the stage where not just the important events like the births, and marriages, and deaths had shaped their story but also the small things: the bucket of colored wooden blocks in the closet that all the children had played with; the ice-cream freezer that Daddy Pop had used to celebrate full moons in summer; the bent and tattered bag of clothespins; the colored metal everyday drinking glasses; the radio; the clock; the ivy that had somehow survived under the watchful care of Wilma, the maid, for years; Daddy Pop's straw fishing hat; the opened and unopened mail on the antique writing desk; the china; the good linens and the shabby linens; the white sofa in the formal living room. Everything would be boxed and moved away because the show was over. Then that song, the one I had been trying to finish for years came to mind, and I had that little magic crystal moment that happens when you write. I finally understood fully what I needed to say. I had my song!

When we recorded "I Just Drove By," Jimmy Day played a steel guitar solo so sweet that it sounded like someone had left the door to heaven open and it had drifted out, and Butch Hancock played a harmonica solo that was almost heartbreaking because it sounded so much like a grandpa on the front porch playing only for the birds and the trees.

Thanks to those guys it became a truly beautiful country record. It was all done live, and I kept the live vocal, even though my voice had cracked a little because I was crying. I really learned something that day about how to make a real record, and I believe it was the moment at which I truly found my voice as a writer and as a singer. I've written and recorded hundreds of songs since, and I might have done as well a few times, but I'm pretty sure I could never do any better. It was my best.

It was the song that hooked Willie, which he later recorded with me—twice. I had been reluctant to think of myself as a songwriter until the day I stood next to the table where Willie and Coach Darrell Royal were playing chess. I heard him tell Coach, "That's a great song." I figured if he thought so, then I had earned the title "songwriter" from someone who knew. A few days later Coach whizzed up in his golf cart and asked if I wanted to go for a ride. He told me my song had just had three grown men "crying on the bus"! Later, the prolific Hank Cochran, who'd had a lot of hits with the likes of Patsy Cline, Ray Price, and Eddy Arnold, stopped me in the studio parking lot and said, "That's a great song, and if I don't know, then I don't know who to ask." (Presumably he had been one of the crying men on the bus that Coach spoke about.)

I knew I had really arrived when Billy Joe Shaver, one of the greatest American songwriters ever, cornered me in the kitchen of the studio and said, "Just about the time I think I'm doing pretty well, some asshole like you comes along with a song like that!" I got him back later, when I had him turn the crank on an ice-cream freezer for two hours, and then we walked into the house and saw the big bowl of peach ice-cream mixture still sitting there on the kitchen counter, because I'd gotten too stoned to remember to put it in the freezer! He was pretty high on tequila and just looked at Gracey. He shook his head and said, "You must be real proud of her." Then he looked at me and said, "That's all right, darlin'; we'll just have a milkshake," whereupon he picked up the giant bowl and drank from it, letting the contents run all down the front of him and onto my clean floor. Then he and Bucky Meadows (who had also been helping crank the empty ice-cream freezer) got in Billy's giant sled of a car and did a few donuts in my front yard before bouncing through a ditch and careening off down the road into the night.

JOE GRACEY—JIMMY DAY

Jimmy Day and I went back to the early '70s, when he was in Willie's band, and I was a progressive country DJ and music writer. I remember the first time I noticed him much; Willie played at a Ford dealer here (in return for a new station wagon so they could get around), and I suddenly noticed what a beautiful sound he created around Willie's voice. I subsequently became a producer and used him every chance I could on sessions. Kimmie and I brought him into our Texas swing band for several years, then he turned around and started a band, and pretty soon we were in it, traveling around Texas doing gigs. We'd play at dance halls down in Bandera that Wills and Willie and Bush had consecrated, turn around and drive back home at 4:00 a.m., and Kimmie would be up two hours later to go to her job in town.

Having Jimmy in your band was pure joy. He was always the one you could turn to to give you a rock-solid intro, even if he had only heard the song one time three years before. You could always lean on him for a great solo, with a perfect handoff into the chorus. His pickup notes would be cues to everybody else in the band, so they all knew where it was headed next.

Sessions were the same. He defined "pro." He came on time, sober, didn't talk about his problems, kept his mouth shut unless asked for his opinion, and played totally usable, brilliant stuff, normally on the first take. He wouldn't write a chord chart; he would just play through the song a couple of times, memorize it (no matter how tough the changes might be), and nail it. He said he learned his studio chops doing demos at Tree Music, where they got paid ten dollars per demo. This encouraged speed and not screwing up, since the more songs you got cut in a session, the more money you got paid.

Later I got to record several records for him. They turned into great projects, with guests like Johnny Bush and Willie and Rodriguez. One of them transmogrified into a Willie Nelson record because Willie came in to sing a song and stayed for four days. Not long after that, Willie and I recorded *Spirit*, so I have Jimmy to thank for that. I considered him to be a soul brother, something far beyond a professional relationship. If I was still a hippie I'd say I'd known him for a thousand lifetimes.

KIMMIE RHODES

We returned to London to play the Wembley festival again, in support of the new record we had done at Sun, *Angels Get the Blues.* As soon as I arrived at the airport, as always, I immediately picked up a copy of *British Vogue* because I love the magazine. To my surprise, I was in it! The label contacted the features editor, Eve MacSweeney, who had written the piece, and told her how thrilled I was. The next thing I know I'm clomping around the *British Vogue* office in my cowboy boots, talking in my Texas drawl to the editor in chief, who invited me into her office and said, "Sooner or later it comes around to everyone. Right now it's come around to you."

Sharon Ely gets credit for this because she was the stylist for the album cover. I had discovered that a dress designed by Christian Lacroix, which I had admired, having seen it in a magazine, was on sale at an outlet store in Austin. Sharon took up a collection from all of our friends to buy it for me. Anthony Roberts did the photo shoot at the Broken Spoke dance hall and used a technique he had invented in which he used colored markers to paint the negatives before developing them.

ONCE I HAD BECOME deeply embedded in Willie World, I found myself involved in lots of crazy and wonderful things, and I learned a lot. I learned to type because I was hanging around the studio office with Lana Nelson and Jody Fischer (Willie's secretary who had become my neighborhood running buddy), and they needed somebody to type addresses on envelopes for Farm Aid. The beauty of that scene, and, really, the fun of it, was that Willie would come up with all these schemes for what was next and enlist the talents of all of us folks who were following him around to see who could be first to grab whatever was left in the ashtray after he left the room. (I had a pretty serious

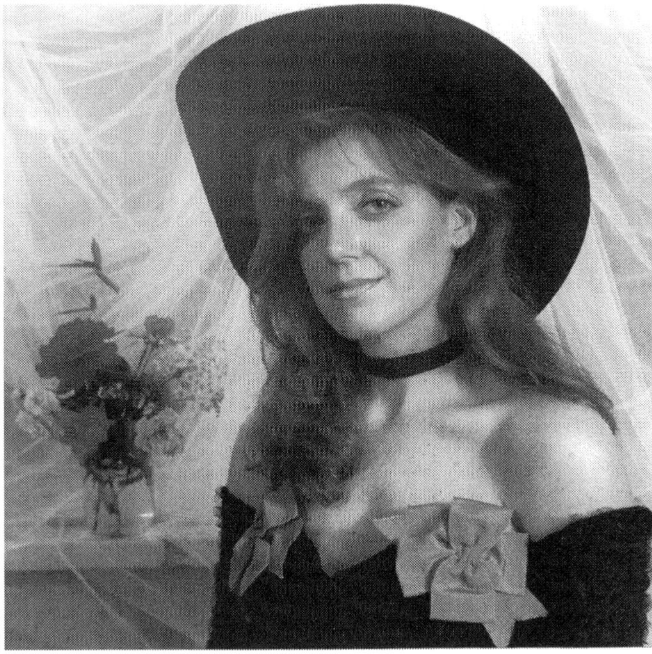

Kimmie wearing Christian Lacroix. Photo by Rob Roberts.

pot monkey on my back until my elementary school–aged daughter busted me smoking with Willie and said, "Mama, I won't do drugs if you won't do drugs." So I thought, "Geez, what kind of a mother am I?!" So I quit and faithfully honored our pact until finally she came to me about thirty years later and told me I was off the hook.)

One evening while Gracey was cooking dinner, I went up to the studio office, which we all called "The Hill," and which had become my favorite hangout. I ran into Bucky Meadows (the zany but very accomplished jazz guitarist who had started playing in my band). He said, "Billy Joe is looking for you. He wants to play you the song he just wrote." We found him hanging around down in the kitchen off the studio, and he played me the song, which was great, of course. About that time Willie walked in, took a seat, looked at me, and said, "Play me a song." I knew he liked "I Just Drove By" because I'd heard that he'd been playing it for everybody on the bus, so I sang that. Then he said, "Do another one. So I sang "Just One Love." Then he said, "Why don't we just go record those right now?" He led me into the studio where, unbeknownst to me, what they were calling their "big guitar" session was in progress, being produced by the legendary session guitarist Grady Martin.

The next thing I know I'm sitting in Willie's chair with his guitar, "Trigger," in my lap playing the songs to a herd of legends—Chip Young, Buddy Emmons, Mike Leech, Buddy Harman, and Pete Wade—while they were all writing charts. It felt like one of those dreams where your teeth start falling out. I had my hair pulled up in a ponytail and was wearing some old T-shirt and jeans and no makeup. What had turned out to be a quick errand up to the Hill was morphing into a major event! Grady listened and said, "Well, those are the two songs we've been looking for."

Everybody went to their corners and started tuning up to get ready to cut the songs. I ran to the phone, called home, and told Gracey, "You'd better turn the oven off and get up here. You won't believe this!" I quickly scrawled the lyrics down and ran back into the studio with them, where a mic had been set up next to Willie for me, and in less time than you can possibly imagine, that stellar band had laid down flawless basic tracks to both songs. One of the most exciting parts of tracking is when everyone gathers in the control room to listen to the playback. There I was surrounded by all these geniuses, standing next to Willie, listening to my songs coming out of the big speakers. Willie knew he had ambushed me, and I think he was really enjoying that. He continued to enjoy it for the next few days because he graciously invited me to hang around and help out with the overdubs and do all the backing vocals on the record.

So it went like this: Willie needed to do vocal overdubs, and he liked to work in the daytime, but during the day Grady was preoccupied with whatever he had going on at the nearby condo where he was staying. Grady knew Willie didn't need him around to do vocals, so he unofficially (and jokingly) assigned me as his "assistant producer," which I took seriously. So I sat at the board with Eric Paul, who was engineering the sessions, and worked with Willie on his vocals. It was a blast sitting there listening to him sing and crack jokes and do the things that Willie does. (Once, I had pushed the talk-back button and heard the words "That was a good one, Willie, but I think you might have a better one in you" come out of my mouth, and I slapped my own hand.) Then the end of the day would come, when Grady would return to work and Willie would go home. They sort of crisscrossed each other, like a tag team. When we would finally all end up together again, Grady and I would dance around the studio while Willie watched and laughed, and we would congratulate each other on how great we were!

So, on the second day, after Willie had worked for hours and left, Grady was supposed to start recording my backing vocals. What he really did, though, was labor over redoing all of my lead vocals, in addition to having me sing on a lot of other songs. Then he got Willie's guitar, "Trigger," and started having fun recording all these great solos on all of the songs that Willie had already played solos on when we had cut the basics. I'll never forget the joy on Grady's face as he came crashing through the control room door with his arms thrown in the air exclaiming, "The damn thing is in there playing itself!!!" So we stayed up all night doing that, meaning that I had now been in the studio for about twenty-four hours. Willie walked in around 6:00 a.m. with his collar pulled up around his neck, his baseball cap pulled down over his eyes, and a coffee mug in his hand.

Grady joked, "Okay, Kimmie, you take charge of Willie," and then he quickly left. Now Willie decided that he's ready to do vocals together. So we launched off into another bunch of hours of recording, during which Willie and I decided we would sing into the same mic on everything with playback coming from the overhead monitors so we wouldn't have to wear headphones, because we didn't like them, which was a really badass thing for us to be doing because of the "bleed."

We decided that duets should be done together, and that must be why they had called them "duets" in the first place. We sang my songs again, and then we sang "Four Walls," which was one of the favorite moments of my life. In the course of all that, Willie had been listening to all of the solos that Grady had played on everything using Trigger. So, of course, Willie had to redo all the solos on everything then.

Grady returned after having slept some, which, as a reminder, Eric Paul and I still had not. He listened to the vocals we'd done, and looked at me, and said, "You went in there and took it away from him. Why the hell did you give it back?!" Willie and I just laughed. (Ours were the vocals that remained on the mixes, bleed and all, by the way.)

A few days later, after some much-needed sleep, I reported back to the studio and was standing in the parking lot with Willie, when Grady drove up, rolled down the window, and said, "Listen to this." He popped in a cassette of Grandpa Jones singing "Eight More Miles to Louisville" and asked if we wanted to sing on it. We said, "Hell, yes," and all headed back into the studio. Grady bragged about my ability to sing "like that, too" on the bluegrass track, like I was a little sister (and admittedly I was the punk kid of the trio). After we'd done that, we sang some background vocals on "Smoke, Smoke, Smoke That Cigarette." Sorry, Tex Williams, but Willie's is the best version ever!

We then started mixing and came to "Just One Love." Willie had been busying himself making notes and writing. He swiveled around in the chair and showed me a hand-drawn "album cover," which was adorable. It showed "JUST ONE LOVE" at the top in big, Sharpie-drawn letters, and he said, "And here's our title track!"

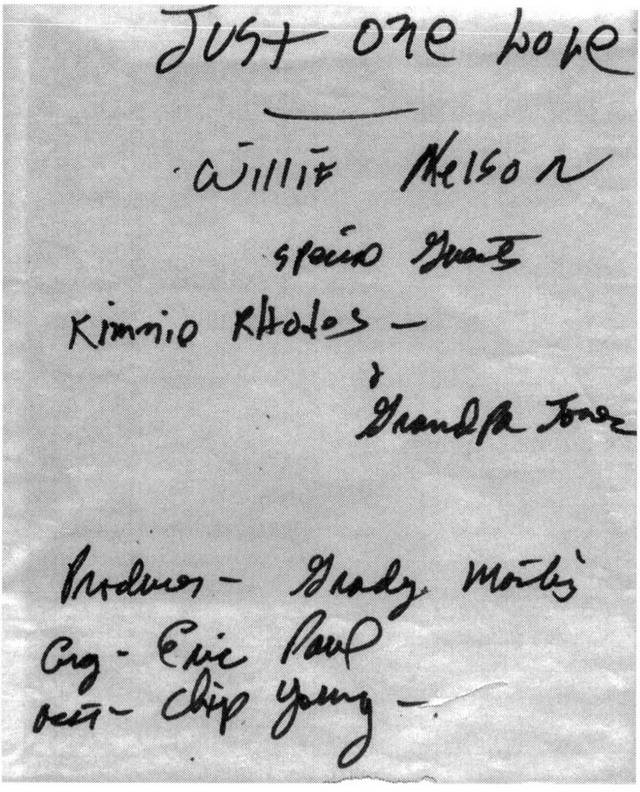

Willie's artwork for the Just One Love *album.*

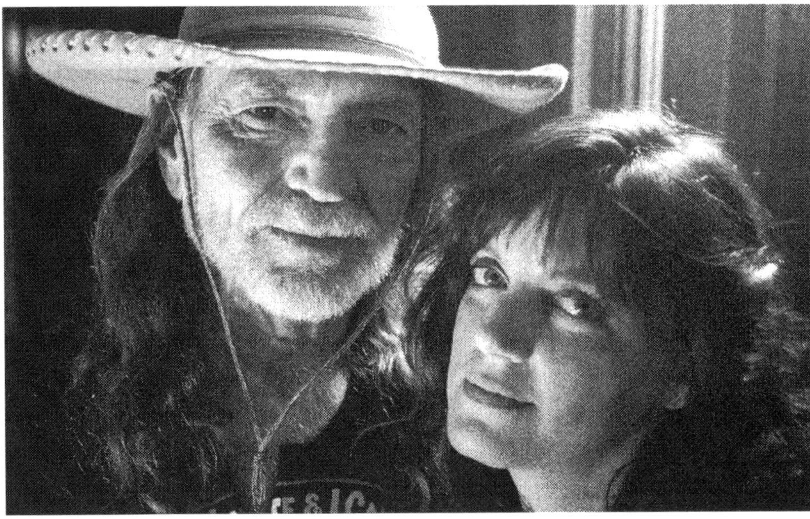

Willie and Kimmie. Photo by Alan Messer.

It was big fun being produced by Grady, although he was crazy and kept hitting on me, which in the normal world might have constituted sexual harassment charges, but for a woman in the music business, it was more like a sport for both of us. He'd make some comment, and then I'd sling something back at him about him being too old and how he might have a heart attack or stroke! Then we'd all snicker, and he'd hang his head like he was weary from trying, and Willie would just sit back and laugh at us. Finally I said, "Look Grady, I'm a married woman, but I'll make you an apple pie." So the last day I brought one of my famous apple pies to the studio. Willie took a bite of it, looked at me, and asked, "You married?" Willie's got the quickest wit of anyone when it comes to one-liners. He always gets the best word in last. I think he got it from hanging around with Roger Miller. I would have loved to have an opportunity to pit Willie and Townes Van Zandt against each other in a "smart-ass-off."

Years later Willie and I also recorded a duet album called *Picture in a Frame*. We just sat down one afternoon with Gracey, Zettner, and Gabriel at Willie's little studio in Luck and recorded songs we knew, including the Tom Waits song that we made the title track. We released it on my label, Sunbird. The day came when I had to design the cover, so, true to the same ease of spirit with which we had recorded the music, I just framed a portrait I had of the two of us, scanned it, and handed it to Gracey, who was doing the layout, and said, "There's your cover." He laughed and said, "Sunbird Design Group!"

RECORDING WILLIE NELSON

I just got out of a Willie session. Larry Butler, the big cowboy who owned all those clubs and who wrote "I Gotta Get Drunk," had recorded twenty-one Hank Williams songs, so Willie decided he would overdub some vocals on the tracks today. He sits down, lights up a giant stick, and proceeds to sing every damn song straight through without stopping, except once, when he sang over a solo. I mean I didn't even stop the machine or take it out of record most of the time, and he never did but two of them twice! They were all damn good except for one you could tell he didn't really like. (It wasn't a very good song, even for old Hank.) Good Lord! After about three hours of this, it was over, and they wanted to know if I was ready to start mixing, and I was as wrung out as if I had been there for fourteen hours. Somebody asked Willie if we were going to mix it tonight and he said, "Why not? Joe don't ever say nuthin'."

Willie has such a weird voice that he has to back up about three feet when he sings loud and then move to an inch away from the mic when he wants to caress a word. He chews them and physically rips them out of his head.

Every time I wonder what I'm doing in this business, something like this session today happens and I remember. Apparently I am supposed to be. Praise the Lord and God bless Texas!

KIMMIE RHODES

Somewhere around this time Willie also started his Cowboy Television Network, which somehow eventually morphed into the Outlaw Music Channel. We filmed weekly shows at Pedernales Studio with Johnny Gimble. I was deemed "The Outlaw Sweetheart"—a title that I was very proud of. Johnny had assembled an all-star band that included Texas Playboys veterans Curly Hollingsworth (piano) and Herb Remington (steel guitar). There were two favorite memories of working on the *Johnny Gimble Show*. One was the day "The Boss" was off the road, because I got to tape my songs with Willie. The other was when the great Floyd Tillman, the singer-songwriter who in the '30s and '40s had not only helped make honky-tonk a genre but had also penned the earliest "cheatin' songs," was a guest on the show. As fate would have it, I had recorded a very smoky, tempoed swing version of his song "Baby" at Sun, and it was out on my album that had just been released. I got to sit between Johnny and Floyd and sing that song as a duet. It just does not get better than that for an Outlaw Sweetheart. We all left every one of those sessions with faces that ached from smiling so big all day, because western swing is such happy music. Wherever those films ended up, they should unbury them and prescribe copies of those shows in lieu of antidepressants. Joe Gracey? Well, he ascended to Nirvana.

I was involved in so many things with Willie and family by this time that it's impossible to touch on all but a few of the highlights. We worked on movies and an old-style television series of westerns where everybody was wearing guns, riding horses, and drinking whiskey in whorehouses. There were writers, singers, actors, and characters like Kris Kristofferson, Rip Torn, and Bud Shrake and Ann Richards, Gary Cartwright, Bill Wittliff, Merle Haggard, Ben Dorsey, Ray Benson, Snoop Dog, and astronauts from NASA. You name it, they were showing up everywhere, in abundance. You never knew who was going to pop up next. Working with Lana Nelson, I got to be on both sides of the camera as an art director for one of Willie's videos of a song called "There You Are." I also worked wardrobe, stand-in, extra . . . the list of job opportunities went on and on. We would get all grubby from working on the set, hammering barn wood on the walls, painting backdrops, sewing, and doing whatever to get the scene just right, and then clean ourselves up, jump into the picture, and be the stars. The majorly savvy Jody Fischer (who had managed Miles Davis and had also pioneered the beginning of Farm Aid, starting with two grocery bags full of letters that had been written to Willie from farmers) was always in the background smoothing the waters and "keeping the wheels from coming off."

At one point Willie and Ray Benson were shooting some kind of television show with Dolly Parton and Gary Busey. I was broke and had secretly missed working on movies, so I was easily roped into working wardrobe on the show. I had sworn I would never work wardrobe again because everybody yells at you all the time, but I agreed to it anyway. The first thing Willie said when he saw me was, "What are you doing here? I thought you weren't gonna do this anymore." I mumbled something about helping out my friend who wanted time off (which was also true), and he just shook his head. Well, this did turn out to be the last time I worked wardrobe, and here's why. . . .

We were shooting at the Broken Spoke dance hall with the huge cast and crew. I had been hanging out for days drawing really good money for basically doing nothing but eating, smoking weed, and watching Gary Busey drive everybody nuts, especially Dolly. (Dolly always had a flurry of hair and makeup people following her around, making sure she stayed the impeccable fantastic creature that she is at all times, so that was entertaining.) The food was good, the pay was great, and I had managed to make Busey understand that I wasn't his nanny, so it was all good until, suddenly, I was under surprise attack. The wardrobe mistress comes charging at me screeching, "Oh, my God, you have to hurry!!! Dolly is about to do the love scene, and we have to have to tape her nipples down so they don't show through the negligee!!!!"

She rapidly explained the exact kind of special tape that was required and stressed that it was needed *immediately*, so I jumped in my car and hauled ass to the drugstore down the street, the whole while trying to calculate in my mind how much it might cost to pay the entire cast and crew of a movie production to sit twiddling their thumbs while I was out running my errand. I shot into the pharmacy and started frantically searching the shelves for this peculiar kind of tape. I guess I must have alarmed the pharmacist, who dashed down from his perch and asked, "How may I help you, ma'am?" I quickly, and in broken sentences, tried to describe this kind of tape, which had not been very well described to me in the first place, whereupon he sensed my panic and offered, "Okay! I can help you! Tell me, what kind of wound are you dressing?!"

At that moment time just sort of slowed down as I stood there staring at his face, while watching my own life pass before my eyes, causing an epiphany in which I became aware that every event that had ever happened to me had now specifically delivered me to this peculiar moment when I was out buying tape for Dolly Parton's nipples. Willie had been absolutely right, as always. I took the tape lying in the pharmacist's outstretched hand, looked at him, and answered, "If I told you, you wouldn't believe me." I strolled to the cash register, paid for the tape, calmly drove back to the set, and handed it over so that art might proceed to imitate life.

GRACEY MEMOIR—BRANSON NEW YEAR'S EVE

We were in Branson, for God's sake, when Willie went up there to see what it was like (he hated it) as his opening act on New Year's Eve. We had this giant country-swing band. The audience had no idea there was an opening act, and the dumb-ass DJ announcer didn't tell them, either; he just said something like, "So let's start the show!" We're behind the curtain, all ready to knock 'em dead and become stars, when I step on my bass cord, pulling it and the jack completely out of the guitar in excruciating slow motion. As the stagehand opens the curtain, a stunned audience is greeted not by Willie, but somebody they've never seen before, and I am on my knees with my back to them, apparently praying over the ruins of a bass guitar. Kimmie looks around, says, "What the hell?," and counts off the first song, sans bass. A big, loud country shuffle with no bass sounds like shit. I'm fumbling helplessly with the jack, like a man trying to stuff his own intestines back into his gut, when, halfway through the song, Bee Spears hands me his backup bass, except that it is a giant old Fender Precision and I have played a Gibson EBO all my life, and to me a P-bass neck seems about ten feet long and each fret a lifetime apart (because the Gibson bass neck is a short-scale and very tiny, almost like an old Bill Wyman bass), so I spend the entire set rattled and searching desperately for the notes and finger placements. Then, either because he doesn't notice my panic, or perhaps because he does and he is a perverse human being, Johnny Gimble insists on keeping up a running commentary the whole set, distracting me and making me play even worse. It was lovely. The next day we all went the hell back to Texas, our dreams of Branson riches shattered.

KIMMIE RHODES

With no label and no budget, we began piecing together an album, which later would become *West Texas Heaven,* but I'd not yet written the title song. Gracey was recording an artist who had purchased a block of time, so once they were finished for the day, we could sneak in and use the leftover night hours at no cost. Having no money for a band, we were cutting tracks with just the vocals and acoustic guitar, jesting that we could "always overdub the band later." Gracey had nicknamed me "Battleship Kimmie" because of my faith and ability to keep sailing in the right direction, knowing things would all work out okay in the end, which they always did.

Willie came home from the road (which was in and of itself a miracle) at the perfect time, and I ran into him on the Hill. I told him I was working in his studio and asked if he'd come sing a couple of songs with me that evening. He had the night off (which was also a miracle), so he said, "Sure." I ran and told Gracey (who was at the board recording the band that was paying for the studio) to get rid of them and set up for Willie as soon as they left.

I hadn't even thought to mention to Willie that it would just be the two of us, so when he walked into the studio and saw two chairs and two mics set up facing each other in the middle of the room and me sitting there in one of them by myself, I swear he took a step back and just stood there for a minute figuring the whole thing out. Then he sat down and I played "Hard Promises to Keep" for him. We cut that in one take, and he played a really terrific solo. He has this knack for learning songs on the fly.

Then we recorded "I Never Heard You Say." Later, Mickey Raphael was in town, and we wanted to overdub him playing harmonica on it, but he didn't have a harmonica in the right key with him. So we slowed the tape speed down so it would be tuned to the harmonica he did have on hand. It took about half the afternoon for him to play it, but when we sped it back up it was absolutely brilliant!

One afternoon not long after that, I came home from the grocery store and found a message from Waylon Jennings on my telephone answering machine. Life had been a lot like an Easter egg hunt of late, with delightful surprises showing up around just about every corner, so I can't say the call surprised me so much as delighted me.

From my point of view, I figured that if I had had the good fortune of having Willie readily accessible and happy to record with me, then I already had something rarer than money and a band. I had no cause to question much of anything. When you're flying blind, life is a bit like a game in which you wait to see what falls into the picture next and have no choice but to trust that things are landing in the right order. I've seen this happen time after time, year after year, and decade after decade until it's become the fun of it, really. After a while you realize you've gotten too far out to turn back anyway, so you just keep following the road you've taken in pace with however fast it unravels.

Once I had played the message from Waylon multiple times (and for the amusement of all the other house members), it began to dawn on me that what he was saying was that he liked my song "I Just Drove By" and had left his number so I could call him back. I screwed up the nerve to dial the phone and was soon speaking with the deep rich voice of my hero whom I'd never met. After some demo mailing and a little more phone calling, one thing led to another, and we decided to record a couple of songs I'd written, "Be Mine" and "Maybe We'll Just Disappear."

Looking back, I marvel now that it never truly occurred to me that we had no more funds with which to produce a recording session with Waylon than we'd had with Willie. I guess I had learned by then that all I really needed was the studio and a song. Willie had enjoyed recording using the "shoestring budget" method and, always the optimist, had even pointed out that no matter what we added later it would be "impossible to ever remove the heart from it."

I picked up the phone and called our infamous buddy, Cowboy Jack, who had a very trippy fantastic place in Nashville, the Cowboy Arms Hotel and Recording Spa, and told him the news, explaining that we needed to use his studio and would find the money to pay the engineer, but would have to swap him something for the studio time. Cowboy had produced earthmoving records on Waylon, including my favorite, *Dreaming My Dreams,* and was happy for me. Once I'd made Jack understand why we would also, due to immediate lack of funds, be recording with no band, he agreed to let us in under the nonnegotiable condition that I hire a bass player to keep us in line. Knowing he was right, I acquiesced to finding the money to pay the Johnny Cash right-hand man, Joe Allen, whom Cowboy suggested, knowing that he was a fan of my singing so he might agree to a modest sum for nailing down the rhythm on my "drummerless" session.

A couple of weeks later, on the eve before the session, we were hanging in a Nashville bar, when in walked Townes Van Zandt. Gracey was writing to him on his Magic Slate, explaining that we were in from Austin to record with Waylon at Cowboy's the next day, and I blurted out, "Hey! Why don't you come sing a song with me?" Townes accepted, and it wasn't until later that I realized I'd just enlisted the Shakespeare of Americana songwriters to record one of my own songs with me the following afternoon, without actually having the song. (So much for "all you needed was a studio and a song"!)

By the time we arrived at Cowboy's the next morning I'd mused over it and remembered a song I'd written recently titled "I'm Gonna Fly." Unlike all the others I'd ever written, I had finished this one without ever really knowing what it was about. When I had reached the end of writing it, I had felt that familiar "tone" that assures me that I've said what I meant to communicate, but this time it had been more like when you wake from sleep and can't remember exactly what you dreamt but know how it made you feel. If that makes any sense, that's why I decided that this song, which was really more of a poem, might be the perfect one to record with Townes. Besides, it was the one I had.

The recordings with Waylon went great, and Cowboy did some dobro overdubs. By then Townes (escorted to the studio by Brother

Bill Gracey, who has another ridiculous story about the roundabout way they got there) had arrived in a very drunken and fragile state, ultra-cool and quietly sweet. We went into the studio, where I timidly showed him the song. The idea was that he would record live with us but it became immediately apparent that Townes wasn't going to be able to keep up, so Joe Allen graciously suggested that we should record the track and then overdub his vocal. Townes was shuffled off into the control room to further imbibe while we laid down the track. My friend, Beth Nielsen Chapman, an incredible songwriter (who, as it turned out, had been the one who had generously pitched Waylon my song in the first place), was at the session, so I invited her to play piano. She played a beautifully simple, childlike solo. Beth and Joe Allen left the room and Townes returned.

He was seated about two feet away from me, and I had placed the lyric sheet on a music stand beside him. He motioned for me to move closer and said, "Okay, here's what I'm gonna need you to do. Put your knees on mine." I guessed this was to steady him in some way. I complied. Once we were settled with both knees touching, he instructed, "Now, when it's time for me to sing a word I want you to point to it." Hearing all of this from the control room, the engineer, David "Fergie" Ferguson, started the playback, and as the track began, I waited through my first verse for the second verse, which Townes was to sing, and then, one by one, I touched each word of the phrase. "The sunbird's song's for what he longs for . . . Other loves may shine as bright but not in my eyes. . . ." Townes sang, but then he stopped and began to cry. Wiping away tears, he said, "This is a beautiful song." In that moment I understood what the song was about, except through his eyes, or ears, as it were.

Forging ahead with a few more stops and a little more crying, and still pointing at each word, in my head voice, I sang along to myself, "Ooohhh, dear, this is sooo aaamaaazing, but I'm afraid weeee aren't geeeetting anything weeee will beeee aaaable to uuuse." Finally we settled in and made two uninterrupted passes and went into the control room to listen back. Not only were both takes entirely usable, but every note Townes had sung was calloused with a showstopping grace that had come from somewhere deep inside his ironic and soulful heart.

We spent the rest of the night laughing and smoking, dancing and drinking, listening to the day's work, and swapping lies and singing songs down in Cowboy's office (which was unchallenged as the best hangout in town). Townes sang his famous rendition of "Fraulein," and at one point Cowboy got mad at Townes because he said he'd made him too intimidated to even play a C chord by badgering him about everything he played (which was true), but he soon returned, and all was well again. Lucinda Williams showed up for her duet several hours late, so that didn't happen, but she hung out with us anyway, as did David Conrad, the gifted songman who was about to become my publisher for the next ten years.

I have no way of knowing for sure, but I've been told that that was the last recording Townes ever did. He died a few months later, leaving me with the memory of a timeless moment that filtered through the guy who was Townes Van Zandt. I sat there fully understanding how a "heart can only make one sound like a whip-poor-will in the midnight."

Once back in Austin, I continued to write for the album. One night while Gracey was cooking dinner, I sat outside the kitchen door at his desk and the song "West Texas Heaven" fell out of me pretty much as quickly as I could write it down. My son Gabriel, who was twenty years old and still living at home off and on, had been playing in the band for a while and was really getting to be a good guitar picker. He came into the

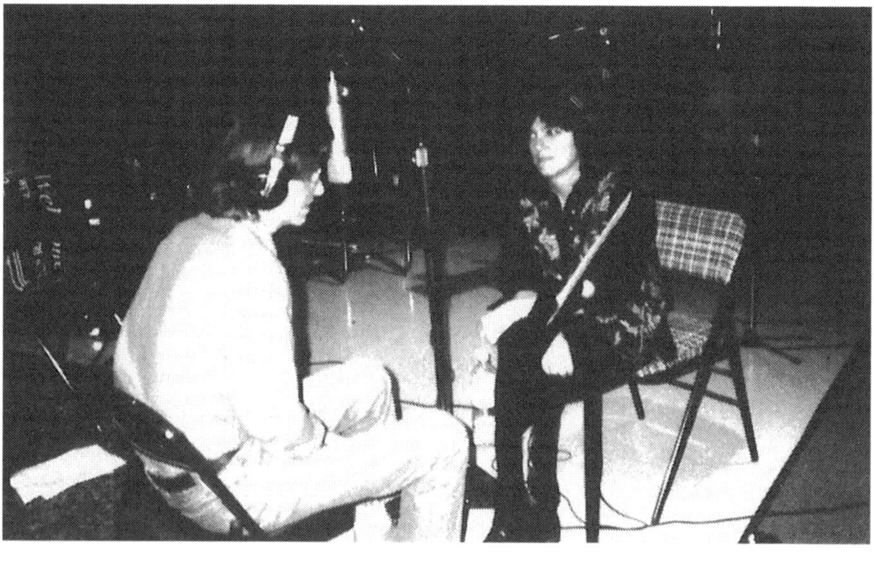

Townes and Kimmie recording "I'm Gonna Fly."

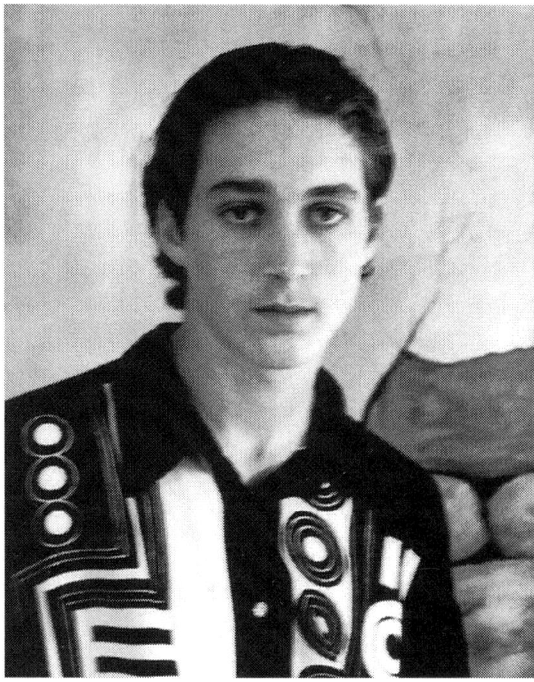

Young Gabriel Rhodes.

office where I was just finishing writing the song. He was the first one I played it for. Soon, somehow, I don't even remember now, we actually got the money for a session to cut enough songs to finish the album at Pedernales Studio. Spencer Starnes was the session leader. When Gabe started trying to get us all to listen to the guitar part that he had created for the intro, Spencer said, "Wait a minute y'all; listen to this. It's really good." So that became the first recording I ever did with Gabriel, who went on to produce many records for me after that. I think the intro he worked up really took the song to a new level and made the record a success. It was also Gabriel's first recording session.

I had been introduced to photographer Alan Messer in Nashville, and he offered to take some photos. Sharon Ely did fantastic styling for the shoot but dressed me up in a bunch of layers of clothing and topped it all off with a full-length wool coat. Alan and I took off for West Texas in his El Camino pickup on a very hot summer day, because he felt that it was important that we should be in West Texas for the shoot, and I believe he was right. He got some fantastic images, but he wasn't really completely satisfied. So Sharon dressed me in the whole garb again a month later and we headed back to the same area and took more pictures. Hot and miserable as it was, this is still one of my favorite photography romps ever because, walking down the abandoned dirt road, I could hear the telephone lines on either side zinging and the cover photo was actually shot in front of a fleabag hotel lit by the headlights of Alan's truck, and the disc image of the moon with the telephone pole in front of it, looking like a cross, was shot in the black of night. Alan jumped out and set up a tripod and stood there waiting for the shutter to open.

I shopped that record all over Nashville, and even with Cowboy, Waylon, and Willie doing their best to get it picked up by a major label, it just wasn't in the stars. It was all too weird and under-produced for Nashville at the time. That was before the term "Americana" existed, and there wasn't even a name for what we did yet, much less a label that would take it. A French label called New Rose licensed it for Europe for three years, which was great because we got to go to France a lot.

JOE GRACEY—THOUGHT ON COUNTRY

I don't agonize over Shania Twain so much for being what and who she is as I do that the hijacking of Nashville by pop forces continues to keep country music from progressing like it should have. Instead of people like Rodney (Crowell) and Kimmie being the new country stars, we have this stagnation into neo and pop camps, neither of which interests me. I really don't want to hear some guy's imitation of George Jones any more than I want to hear Shania. I want to hear something new and vital, like George was when he hit his stride. I'd say this was the missing ingredient right now rather than some tired "returning to our roots." Like Jack Clement once said to me, "Let's do something old and familiar in a new and different way."

KIMMIE RHODES

Waylon kept on trying to help find a label to sign me. One day I checked in with him from the pay phone of a laundromat because my washer was on the blink at home. It felt surreal to be standing there watching the clothes spinning around in the suds, talking to Waylon. He asked, "What are those places like now? I haven't been to one of those in years." I looked around and said, "I think there are a lot of homeless people living here." I had sent him my concept idea "Small Town Girl" in its very early stages, and he said, "I think this is great, but could you send me something else? This reminds me of trying to get anyone interested in *Red Headed Stranger*. They just didn't get it." Hearing him say that made things seem even more surreal.

Looking back on my friendship with Waylon, it was kind of like being on friendly terms with a cartoon character. He could say some of the damndest things and not even know he was saying anything weird. He took to calling me every time he was coming to Austin with about a five-minute warning before his arrival. One day we ran all over town doing all kinds of things. One of his requests was to take my daughter, Jole, to a western wear shop to pick out matching shirts for them to wear to the show in La Grange that night. (Waylon loved kids, and he called Jole on her birthday every year.) Jole picked out these goofy-looking Looney Toons shirts with Daffy Duck, Bugs Bunny, Porky Pig, and the Tasmanian Devil dancing across the yoke.

Then he decided he wanted to go eat "the best hamburger in town." Now, I knew for a fact that Waylon was on a very strict diet because every time I'd ever eaten lunch with him at his house he'd had a special box lunch with healthy salads and carrot sticks, and the like, no matter what the rest of us were eating. I tried to talk him out of it, but he insisted, so I took him to this famous Austin place on the Drag down by the university called Martin's "Kum-Bak" Burger, which had been there since 1926. It got the name because the owners always stood by the door and said, "Come back," when you left. All the locals just call it Dirty's and go there to eat good old-fashioned greasy burgers and fries. Then we all headed to the bus to go play a show in La Grange, after which Waylon and the band would be heading on to Littlefield, his hometown in West Texas, to play the annual Day for Waylon celebration.

On the way to La Grange, dressed in his Looney Toons shirt, Waylon started having indigestion but figured he'd be fine. He played a dynamite show and brought me on to duet on the Rodney Crowell song, "'Til I Can Gain Control Again," and a very good time was had by all. Afterward, Waylon was starting to feel worse and worse but was too gracious to go lie down, insisting that he wanted to visit with us until they dropped us back at our car in Austin. As we said our goodbyes, he assured us that he'd be fine and would get plenty of rest on the way to Littlefield. The bus took off, and we drove home and went to bed.

The next morning I woke up and went into the kitchen to make coffee. I turned on the television to check out the news. The picture popped on with a big publicity shot of Waylon in full regalia and the anchorperson said, "Country singer Waylon Jennings was hospitalized this morning in Nashville, Tennessee." I yelled back to the bedroom, "Oh, good lord, Gracey! We've killed Waylon Jennings with a hamburger!" It was crazy! Plus, how did he get hospitalized in Nashville just a few hours later? They had certainly been headed to Littlefield when they'd left us just a few hours before. We kept an eye on the news. Since they never reported that he died, we figured everybody was in the clear. A week later I walked into a party at Beth Nielson Chapman's house in Nashville, and sitting on the ottoman in the living room with his back to me was Waylon. I walked up behind him and pecked him on the shoulder. When he looked up at me, I grinned and said, "See there? I told you those were great hamburgers!"

He jumped up screaming, "You little shit. You little shit!" (That's what he always called me.) When I asked him what on earth had happened and how the hell he gotten to Nashville faster than was humanly possible on a bus that was on the way to Littlefield, he explained it like this, "Well, by the time we got to Littlefield I was feeling so bad I just had them take me on to the emergency room. It was the wee hours, and there was nobody around but a nurse and this doctor from India. He had no idea who I was but the nurse on call did, so she told him. I'm lying there on this table and he bends over and gets right in my face and asks, 'Did you know Elvis?' So I started screaming, 'Jessi, get me out of here! I was born here, but I'm sure as hell not gonna die here!' So they called for a helicopter and had me airlifted back to Nashville."

One time he blew into town with Jessi Colter to do a talk at the

University of Texas. This time we assuredly did not eat hamburgers, but as we were driving along, he spied this giant taxidermy store that had all kinds of cowhides and flags and furniture made out of horns and crap displayed out front. He pointed and said, "Stop there." We went in to browse around and got separated from each other, but I could hear his distinctive deep voice here and there. Finally, we bumped back into each other standing in front of the full-sized giant stuffed bear. As we stood there gawking at it, he said, "This guy'd kill and stuff anythang. Let's get outta here." We got back in the car and started driving, and he asked, "If you could be anywhere in the world you want to, where would you be? I thought and answered, "Austin. That's why I'm here." I asked him the same question, He thought for a second and replied, "Arizona. That's where I'm the happiest."

After tooling around town, we headed to the University of Texas so Waylon could give his lecture about "being in the music business." He got kind of nervous once we were there and he saw that it was one of those giant classrooms that fans upward with all these individual desks, with him alone down below as the object of everybody's undivided attention. He made mention of the fact that he probably should have prepared something to say but decided he could just start into it and figure it out as he went along. They brought him a podium to stand behind and then he became more relaxed and started kind of clowning around swaying back and forth with his arm resting on it and acting all official and everything. Gracey, Jessi, and I took seats down front, and all the students arrived. Waylon greeted everybody and headed off into some spiel, which was really pretty informative actually, about how to be in the music business. I looked from Waylon with his dramatic jet-black hairdo and lawless-person country-western clothes, looking every inch the singing star, up toward these students, hoping to see it through their eyes. It was a really pedestrian setting, and all these wide-eyed students are sitting behind these desks, notepads and pencils at the ready, in awe of this legend standing before them, clearly expecting to walk away with some real knowledge of how to get their songs heard or published or get a record deal or some such nonsense.

In an effort to impart some sort of truly useful information, Waylon started talking about his early days of trying to make it when he had lived in Arizona and said something like, "Stay right where you are and make so much noise they'll come to you." This triggered more reminiscences as he meandered all the way back to the days when he was playing bass with Buddy Holly and the Crickets and, seemingly apropos of nothing, but fascinating nonetheless, he strayed into some really intimate territory, as he began to revisit the night of the fatal plane crash that killed Buddy, the Big Bopper, and Ritchie Valens. (He couldn't recall Valens's name, so he said, "What's his name? Uh . . ." and, snapping his fingers, called him the name of his hit, "La Bamba.") He said, "The last thing Buddy said to me, joking, of course, was, 'I hope you die in a car wreck.' So I said to him, 'I hope you die in a plane crash.'" He became pensive, and there was this touching pause as he relived it and then confessed, "It took me years to get over that."

Then he launched off into the story of what happened, recounting how Buddy's band had arrived to the news that the stars on the plane who should have arrived before them hadn't made it because of the bad weather. They were in shock and just wanted to go home, but apparently the promoter convinced them that the thing to do would be to comfort the fans . . . the show must go on . . . yada yada yada. . . . So they went on and did the show. Then, as his tone shifted, building from tenderness more and more toward anger, he said, "After the show, the promoter comes back to us and says he's not gonna pay us now because the contract says Buddy Holly, and Buddy didn't show up!" Jaws and pencils dropped. His thoughts sobered to the present, and he looked up at the students and declared, "And that's what I think you all really outta know about being in the music business. C'mon, Jessi, let's go." And we left.

Waylon was an early riser. He liked to call me up about 6:00 a.m. and shout, "Little shit! What are you doing?!" I'd say, "Uh . . . sleeping?" He'd say, "Wake up, little shit! I wanna talk to you about something!" When we would write, he liked for me to come over about 8:00 a.m. I'd show up at his and Jessi's house in Nashville, which had the big orange "General Lee" Dodge Charger, from the *Dukes of Hazzard* show, parked in the driveway, and they'd welcome me into the living room, which had the gold harp he was planning on learning to play someday. Or he would lead me to a bedroom that had a big vibrating massage chair someone had given him. With Waylon manning the controls, I would be treated to a demonstration. It was, like Cowboy's place—which had the swimming pool with the remote control boats and the paintings of heavenly clouds on the walls as you ascended the stairway up to the studio—a fun place to be.

The first time I wrote with Waylon, I came in with this idea for a song called "Lines," so we spent hours talking our way to why we truly write songs, and wrote this philosophical song about that. Imagine having the opportunity to sit there with him and have that conversation and come away with a song that he recorded! The day he was in the studio recording "Lines," I went there after leaving a meeting in which I had to turn down a major Nashville label deal because they wanted me to do something that was completely wrong for me artistically. I buried my face in his mighty chest, and he patted me on the back and said, "Don't you ever sing a song you don't love." I mumbled, "I guess, apparently, I can't." Then he did it . . . that thing where he says one of the damndest things. He said, "I hated 'Luckenbach, Texas' the minute I heard it, but I did it because I knew it was a hit. And now I have to sing that son-of-a-bitch every night of my damn life!" Last time I saw Waylon we did a gig at Luckenbach with Willie, at one of his picnics. Daddy Ray was there and I was really proud to be able to introduce him to Waylon and Willie and, most important, his hero, Ray Price.

Once when I was visiting Waylon, he searched the house for about an hour until he finally found what I presume was the only remaining copy of his first 45 rpm record, which was produced by Buddy Holly. He signed it to Jole, because he knew I had named her after the song he had recorded, "Jole Blon," even intentionally misspelling her name in the Cajun way.

The Texas Palo Duro Canyon is considered to be the second-largest and longest canyon in the United States. It was formed by the Prairie Dog Town fork of the Red River, and its highest elevation is 3,463 feet above sea level, and its deepest point is over 800 feet from the rim. If I remain unable to find that 45 single that he so graciously entrusted to my safekeeping, hopefully buried in the rubble of my life's archives, I plan to travel to the Texas Panhandle and throw myself off into the desert abyss. . . . You have my word.

Meanwhile, thanks to a whole slew of synchronistic events, including, but not limited to, a fiasco that involved some artist development demos (that I hope never see the light of day—don't ask), life led me

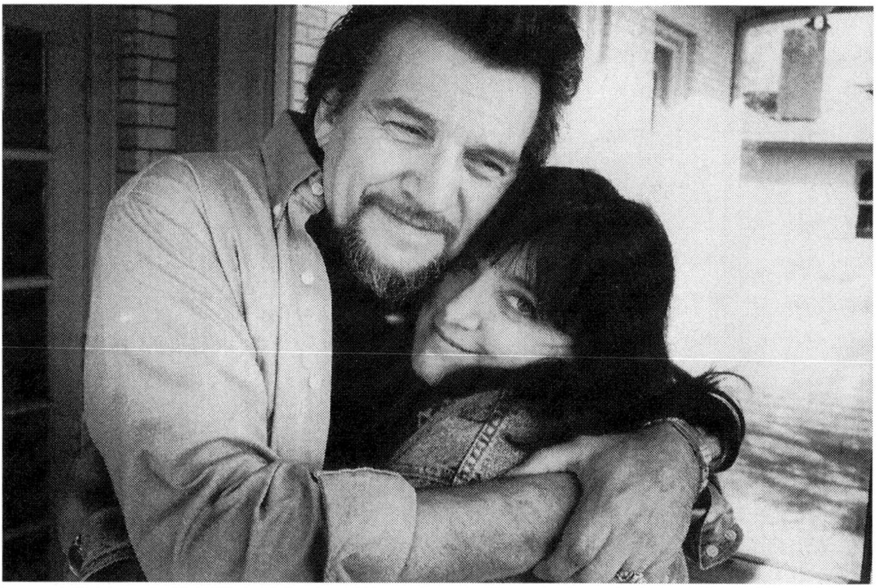

Waylon and Kimmie in Nashville, Tennessee. Photo by Alan Messer.

to my beloved songman, David Conrad. David was president of Almo/Irving Publishing, a division of Rondor Music, the largest and "bestest" indie publishing company left on earth at the time.

I was kind of a wild card lyrically and melodically and had no knowledge of, nor did I aspire to learn, the Nashville formula rules. I was a stranger in a strange land. We agreed early on that David shouldn't sign me to a publishing deal. He didn't want to, and I didn't want him to, based on the fact that I didn't live in Nashville and didn't plan to move there. I had a family and had been blissfully toggling between the jubilee of Willie World and the splendor of tours that ended in Montmartre, so Tennessee just didn't appeal to me. I was a native Texan and a cosmic cowgirl through and through. It was before the Nashville "hat acts" came along and complicated things by hijacking Texas fashion, so I still wore cowboy boots and hats and bandanas with my trendy all-black Parisian clothes.

One afternoon David and I were in a parking lot on Music Row, and a rival publisher walked up to my car window. David introduced me, and the publisher guy said, "Hey, I like your songs; you writing for Almo now?" David said, "Well, she ain't writing for anybody else," rolled the window up in his face, and drove off! I was thinking, "You know, I'm really starting to like this cat." Finally, one day David called me at my home and said, "Look, I want us to negotiate a publishing deal contingent upon you agreeing to never move to Nashville." I said, "Okay."

The month before Wynonna recorded "I Just Drove By," Gracey and I had typed up a sort of form letter, explaining to our creditors that we "intended to pay but just couldn't right now." And then, whether we owed them a hundred or a hundred thousand dollars, we put a ten-dollar bill in each envelope with a note saying that we "hoped they would accept that in good faith." One short month later I had not only the Wynonna cut, but Trisha Yearwood had picked up "Hard Promises to Keep." With a publishing deal on the heels of all that, we were looking at around a quarter million in the pipeline to pay the bills with, so I had no real reason to think that what I was doing wasn't working.

One afternoon while our deal was still in the works, David took me to lunch. Having listened to the songs I had sent him, as any good song-plugger would, he had made notes. When we discussed "West Texas Heaven," his notes read that it was just too deep to understand for him to be able to pitch to the market. I assured him that it was okay because it was the title track of my record anyway and I would be releasing it soon. He said, "Look, I'm saying to you that if you would consider tweaking the song a little, I might have you sixty thousand dollars by the time the sun goes down." I didn't know what to say because I didn't want to jeopardize the good thing we had going, but I actually had no idea what I'd do at that point to change it, although I must say that the money sounded good. At that impasse in the conversation the waitress arrived with my sandwich, and I said, "I don't want sixty thousand dollars. I just want to eat my sandwich."

To David's credit (because I was hardheaded to the point of stupidity), he understood and perhaps admired the world I'd come in from enough to embrace me as "different." Maybe he was even amused. At any rate, thank God he put up with me! He promised me that he could help me "take my place among the other respected songwriters in Nashville," and that's exactly what he did. I lived a double life for around ten years, commuting between Austin and Nashville. With their encouragement, help, and support I was able to pay my bills and focus on writing hundreds of songs. I had, for the most part, written songs on my own to that point. I also began to appreciate the fun of the cowriting "hang." One of my favorite songs, "Love and Happiness for You," was written on a snowy day with Emmylou Harris, as we stirred the fire and, as she put it, "finished each other's sentences." Then there are those guys like Gary Nicholson and Kevin Savigar, with whom I've written whole catalogues of songs because every time we find ourselves in the room together, a song just happens. It just becomes part of the conversation.

When in Nashville, I lived at Beth Nielsen Chapman's house for the most part and helped raise her son Ernest, who called me "Sub Mom," so I called him "Subbie." I had taken to renting a convertible for weeks at a time and was kind of racking up a healthy advance on travel expenses, so one time I came to town and rented a cheaper car. I went to pick David up after work to go to dinner, and he asked, "Where's the convertible? It makes me look good when you're driving me around in the convertible." So I drove out to the airport the next day and got my "by God" convertible back and picked him up after work. We drove around town with the top down and the killer collection of classic country music that Mark Knopfler had sent, blasting ear-bleedingly loud. Did I say I love David Conrad?

Sometimes when you meet people, if you're actually listening to what they are saying, in the very first conversation they will tell you exactly what's going to happen in the future. The first time I met Lance Freed, who was the hip and fearless leader of Rondor/Almo/Irving, he said to me, "Your songs are picturesque, like little movies. We'll work with you here in Nashville, but eventually I'd like to get you out to L.A. to write for films." And that's exactly what happened. Shania Twain and Garth Brooks hit the music scene, and the "Nashville sound" changed once more. I went out of style, so Lance, Derek and Eden Alpert, and Barbara VanderLinde became my angels and took me under their wings. They started pitching my quirky songs to L.A. pop stars and filmmakers and got some good things going for me in Hollywood. They introduced me to legendary producer Bones Howe, who produced some great tracks on me that later were released on my album

Lost and Found. As all good things must come to an end, the party was finally over. Universal bought Rondor and decided not to keep me on when my option came around next time, but those were some of the best days of my life.

JOE GRACEY—"NO MONEY TO PAY FOR DINNER"

I read recently about somebody, I forget who, who had a Garth cut, and every time he sang it, he thought of appliances dancing around the room.

When Wynonna decided to cut Kimmie's "I Just Drove By," we were teetering on the very verge of disaster, money-wise, and suddenly we had this advance check for five thousand dollars in our hands, and we were up there in Nashville, on the way home from one of our low-budget tours of Europe, to pick it up. I stuck it in my pocket, and we decided to go celebrate at a local haute cuisine joint there. We had a few bottles of champagne and burgundy and ate like dancing pigs, and, at the end of a long, happy evening discussing our newfound fortune, we realized we had exactly three dollars on us. We called the waiter over and explained that we had just returned from a European tour and we were temporarily embarrassed, and he said, "What do you have?" I said, "Well, we have three dollars, a hundred francs, and this check for five thousand dollars. Take your pick." He was less than amused by this, especially since I was dangerously close to being tight. He called the manageress over, and she said, "Sir, what have you got?" I said, "Well, I have three dollars, a hundred francs, six marks, and this Visa card." So she tried the card and, of course, it was maxed out by our tour, as it always was. She returned, less amused than before, tossed the Visa in my face, and said, "What is this about a check?" I said, "Madame, one of Nashville's finest publishing firms has just issued us this advance check for five thousand smackers on account of Wynonna Judd is gonna sing this little lady's song. Can you, like, take the three hundred dollars we owe you out of that and give us the rest?" I showed her the actual check, but this seemed to unsettle the waters even worse for some reason.

By now we had a semi-hostile array of manageresses, owners, and waitpersons gathered around us, and none of them was amused. A sweet little old southern widow lady sitting next to us offered to bail us out because she liked our style, but finally Kimmie, who was still sober, remembered that I had a brother who lived in Nashville who is a big mogul and could surely rescue us somehow from being thrown in jail, as was now being bandied about. They called him and said, "Sir, do you have a brother who is habitually drunk on French red wine and who would come in here and run up three hundred dollars in wine and food and try to pay us with a five-thousand-dollar second-party check?" He said, "That's him," and they used his American Express to pay our tab. I need to pay him back, that reminds me. Anyway, when the money from the Wynonna cut started to come in, we paid all our overdue bills, and, with what was left, the first thing Kimmie went out and bought was a decent vacuum cleaner. She named it "Wynonna."

KIMMIE RHODES

While I was busy writing songs like crazy, Gracey had produced a record on an Austin artist, Calvin Russell. I had done some backing vocals on that song, which had become a major hit in France; everybody there was crazy about it. French recording artists started pouring in to record with Gracey to get that "Austin sound." This led to a stream of French artists that flowed through the house for about eight years or so. We were finally able to make a living and were having a great time doing it because it was what we would have been doing anyway, except at that point we were getting paid.

There was this one French artist named Dick Rivers, whom we all called "Uncle Dickey," and who was known as "The French Elvis." He'd been a star since he was a kid. Before they were famous, the Beatles even opened for him on a tour of Europe. Uncle Dickey had a tremendous voice, and Gracey loved recording him. He spoke great English and had a cool accent. His wife, "Aunt Babette," was a gourmet cook whose superpower was to keep everybody stuffed on great French cooking every night. At the end of every evening, after the session was over, everyone would come to the house and we'd have a three- or four-course meal on china plates and wine at a big candlelit table outside under the trees. These dinners could last up to four hours.

One week, the acclaimed drummer Jim Keltner was around to track basics. A few nights in he said, "You people party more than the Rolling Stones." That, of course, gave everybody pause until someone spoke up and said, "But we're just having dinner." We did this every night for a couple of months or so during a year. Then we'd take our movable feast to Paris and finish the overdubs and mixes for a few more weeks. Paris became our "stomping grounds," and we'd end every tour there and hang around until we'd spent all our money and then go home.

There was another really cool, poetic gypsy guy named Fred de Fred, who came to Texas and made a record. He usually showed up whether he was over to make a record or not. He was just part of our big family. He only packed about five articles of clothing for a month-long trip to the States, and one of his main outfits was a brown "shark" business suit with no shirt. I thought that was just cool as shit. Fred wasn't just playing at being a bohemian. He was one. Fred inspired me to start speaking French. I was afraid someone would laugh at me, but Fred, who spoke the worst English you've ever heard, never let that slow him down one bit. I was the only one who could really understand Fred, so I would translate for him, even though he was speaking English, because I could "speak Fred." I placed Fred under my protection because I thought he was younger than me, although I found out years later he was my age.

Looking back, I have to wonder what the neighbors must have thought, but at the time I was completely oblivious. Everybody was working long hours in the studio, so when I wasn't in Nashville writing songs, I'd hang with Fred, who enjoyed being outdoors as much as I do. We went to Target and bought an inflatable kiddie pool for the front yard, some plastic flamingos, and some reclining lawn chairs, and I put a message on the answering machine that said, "Sorry, we can't come to the phone right now because we're probably out by the pool." I could be sighted most days lounging in the front yard by a baby pool with a really hot-looking French guy while my husband was at work.

One day we were all up and stirring around and finally, around midday, everybody realized that nobody had seen Fred de Fred yet, so we searched everywhere but just couldn't find him. Finally, I looked in the front yard and found him lying flat on his back with his arms and legs spread, roasting in the July sun. I roused him, brought him inside, and asked him what on earth he was doing out there. He said he had passed out while looking at the stars. I was only concerned with Fred's well-being at that time, but looking back, I wonder why people driving down the street either didn't notice or think it strange that there was what appeared to be a dead businessman lying on the lawn. I'll always love Fred for being so good to me because even though he had zero money, when everybody else in the gang was taking off for France and I couldn't afford the flight, he took what was left over from his recording budget and bought me a plane ticket so I wouldn't be left behind.

We were like these Hemingway characters who all traveled en masse and drank and ate together every day for years. One of our favorite pastimes at meals was to teach each other the finer points of colloquial sayings and the French and English equivalents of filthy language. Sometimes we'd go nuts and erupt into these big dramatic fights and cry and scream at each other, and by the next day we'd be singing songs and laughing at each other's misuse of the newest dirty words we'd memorized. Jole, who had been charging a quarter for dirty words in English, soon learned the French versions, so her money jar started filling up pretty quickly.

Jole's first trip to Disneyland was when we played Uncle Dickey's sixtieth birthday party. We got to stand on the starting line with the "President" of Euro Disney and help Goofy wave the flag. That was the trip during which I accidentally ran up a thousand-dollar phone bill because everything was free except, unfortunately, dialing out, whether you had used your credit card to make the call or not. Jole was so affected by this lifestyle that by the time she reached college age, she went on to major in French, theater, and costuming and finally became a burlesque star, a fearless advocate for women's rights, and, above all, a true artist who fully trusts the magic of believing.

In 1996 more good things happened all in a row. A Houston label, Justice Records, owned by a soulful guy named Randall Jamail, signed

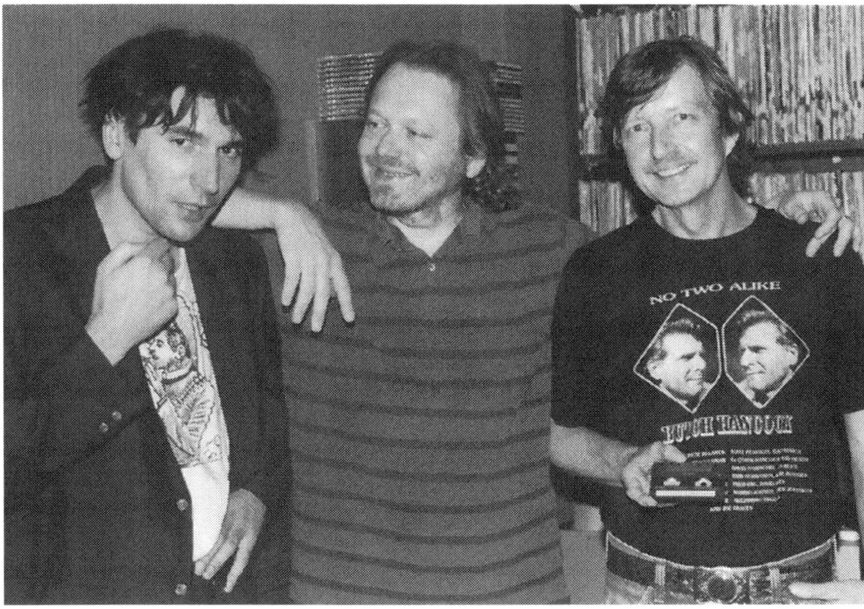

Fred de Fred and Joe Gracey with Larry Monroe, KUT-FM, Austin, Texas.

Willie, Billy Joe Shaver, Kris Kristofferson, Waylon, and me, with *West Texas Heaven,* meaning that I would finally have distribution for that record in the USA. They had a really fine in-house publicist, Hope Edick, who went right out and proceeded to get me a load of great press for the album. *USA Today* placed it on their front cover and shoved it under the door of every hotel room in America. Then they later listed it in their Top 10 records of the year, among all the big Nashville acts. Sony Pictures was featuring my song "I'm Not an Angel" in the body of *Mrs. Winterbourne,* but since there wasn't a soundtrack planned for the film release, they asked if it could be tacked on to *West Texas Heaven,* which gave us the added bonus of a major motion picture to brag about in the press. The Willie release on Justice was *Just One Love,* the album that we'd recorded with my song being the title track.

We were all booked to play *Austin City Limits* for a taping that was later released as the *Live from Austin City Limits Outlaw Country* album. It was an exciting day, and I managed to get Gabriel in on the act to back me up on guitar. In the elevator on the way to the stage (which it so happened that when the door opened, you were, in fact, on the stage), Willie and Waylon got into a heated discussion over the previous night's events. From what we could gather in the short ride up, they had been playing a show together, and Waylon, for whatever reason, did his set, and, instead of staying around to come back on with Willie, decided he was finished and left, only Willie hadn't "gotten the memo." He looked up and saw Waylon's bus disappearing up the road and into the distance. The rest of us had "no dog in that fight," so were just watching and thinking, "Hmm . . . wonder what's gonna come of this when we arrive at the stage in a couple of seconds?" because they were nowhere near a resolution.

The doors opened, they went out, sat down, and continued the argument, so the video actually starts with that. It started to dawn on me why the producer had made some aside earlier like, "We're gonna sit you beside Waylon to keep him calmed down." But everybody cheered up once the music started, and we all had a good time. Kris, besides being his marvelous self, just sat there and took it all in and chuckled, Billy Joe testified and sang gospel songs, and I unveiled a song, "Espiritu Santo Bay," which I cowrote with Walt Wilkins, so I gave him a shout-out without knowing he was in the audience. I, of course, also sang "Just One Love" with Willie and "Lines" with Waylon. Waylon and I had never been able to agree on whether the lyric should say "highway to heaven," which is what I wanted, or "highway to nowhere," which is what he'd sung when he'd cut the song. When I sang "highway to heaven," he jumped and laughed a bit. You can see that when you watch the video.

We played a lot of shows, with Willie to promote both of our records, and toured Europe with him. We rode the band bus, so we were kind of "fresh meat" the first night. Gabriel was along for that one, too. Bee Spears, who was an infamous prankster, started hitting on Gracey, rubbing on his leg and acting like he was "gay" for him. He looked at me to see how I would respond, and I just shrugged and said, "Um . . . can I watch?" He smiled and acknowledged that I had already passed the test. Paul English (whom I adore by the way), not knowing that I had been raised by hustlers and gamblers and seen way too much before I was even in first grade, sat down beside me and started telling me tales of whorehouse shoot-outs in Fort Worth and similar incidents. I just said, "Wow, cool, man. . . . I'm really sleepy. I think I'll check out my bunk." So

I climbed into my new crib. It's no secret that Paul has a seriously checkered past and carries a gun and the story of how he solved the problem of the rainwater that was collecting in the tarp over the stage at Willie's picnic by whipping out his pistol and shooting holes in it is a page torn from Texas Musician Folklore 101. If you really think about it, there's no telling whom all Paul might have saved that day by thinking fast!

Gabriel had gone up to the top of the bus to the sitting area to watch the world go by and had failed to locate his bunk. By the time he climbed down he realized everybody had already gone to bed, and he still didn't know which bunk was his; the curtains on all of them were drawn. He finally thought he had found one that was empty but reached inside and started feeling around to be on the safe side. He grabbed what he thought was a skeleton, and it really freaked him out, but it got even worse when it turned out he had actually grabbed Paul by the arm!

The whole tour was such a blast! We opened a string of sold-out shows all over Europe. Willie would bring me back on to do "Just One Love," and they even had guitar picks and backstage passes printed with my song title on them, which was thrilling. Bee was an angel and "hosted" us through the tour and hung with us on the rare moments off, but he kept teasing Gracey and flirting with him the whole time. Gracey was a good sport about it, but being a "meat and potatoes" guy from Fort Worth, he was still pretty embarrassed and blushed every time Bee made "an advance." By the time we'd gotten to Germany, Bee had nicknamed Gabriel "Schnitzengruber." He called him that for the rest of the tour. One morning, I woke up in the wee hours because the bus had stopped. I looked out and saw Gabriel smoking beneath my window between our humongous bus and a gas pump. Bee caught wind of that and said, "What are you trying to do, Schnitzengruber, blow us all sky high?!!

Finally, on the next to the last show of the tour, we all rode the early morning ferry from France to London. Once ashore we reboarded the bus and climbed up to the sitting area at the top as we rode into London, all excited to be playing the Royal Albert Hall. That evening, just as we were being announced to go onstage and heard "Ladies and gentleman, Kimmie Rhodes!," Schnitzengruber looked over to see that Bee was detuning every string on his guitar.

That was the only gig of the tour that I didn't get to go back on and sing with Willie, because we had cabs waiting to rush us to the Weavers Arms pub, a regular gig on our circuit, one that paid enough to cover our expenses for the entire tour. It was so ironic to hurry from the biggest classiest sold-out theater that we'd played in London since Wembley, to the crème de la crème street-level venue where we actually made great money. Most people think you're getting rich and don't really understand the "tour support" thing for a touring band at our level but anyway. . . . It reminds me of the story about the guy who follows the elephants around at the circus cleaning up after them, and someone comes along and says, "Man, why do you do this? Why don't you get a real job where you make money and don't have to shovel dung?" The guy looks at him like he's crazy and says, "What? And leave show business?!" But that was us. . . . What an honor and a privilege, and we loved every single minute of all of it. Needless to say, it gained us many new fans overseas, which is what we were all about.

The last night we were at a big rowdy joint in Luton, the Palace. It's such a famous shithole that it was even mentioned in the movie *Spinal Tap*. It felt more like a Texas honky-tonk than the other arenas and theaters we'd played during the tour. The back stage was tiny, and about fifty or so of us were squeezed into this little smoky ten-by-ten-foot area just off the stage, drinking and joking around. There was this door that led into a little bathroom. We were so packed in there that you had to shuffle everyone around to open the door. Gracey decided to use "the loo." Just as he was coming out, Bee shoved him back in, jumped inside with him and slammed the door and started banging against it yelling, "Oh, Gracey, Oh, Gracey, Oh, Gracey!! Ohhh!! Ohh . . . aaahhhhhh." Then he opened the door and shoved Gracey out into the mass of laughing hyenas. Gracey was beet red but his sense of humor was still intact, because it really was funny! Bee came sauntering out after him acting like the cat that had just eaten the bird. He was maybe the most lovable asshole who ever lived.

About the time the French people stopped coming to Austin, the silliest man in show business, playwright and comedian Joe Sears, moved in two doors down from us and declared me his new writing partner. So we wrote plays and enlisted all our friends to play all the characters

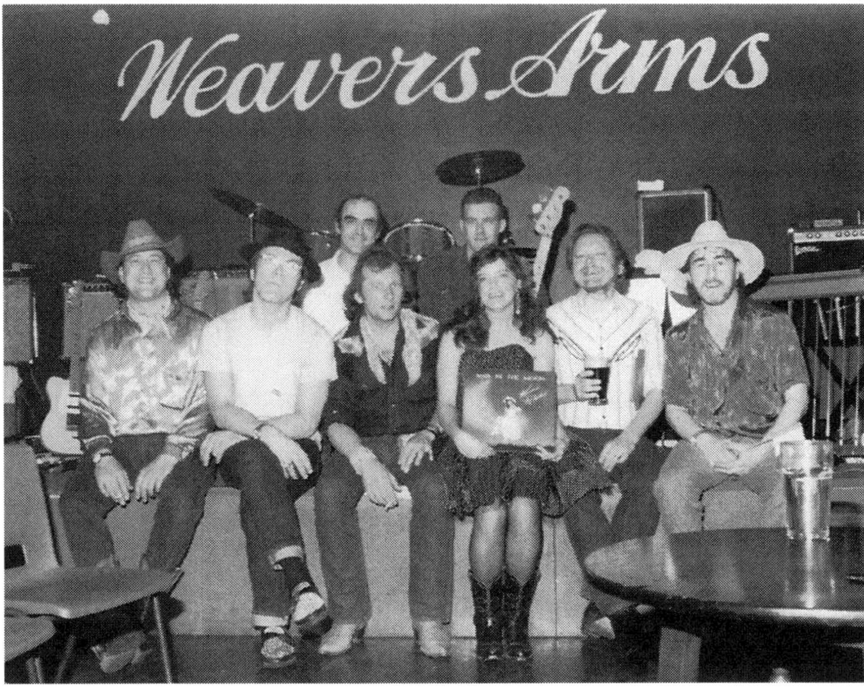

Kimmie and "Her Band" at the Weavers Arms in London, England. Left to right: Bob Loveday, B. J. Cole, Maurice McElroy, Wes McGhee, Kimmie Rhodes, Joe Gracey, Dermot O'Connor.

and romped around doing that for about six years until we wore everybody and each other out and almost went bankrupt. Still, it was probably the most imaginative era of my life, creatively. We formed this community theater company and called it "Stone Soup Productions." We played everything from clowns to dancing skeletons to red ants. Joe and I would sit on the front porch and, as Gracey put it, "Dream up God-knows-what for us all to have to do next." I worked with Joe as his musical director for three summers in Tahlequah, Oklahoma, on a big outdoor drama called *Trail of Tears* for the Cherokee Nation. Gabriel composed and recorded a brilliant score for that play, which opened some doors to other record production opportunities for him.

It took about ten years to complete, but Gabriel, with the help of Willie's carpenter, John Lacey, built a studio out behind our house so we could make demos and records without having to first set up a

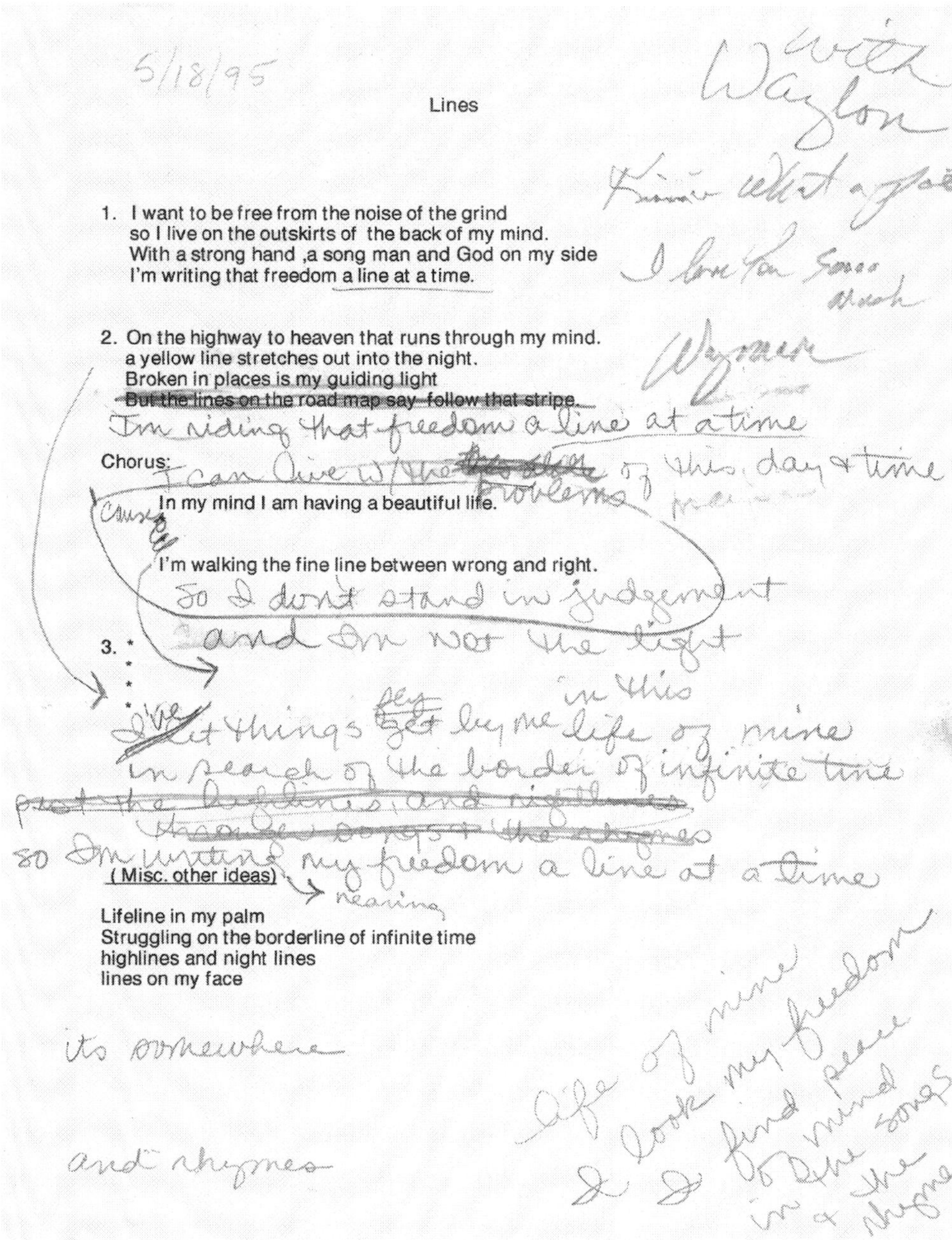

5/18/95

Lines

1. I want to be free from the noise of the grind
so I live on the outskirts of the back of my mind.
With a strong hand ,a song man and God on my side
I'm writing that freedom a line at a time.

2. On the highway to heaven that runs through my mind.
a yellow line stretches out into the night.
Broken in places is my guiding light
~~But the lines on the road map say follow that stripe.~~
I'm riding that freedom a line at a time

Chorus:
In my mind I am having a beautiful life.

I'm walking the fine line between wrong and right.
So I don't stand in judgement
and I'm not the light

3. *
*
*
*

so I'm writing my freedom a line at a time

(Misc. other ideas)

Lifeline in my palm
Struggling on the borderline of infinite time
highlines and night lines
lines on my face

its somewhere

and rhymes

With
Waylon

Waylon autographed work copy of the lyric to the song "Lines," written with Kimmie.

makeshift studio either in our bedroom or the living room. Once we had a studio, we were rocking and released lots of albums on our own label, Sunbird Music. Following the Cowboy Arms Hotel and Recording Spa Band rules, which Gracey taped to the wall, we've been making records back there ever since. I love it because I can overdub background vocals without even having to change out of my pajamas.

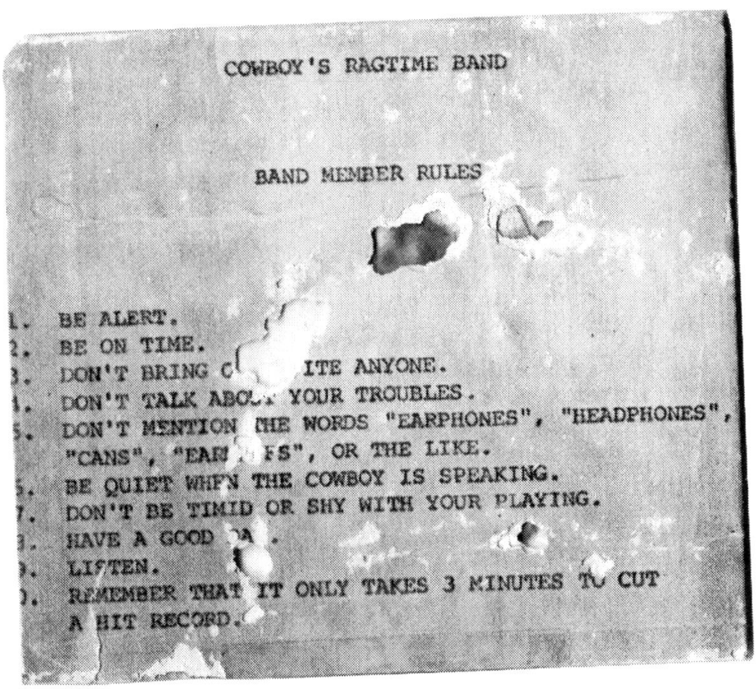

COWBOY'S RAGTIME BAND

BAND MEMBER RULES

1. BE ALERT.
2. BE ON TIME.
3. DON'T BRING C[illegible]ITE ANYONE.
4. DON'T TALK ABO[illegible] YOUR TROUBLES.
5. DON'T MENTION THE WORDS "EARPHONES", "HEADPHONES", "CANS", "EAR[illegible]FS", OR THE LIKE.
6. BE QUIET WHEN THE COWBOY IS SPEAKING.
7. DON'T BE TIMID OR SHY WITH YOUR PLAYING.
8. HAVE A GOOD [illegible].
9. LISTEN.
10. REMEMBER THAT IT ONLY TAKES 3 MINUTES TO CUT A HIT RECORD.

Cowboy's Ragtime Band Rules.

8

THE WHITE MOTH

KIMMIE RHODES AND JOE GRACEY

KIMMIE RHODES

MD ANDERSON, the great cancer hospital in Houston, Texas, part of, but seemingly apart from, the whole world, is like an intricately syncopated trinket thing that clicks on perpetually day after day after day, churning out both the survivors and the dead, regardless of the fact that it operates on the outskirts of happy, normal, cancer-free existence. Here, the minions of God, ranging from lowly janitors from Nuevo Laredo to brilliant surgeons from Beijing, join forces with a common intent: to give hope to the living as well as the dying, moving ever forward in their mission, to be, as their motto says, "Making Cancer History." We valet-parked our car with the smiling "parking angel," Bertha, a four-foot-tall attendant from Chile, and passed through the war zone of misfortunates, who were also from multifaceted walks and cultures but in various stages of cancer treatments, evident by wheelchairs, bandages, gross disfigurements and metal poles hung with plastic bags of caustic-looking liquids.

Everyone is somebody, and the ego must work with what it's been handed. We take that material and use it to build who we are and, good or bad, that becomes our contribution to society. Some of us become rock stars, some blue-collar workers, parents, teachers, prison inmates, billionaires, and so on. Joe Gracey Jr. ("Gracey") was the hip Texan singer who had lost his rich voice to oral cancer in his late twenties and had proven that, sans dulcet tones, it is still possible to fill the world with music as a record producer and star-maker, and that, miraculously, without a tongue or larynx, and while breathing through a hole in your neck (in medical terms, a "stoma"), you can still taste and become a gourmet cook and food writer for a prominent New York magazine. Gracey's status was based on being the legendary disc jockey who had licked an aggressive head and neck cancer and thereafter enjoyed thirty years of living, even without the physical ability to speak. He was cherished as a charming and witty friend and a wise and beloved husband and father. Unlike society, cancer doesn't really care who you are.

The big glass entrance doors of MD Anderson slid shut behind us for what would become almost four years, as we joined the suffering, hopeful in the wonder of a vast air-conditioned realm that was decorated with sparkling tropical fish tanks, original paintings and sculptures, and flower gardens. And the battle began.

We had gotten past the dreadful wait between the dental hygienist finding the small tumor during a routine cleaning and the disappointing biopsy results that read "squamous cell carcinoma," meaning that his cancer had returned. Naively, I had felt relieved, thinking our worries would soon be over, when I received the call saying he had been assigned an oncologist and giving me instructions on how to set up an appointment for him at MD Anderson. I had cajoled Gracey (who just loved women) by teasing, "Good news! You'll be fine because a female doctor is in charge!" He made the familiar sound of sucking air through his teeth, which was his comedic, though mute, way of saying, "Yikes!"

Now the day had arrived, and we waited nervously in the bright, sterile light of the inner sanctum of the Head and Neck department, bemused that the same patient number from thirty years before had been located by the friendly woman at the check-in area who had marveled that the number was so much lower than those of the present time. Suddenly, a tall woman, bent toward the feminine side of androgynous, burst through the door, followed by a small herd of interns, gleefully exclaiming, "Dr. Jesse! Dr. Jesse!" (the name of the groundbreaking doctor who had saved Gracey's life thirty years prior). "He is an icon around here! Maybe we can get you talking again!" She plopped her lanky body down on a stool, fixed her intelligent playful eyes on Gracey's, and continued saying positive things like, "Don't worry; we'll build a team to get rid of the cancer. You'll probably even have better mobility in your jaws. We can get you with a dental oncologist to improve those problems with your teeth [deteriorating from past radiation damage] and help you breath better" . . . and, finally, "Once you have met with a speech pathologist and the tumor is removed, we'll fit you with a tracheal esophageal prosthesis, and you'll be able to talk again." In the stunned silence you could have heard a jaw drop.

Ironically, we topped the first hill on the carcinoma roller coaster that day, thrilled with the possibilities and delighted that in our excitement, we kept forgetting that he still had cancer. We even thought that maybe it was a blessing in disguise because he wouldn't have discovered the tracheal esophageal prosthesis (TEP), had his cancer not returned! Forever needling him to finish the book, *Radio Dreams,* which he had begun to write, I pointed out that he would have the perfect happy ending, one in which he had regained his speech! However, he would soon be run through a grueling battery of tests, followed by a nine-hour ordeal, which included intensive plastic surgery, followed by a very long and painful recovery and rehabilitation process.

Once the surgery to remove the tumor was accomplished, tests, scans, evaluations, and more surgeries were to follow, as day after week after month passed until more than two years had blown by. Very, very, long story short, the rainbow at the end of that storm wasn't quite as bright as had been expected, though the scans after the initial surgery were showing clean, and the team had determined that neither radiation nor chemotherapy was required. The dental oncologist had done the impossible by designing a full set of nice looking dentures, made specifically to snap onto screws that had been implanted into Gracey's fragile jawbone. This was after the dental oncologist successfully accomplished an unpredictable surgery to trim away half of the bone under his upper gums to allow for an ample mouth opening. Unfortunately, even with that, his upper and lower teeth would only part about ½ inch, so he had been fitted with a torturous device designed to stretch his jaws, which had become stiffened by scar tissue. He had to wrangle the device between his upper and lower dentures, and, cranking it wider each time, wear it for a couple of hours a day.

Finally, Gracey was pronounced basically cured, and it was during this time period that he flew to Paris to meet up with me at the end of my promotional tour. (With the help of our son Gabriel, I'd somehow managed to write and record a batch of understandably poignant songs and had released a record, *Dreams of Flying*. It was the last album of mine that Gracey would mix and master.) I had only been in Paris for four hours, and we were drinking champagne at our favorite café in St. Germaine, when we received a call that his mother had suffered a massive stroke. We returned home, and a few weeks later dear Mary Ann, who had been having "visitations"—visions of her father, Daddy Pop—saying that he was coming to take her on a vacation, finally decided to take that trip and so passed away. It seemed that at every place where life might turn a corner and improve, things just got worse.

One day early on in his second bout of cancer, we'd had an appointment with the speech pathologist to do a test that would determine if Gracey was a candidate for the TEP, which would effectively make his esophagus able to function as a larynx by rerouting the air. She inserted the necessary device through his nose and did a few other odds and ends of things and said, "Okay, say something." Always the joker, especially when nervous, he produced an "aaarrrggg" sound. We all laughed, and then she said, "Say something to Kimmie." He looked at me and for the first time in the many years we'd been married he audibly, though with a very low and gurgling voice, spoke the words, "I love you." Hopes soared, and tears were shed.

All along, the plastic surgeon on the team had strongly protested any attempt at a speech prosthesis, feeling that the absence of a tongue would be too much of an obstacle. He insisted that the quality of speech would be poor in the end anyway and not be worth the possible damage to the delicate reconstruction. But the possibility of regaining his voice was irresistible, so Gracey naturally sided with the opinions of the

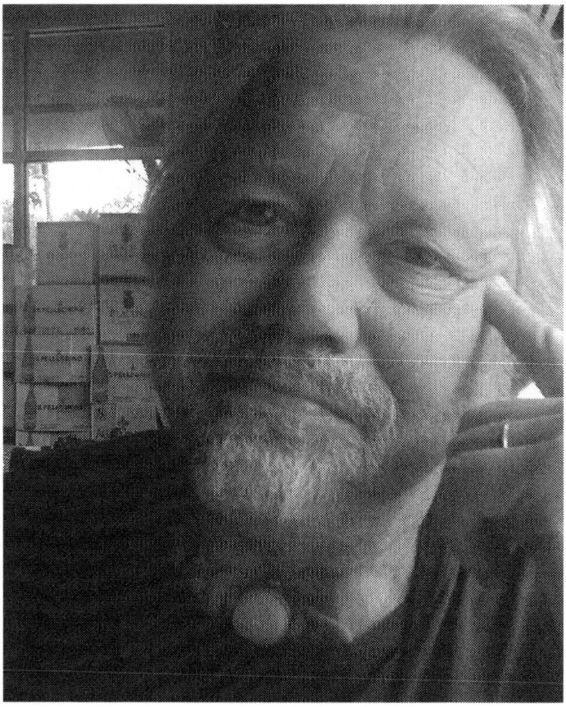

Gracey with the TEP, 2010.

speech pathologist and the head oncologist surgeon who, without the blessing or even knowledge of the plastic surgeon, finally performed the short operation to prepare him for the TEP. Following the surgery, the first attempt to install the apparatus, which was supposed to have been a routine office visit, had resulted in a near heart attack and rush for an EKG, but, finally, a week or so later, the device was in place, and Gracey began to practice speaking words formed using only his lips.

The plastic surgeon had constructed a hump of skin in the floor of Gracey's mouth, which everyone had hoped would aid in chewing by pushing food against the roof of his mouth, but, in fact, all it had really done was make it physically impossible for food to make the ninety-degree climb over the mound of tissue and down into his throat. Because of all the reconstructive surgeries past and present, it had become difficult to know where Gracey's carotid artery was located, and with one wrong slip of the scalpel he might die instantly. So, understandably, the surgeon refused to try to correct the situation, pointing out that Gracey was lucky to be alive, which was true. Also, as predicted by the plastic surgeon, the TEP had rendered only a rumbling of barely audible words, which Gracey found so unpleasant, having once enjoyed an extraordinary timbre, that in the end, he only ever used it to get laughs by cursing me and to scare small children. As he put it, "It sounded like a swamp monster." There was also a nerve-racking weekly maintenance I had to tackle. If done improperly, a piece would fall into his air passage and cause him to suffocate unless I was able to quickly fish it out with these long tweezers we were given as part of "the gear." Neither of us enjoyed that very much!

Finally, after the eight major surgeries involved in the multiple attempts to make it to where he could continue to eat and speak, all that seemingly remained was to be grateful to be alive . . . barely. In the aftermath, kicking the morphine addiction wasn't so bad because he'd never liked the drug much anyway, but he did have to overcome a rather powerful codeine habit, so the annoying restless leg syndrome from a too-rapid withdrawal had taught him to wean himself slowly between surgeries. The worst problems at that point were severe clinical depression and a feeling of detachment that seemed to be insurmountable, even for his invincible spirit. On a liquid diet of bad-tasting nutritional shakes, the too-familiar arduous task of lifelong reinvention had become tiresome, and the dream that a miracle had come along to return his longed-for voice was dead.

We watched as the beautiful, courageous man we all loved and admired struggled for the strength of spirit needed to rise once more from the ashes. I believed he would and did my best to help. During a few months of recovery, we were able to go home, but we would return to MD Anderson every couple of weeks for checkups.

Throughout the skirmish against cancer and its setbacks, we had cheered ourselves on by scheming up one of our romps through France as soon as he was strong enough to travel again, but by then all the disappointments had caused him to "lose his place," and his incredible knack for re-creating himself had all but vanished. I started encouraging him by saying, "I know who you are now! You're the guy who lives in the south of France! You can write while you heal enough to eat again!"

I began searching online every day for houses, showing him ones that seemed to have potential. One morning an e-mail arrived with photos of a thousand-year-old stable being renovated by an acquaintance in an ancient Cathar fortress village where we had already made friends, having visited there many times over the years. A few days later we jumped on a plane to have a look, and while there, agreed to the purchase on the condition that we could hire the person selling it to continue to conduct the renovations for us. We flew back to Texas feeling that at last we were returning to life. Looking back I realize that I should have received the "What on Earth Are You Thinking?" award for taking on the renovation of an ancient stable with dirt floors by way of text and e-mail during all of this, but as the old saying goes, "Hope springs eternal." Besides, it was a great diversion, and there is no rule that says you have to think about what's worrying you all the time. In fact, it's better if you don't. I could, however, write a book about the experience that would make "A Year in Provence" read like a Dr. Seuss ditty . . . but that's another story.

Gracey was so inspired to live again as a foodie, writer, and chef that through his incessant pleading, the wearied plastic surgeon finally caved in and agreed, sighing, "I'm the only one in the world who would touch you." A pregnant pause followed, in which they just sat looking at each other. I translated as Gracey signed, "Is there really a chance I could die?" to which the reply came, "No, I can do it." Gracey grinned and snapped his fingers and signed, "Okay." The surgeon's only condition was that the TEP be removed forever and that the notion of speaking again be abandoned. So Gracey bravely, yet perhaps foolishly, decided to undergo another long and treacherous repeat of the "free flap" surgery. (I watched this type of scene play out over and over again as various doctors, charmed by Gracey's tenacity and stubborn will to return to the grand life he envisioned, "rolled up their sleeves" and accomplished the impossible.) The operation was a success, and, on the final visit, the plastic surgeon laughingly advised, "Once you are healed, just make sure to cut your steak in small pieces and wash it down with lots of great French red wine!"

So infectious was his desire to "conquer all" that I also supported all of his decisions to try any and every chance for improvement, although I will say it made for many long days in the MD Anderson waiting room. Surprisingly, the stress had been so intense for such a long time that, strangely, I lost my ability to feel anxious somewhere along the way. I had finally been in the belly of the whale for so long that I'd become sort of numb, and there was a weird normalcy to it all. I imagine that this must be what happens to soldiers who have been at war for extended periods. I was resigned to a routine in which I would settle into a quiet corner with my pillow and laptop and just wait for the nurse, who would come and take me into a small private room and give me hourly updates. Some of the surgeries went on for nine hours or more and involved multiple surgeons, followed by a recovery period of up to three weeks in critical care before Gracey was finally moved to a regular hospital room.

The critical care nurses were kind, special people, with their own brand of calm temperament. After the first of these many surgeries, I arrived by Gracey's bedside to find him scribbling unreadable squiggles on his Magic Slate, and when I asked him what he wanted to say, he weakly finger-spelled in sign language, "Please, tell them I'm in horrible pain." It was not only heartbreaking; it was eye-opening. Against visiting-hour rules, the nurses hid me in his room and allowed me to sleep beside him in a chair that made into a bed. They would let me know when the coast was clear, and I'd run out to the restroom and quickly make a phone call to a family member who could then pass the word along as to how things were going. During these postsurgery periods in the critical care unit, our faithful friend, Susan, would show up every morning at visiting hours and bring me an extremely welcomed large café latte, a muffin (my breakfast), a big chocolate chip cookie (my snack), and a ham and cheese croissant (my main meal) every single day.

Hours didn't matter in this unique world, and time became irrelevant and didn't really seem to pass or not pass. An oxygen mask is harder to keep attached to a man who breathes through a hole in his neck. I watched it constantly, and when I slept, I learned to use the various beeping signals of the machines like an alarm clock. If the beep changed, I woke up. Sleep wasn't a thing that necessarily happened at night. I just slept whenever things felt safe. I became focused, hyperalert, like the German shepherd of all things pertaining to his care, as I grew more and more stalwart by the day. I had no idea at the time that this was the no-man's-land I now know ran pre–post-traumatic stress disorder. I didn't dream. I didn't write. I didn't talk. I didn't have a lot of thoughts. I didn't do much of anything except read books that I didn't remember.

Finally, after the last surgery, following a long recovery, Gracey became strong enough for me to take him down to the lush indoor park (complete with the recorded sound of crickets) in a wheelchair, where he would walk a bit. It was a really encouraging and hopeful time for us, and we started to talk about our new house, which was almost ready for us in France, and make plans for the future again.

Finally the wounds from the plastic surgery had completely healed, and disfigurements from the more primitive surgeries done in the '70s had been erased. He was looking great and feeling much better. He was even able to drink some wine but was still having unexplained "dysphagia," which is medical-speak for inability to swallow, although all the CT scans were showing clean.

He had begun exchanging e-mails with Roger Ebert, the famous American movie critic who had suffered a failed "free flap," the same procedure Gracey had been undergoing. It turned out that he and Gracey even had the same plastic surgeon at MD Anderson in common. In a widely publicized appearance, Ebert unveiled his new voice, testing it on his wife, live on *The Oprah Winfrey Show*, and using the famous gesture he had employed to critique films throughout his career, he gave it the thumbs-up. Inspired by Ebert's courage and grit, Gracey gained stamina. He started communicating with the Scotland-based company CereProc, an advanced voice synthesis company in Edinburgh that creates customized text-to-speech software. Instead of producing flat computerized voices, their products' voices, as advertised, included realistic, animated, and emotional dimensions by using archived recordings. Suddenly the house was filled with the sound of his voice, as Gracey began resurrecting copies of shows from his radio days, sifting through them and choosing the vocal inflections that would be needed to customize the program for him.

He also bought a cool-looking Paul McCartney Höfner bass guitar and started practicing so he could join us on the road again. Now all of our days were spent making plans for a new life—one in which we would wine and dine and entertain friends in our new French home. We visited a couple of times and closed the deal on the house, and together we bought a really nice restaurant-style gas stove and appliances and furniture. Passing through Paris, we loaded up on the culinary gear that Gracey had always dreamed of buying, copper pans and good knives from the famous E. Dehillerin Restaurant Supply. At our favorite market in Saint-Rémy-de-Provence, we picked out traditional quilts and tablecloths. We commissioned an excessive amount of colorful pottery from the nearby Poterie Not Frères and dreamed of the many cassoulets Gracey would bake in the fireplace that we had built just for that purpose. We scoured the local *brocantes* (antique and flea markets) and bought a chandelier for the downstairs bedroom, corkscrews made from grapewood, wine glasses, and Laguiole steak knives. Gracey bought the shutters, which we had always dreamed would be painted blue and hanging on the windows of the house in southern France that we had always known would someday be ours. Exhausted but joyful he drank wine and proudly watched as I painted the shutters French blue and the hutch in the kitchen a lovely bright yellow.

We decided to drive over to Pézènes-les-Mines, an ancient village just up the road, to celebrate Gracey's sixtieth birthday on November 11, 2010. He had been trying to eat solid foods again with a little success since the last surgery, to improve his swallowing, but during lunch he began having dysphagia and was unable to swallow his last bite. We sat in the car for a long while waiting for him to feel better, and during that time decided that we'd better discuss the incident with the plastic surgeon the next time we saw him because clearly, something still wasn't quite right.

We passed through Paris on our return to Texas and had a fantastic time at the Fête de Noël on the Champs-Élysées. Back home, we celebrated Christmas with our family, and early in January we returned to MD Anderson for routine checkups. The plastic surgeon ordered a procedure called a barium test, determined that the issues with swallowing were definitely not related to the latest reconstructive surgery, and recommended that Gracey see a gastroenterologist for an endoscopy, an exploratory procedure in which a small camera is run down the esophagus.

Having graduated from the University of Texas at Austin, like his parents and grandparents before him, Gracey prided himself on being able to contribute to the research program at MD Anderson because it is a University of Texas teaching hospital. It is very rare for anyone who had survived a head and neck cancer since the '70s to have it return, so his case was considered important because he was one of the few remaining specimens still living, whereby surgeons could study the past operational procedures that had become not only considered to be obsolete but almost archaic.

The protocol at MD Anderson is that first an intern enters the room unassisted to see the patient, in order to gain experience and "practice" medicine. Flashing his big, toothy grin and unprompted, Gracey delighted in stripping off his shirt and proudly displaying his shockingly extensive scaring, explaining how his still-connected shoulder tissue had been wrapped around to re-create a trachea, which had been removed (along with his tongue) to form "a gullet" back before the "free flap" procedure used now in which loose tissue is hooked into nerves and veins using microsurgery. If not arresting enough, he would then enthusiastically strip down to his boxer shorts to reveal the areas on each thigh where tissue had been removed and grafted to the shoulder area, leaving rather immense waffle-textured scars. We found this part of office visits to be interesting and sort of "part of what we got" because we later enjoyed discussing whether we thought that day's intern would turn out to be a good doctor or was just "wasting Daddy's money," and we liked tossing around ideas about small or large towns where they deserved to find residency based on their performance. One day an untactful "whippersnapper" whose bedside manner was still in the awkward stages yapped on and on about how he couldn't believe Gracey "hadn't died by now like most people his age." Gracey suggested, "That kid should be offered a practice in Littlefield, Texas."

So, on this one particular follow-up visit, we were taken aback when, without the opening entertainment provided by a student, the normally cheerful female surgeon with the perennially positive attitude (who by now had become a chum) walked into the room wearing a very grim look. She explained that she had news that she didn't want delivered by an intern. She then showed us a CT scan, which caught the top of a mediastinal lymph node that was showing unusual activity, about which she said, "This probably means you have cancer somewhere in your body and we have to find it and get rid of it." Following the advice of the plastic surgeon, we booked an endoscopy and prayed for deliverance. A few days later, the endoscopy, which renders detailed full-color photographs, showed a very angry large red tumor lodged in the lining of Gracey's esophagus.

A new team was quickly assembled, this time headed by a gastroenterologist oncologist, along with one of the leading esophageal oncologists in the world. Looking at a PET scan with us, he turned to Gracey, and, with a long Texas drawl, diagnosed, "That thing's been there for a while. Now, you've had cancer most of your life, so you know how this goes: This could well be the one that gits ya." Gracey pulled a large bottle of hydrocodone from his coat pocket and took a big swig. Because the countless CT scans had stopped just above the location of the tumor, it had metastasized to fourth stage undetected. It was a blow too sad for words. So we reported for duty once more, this time gazing longingly at the head and neck clinic just down the hallway from Gastroenterology, wishing to return to the good old days.

There would be no more lovable, cheerful lady surgeon. For the first time we heard the phrase "palliative care," which we not only didn't like but didn't appreciate hearing incessantly from the strange new doctor, who had a bedside manner second only to the Grim Reaper. The survival rate for fourth-stage esophageal patients is a mere 5 percent. So while Gracey checked out of reality by playing video games and researching how to turn our Mazda Miata into a race car (which had become part of his next personal reinvention plan), I stayed up most nights eavesdropping into the online chat rooms of fourth-stage esophageal survivors (yes, they exist) and began scouring the Internet for medical papers on the results of immunotherapy treatment to keep my hopes up. Meanwhile, the gastroenterologist just kept on insisting that Gracey should give up and die. So one day, annoyed beyond tact, I told the doctor that we truly understood that we all—even himself—would not be leaving this world alive, and that since my husband was sick as a dog and had no hair or fingernails left, it was pretty clear to us that he might not make it, but since Gracey was still trying to get into the Lucky 5 Percent Club, it would be helpful if he'd just get onboard for the time being. Gracey liked that, so I got to keep my job as head of the "Oh, By the Way, He'd Like to Try to Live" team. Gracey even wrote a poignant letter to him, explaining his position.

Whether time proves them right or wrong, some wise and well-meaning friends try to help by encouraging you that it's okay to stop trying to live . . . but I guess you had to be there. Saying goodbye is just not that easy for some folks. Gracey refused to talk to me about dying, but he did tell our friend Bobby Earl that he didn't fear dying but regretted that he might not be around to watch his grandchildren "turn into insufferable teenagers." He told our friend Colman, who was his editor at *Saveur* magazine, that if he did not make it, he would "miss the oysters."

The irony of cancer and why it has been so hard to cure is that it is not an alien virus or disease that comes from without. Cancer *is* us on a molecular level, an abnormal growth of our own cells, but fortunately weaker ones. In order to illustrate that point for me, one day an oncologist turned over a prescription pad and drew a sideways T—a picture of a three-inch horizontal line that stopped at a vertical line, which he described as "the wall," which, in other words, meant death. It's a real crapshoot. The way he described it, apparently, chemo destroys in stages a pre-calculated number of cells. Then, before those cells are rebuilt completely, the patient is hit again and yet again with more doses as we move on down the line, marking the rounds of chemo, drawing closer and closer to "the wall." Stopping ¹⁄₁₆" short of the dreaded abrupt end of the line, one has been almost completely slain except that through the miracle of regeneration, the lion's share of the whole body is now "brand spanking new," and the oldest, weakest cells have hopefully died. Past that ¹⁄₁₆" is the place where grace goes into overdrive and hope must morph into whatever we are able to conceive, where cancer is finally left behind in a mess of cells, but the spirit is free to fly. *But* . . . we still had ¹⁄₁₆" of a line left, so having spent most of his adult life being the guy who had licked cancer, true to his persona, Gracey decided to go for it!

After several rounds of chemo concoctions and even a few shots that cost eight thousand dollars a pop of the latest cancer treatment called monoclonal antibodies, which somehow miraculously cause the immune system to recognize cancer cells as foreign objects and therefore attack them, various alternative practices, including meditating with a real live guru from India and taking innumerable baking soda–lavender oil baths by candlelight, most of the lymph nodes scanned clear with cancer no longer showing up in the vertebrae. This was *very* encouraging, and Gracey felt that it made the hair and fingernail loss, the numerous hospital visits where he nearly died from complications of low white blood cell counts, and even the incident where the cocky dumb-ass resident physician, ignoring the warnings of the very competent night nurse, almost killed him by letting fluid build up in the lining of his lungs, seem maybe worth it after all.

So that we might "ever return home again," I had attended two required mock-up classes but failed the final real-world exam (given by an RN), where I was tested to see if I could be trusted to maintain a sterile area and change the dressing around the portal tube inserted in Gracey's upper chest, which delivered the toxic chemicals to about ½" above his heart. After accidentally barely grazing the sterile area with my shirtsleeve, the nurse, not so calmly, instructed me to wash my hands and start over, because even the slightest mistake could cause a fatal infection. At that very moment I realized that I was a songwriter, not a nurse, and we all mutually agreed that we'd best keep living in the boutique five-star hotel down the street so that Gracey might continue to don his white linen suit (he'd taken to dressing like Mark Twain by then) and aviator Ray-Bans and enjoy riding the limo with the longhorns for a hood ornament to the clinic in order to have his dressing changed by someone who would not accidentally kill him. So we lived in a gorgeous suite at a grand hotel (paid for with donations collected by loving friends in order to help balance the unpleasantness of our lives being highjacked by cancer) with fountains, swimming pools, chandeliers, flower arrangements, massages, pedicures, and fine art exhibits at the museum across the street. The staff at the hotel called us "The Graceys" and gave me free meal vouchers, and every evening before sundown we walked around the block and then sat on the bench in the park, assuring each other as we always had, that this too would pass and we *would* win and go to our new home in France, which was waiting for us; we *would* make a triumphant return.

One morning Gracey had gotten up early to go to the clinic for a CT scan always taken before we went to review the results of the latest round of chemo with the doctor later that day. Half asleep in the plush king-sized bed with crisp sheets, I had a vision, dreadful because I had seen it once before, while caretaking my friend, Jody, who was dying of lung cancer. In the state between wake and sleep, I saw a large white moth fly through the wall above the television and flutter all around the room. Disturbed, I awoke and then dropped back into sleep, when, again, the big moth entered through the same place in the wall and flapped around the room. I knew well in my heart, despite denial or any belief in an ability to actualize an outcome by keeping the faith, that this was an omen of death. If you think I'm crazy (which, in fact, I probably am) Google "white moth death omen." To date it shows 16 million results.

We had an especially gloomy visit with the doctor that afternoon, and for the first time, the unfathomable prospect that Gracey might not make it crept into my consciousness. Returning to the hotel from the clinic he pulled my latest CD, *Dreams of Flying*, from his pocket and, stumbling a bit (as his role model, W. C. Fields might do) and laughing his charming, wheezy laugh, handed it to the doorman from Tanzania, who had become our friend. This thing he had done for me since the day I met him—promoting my music, never giving up, and always believing in me—he was still doing now, in the face of the worst possible circumstances, and that is most certainly when the initial tiny crack in my armor appeared. Back in our room, for the first time since the ordeal had begun, I sobbed into the well of his shoulder and thanked him for everything he had done for me through the years.

I had begun experiencing a separation anxiety that was familiar to me because I remembered feeling that same singular sadness when my family moved away from my childhood babysitter when I was five years old. Later that afternoon, lying alone on the grass in the museum park, I dreamed that my own self as a five-year-old child walked up and stood above me. The child-me said, "I'm sorry you're sad." I said, "Thanks, I'm sorry you were sad, too." The child-me then said, "What should we do now?" The adult-me replied, "I'm not sure. What would you like to do?" The child-me replied, "Would you like to sing songs?" The adult-me answered, "Yes, very much."

But finally the chemotherapy, along with monoclonal antibody treatments, ended, and the radiation treatments began, and as things progressed, the news got better. There was no cancer showing in the vertebrae, the lymph nodes were clearing, and the tumor was finally shrinking, although Gracey had sustained some lung damage due to the radiation. We made plans to leave for France as soon as the treatments had ended. A few days before we left the country, we looked at scans with the radiologist and were amazed that the tumor we had been bombarding for months was nowhere to be seen! The grim doctor left to become a full-time professor, and we had been assigned a wonderful new gastroenterologist who looked at the scans with us and said that some very small spots in his lungs that were showing up were probably cancer, which the radiotherapist assured us could easily be zapped. It was clear to us that Gracey still had cancer in his system, but the great news was that we were finally hearing the word we had longed to hear, "restage." The new gastroenterologist said, "We've done all we can do for now. You need to rest and let your white count rebuild itself." She said, "Go rest and have fun and come back, and we will restage your cancer and make a new plan for continued treatment." So at least, for the time being, we could breathe and be grateful for a chance to resume our lives.

The following is a letter Joe Gracey wrote at the request of his speech pathologist to a patient who was about to permanently lose his voice to cancer and was preparing to undergo a total glossectomy and laryngectomy at MD Anderson.

Hello,

Our speech pathologist told me about you last time I saw her. I assume you will be having a total glossectomy (tongue) and laryngectomy (larynx) like I did thirty years ago. Couple of things I can tell you based on my experience, for what it may be worth:

1. Squamous cell carcinoma is very slow to spread, if at all, so your chances of long-term health are extremely good. I am living proof of this.
2. Not being able to speak has its advantages as well as its frustrations, of course. I do miss singing, which is a *&&^%$%$ drag, but on the other hand, I almost never say anything I wish I hadn't said, because by the time I write it down I have edited myself. And, people think I am wise because I don't rattle on about stuff like most people. I am not.
3. Now they have ways to give you a pretty good voice back, such as TEP, which I am myself about to try out, and which seems to hold real promise for most of us.
4. You will still be able to eat and taste food. The only flavor I don't really taste is sweet, which means I don't care much about dessert, but I still love and enjoy ice cream. This is because most flavor actually resides in the sense of smell, not in the tongue. I'd say about 95 percent, in fact. At first it may not seem that way to you, but as time goes on you will begin to sense aromas and tastes more fully. I also seem to have some residual ability to taste bitter and even sour, because I have the feeling that there are a few taste buds that reside in other parts of the mouth and throat besides the tongue. So don't mourn the loss of food and its pleasures. . . . They will still be there. In fact, one of my jobs is as a food and travel writer, and I love good wine and food.
5. You will have to get used to the whole thing, of course. I live with a certain amount of frustration, and I think you have to go through a period of mourning for the loss of your voice, but life does go on and eventually you figure out ways to cope. Therapy is good. A supportive spouse is good. A sense of humor and a willingness to adapt and not sulk or throw tantrums is good. I wish I had something wise and terrific to tell you that would fix everything and make it okay, but I think the thing to remember is that the human spirit is very able to handle setbacks and problems, much more than you may know right now. I would rather have lost my voice than my sight, or my hearing, or my

> legs. It is, in fact, almost a minor handicap when you get right down to daily living, as far as I am now concerned. There are many ways to cope, and deal with it, and laugh at it, if you just plow ahead and figure it is just a minor test of your will to live fully and well and happily.

I wish you all the luck on earth, and if meeting me personally would help you, of course we can do that. I am out here in Spicewood, west of Austin on 71. I am, in fact, going to MDA to have some more stuff done, the TEP insertion and some dental work, from the 13th to the 23rd, so perhaps we can even meet there before they haul you in for your fun and games.

Yours sincerely,
Joe Gracey

P.S. The MDA team is the greatest on earth. Lean on them—they can help, too.

The following is a letter written by Joe Gracey to his gastroenterologist oncologist, hoping to encourage the doctor to stay positive and not give up the fight.

I first had cancer thirty-three years ago, when I was twenty-seven. They told me I "had an old man's disease," squamous cell in the base of the tongue, something usually the result of a lifetime of tobacco, alcohol, etc. But this was "curable." My surgeon grabbed a scalpel and plunged in there (at my insistence, we did it in stages to try to save my tongue since I was a celebrity DJ, a singer in the UT opera, and about to have a singing career in Nashville), and over twelve months and seven surgeries, he installed pedicle flaps and radiated the tongue, but ultimately had to do a "commando" procedure on me and take the larynx and tongue in the end. I struggled with both the fear of recurrence and the fear of losing everything I had worked toward, and for three or four years, my therapist was booze and late-night plane flights to Nashville to put a life back together.

But, I was "cured." I found a new life as a record producer and small label owner and studio engineer. I produced Stevie Ray Vaughan, Willie Nelson, and many others. I had my first gold record in France and began producing a string of French artists in Willie's studio, using my Texas studio players to give them that "Texas sound" they craved.

I met Kimmie Rhodes, a young woman who was a burgeoning poet and singer, and with whom I ultimately fell in love and married. We are still married, thanks to our shared sense of humor and love of life. We have toured the US, Canada, and every nook and cranny of Europe and the UK, playing her songs (and a few of mine) and making friends and eating the local foods with the local wines. I began to write features for *Saveur* magazine in New York as I discovered things of interest, and I wrote about Texas foods for people who had never had a real enchilada.

Kimmie and I shared an unquenchable thirst for the next town, the next interesting new friend, the next crazy dish we'd never heard of, a wine or spirit or tea or salt new to us. We'd rent a convertible, throw our guitars over the back, and head out for places we'd never been to play her platinum and gold-selling songs for intense European fans who knew more about us than we could ever remember. We taught cooking classes and wrote a cookbook.

Thirty years . . . children, couple of grandchildren, as my grandfather would say "eating your white bread now." I was immortal, a survivor, I had crushed and killed and stomped on cancer's head and heart. We recently bought a little house in the south of France and are renovating it and were about to spend a lot of time there, where we are in love with the food, the air, the vines, and the "joie de vivre." Life thrives in our little corner of France, and we long to be there.

Then three years ago a surprise squamuous cell tumor showed up in my mouth again. This was like a repeat performance. My head and neck surgeon galloped in and cut it out, and my plastic surgeon and I wrestled the swallowing issues (and each other) to the ground until I could—by God—eat again, no matter how many flaps or surgeries or appointments it took. I was cured, walking out the Discharge Door in January, when my oncologists said, "Um, wait a minute. There is something on the CT we don't like the looks of," and now here we are.

There is little talk of "cure" in this new department I find myself in. No talk of "We'll just cut that baby out, and you'll be home in a month." I heard the word "palliative" for the first time in my cancer life. My first reaction after fear and shock was "Hell with palliative, let's wipe this thing out!" Then I began to understand better how this works; chemo is a kind of ongoing changing world, in which both your medical progress and your own wishes and feelings steer your next set of choices. But here I need to make myself clear: I have a life full of living left and I want to beat the bloody hell out of this cancer and go on full-blast. I want to watch my grandchildren zoom, firefly-like, around my yard at sunset, play bass guitar on our tours, and hold court at our house in the Languedoc over a glass of cool rosé wine while we slow-cook a lamb and goose cassoulet in the fireplace. I do not have any room in my desires for anything less, unless I have no choices left.

I just bought another bass guitar and I am learning how to play it with the three good fingers I have on my left hand. I am about to buy a convertible for the new house so Kimmie and I can go whizzing over those great little two lane roads on the way to turn in our homegrown olives to be made into a year's worth of olive oil. I have an offer to write food and travel from my old editor at *Saveur* again. I'm ready to go on the attack. What's next? Now, with your help, I'm ready.

The following are excerpts from Joe Gracey's blog posts, which tell the story firsthand of his journey through the return of cancer. The full content, related photos, and other blogs written by Gracey from June 29, 2007, through August 20, 2011, can be found online at www.graceyland.blogspot.com.

March 20, 2009

What? Again?

I figure it's time to talk to my friends and readers who may be interested in what I've been up to lately. The quick answer is I learned that I have cancer. Again. After thirty joyous years of being a proud "survivor," I'm back being a "patient" again.

As I have written about here in the past, my first experiences with cancer and recovery actually led to some good things, like my intense interest and pleasure in food and wine and "life its own self," to quote the sainted Dan Jenkins. Most of my cooking and eating experiences since 1979 are the outgrowth of those battles with cancer and the aftermath in which I began to reprioritize my new life.

Since then, my wife, Kimmie Rhodes, and I wrote a quirky little cookbook/novella, *The Amazing Afterlife of Zimmerman Fees.* We teach cooking classes at Central Market in Austin, and we have been known to cook for parties and dinners for money, and to be serious about it. I have written for *Saveur* magazine and others. We cook for our own pleasure and the pleasure of our friends and family and guests, as another expression of our artistic personalities. Cooking is fun, is expression, is life, family, reunion, reinforcement. And, as one of my writer heroes Jim Harrison says, "Eat or die!"

So to find out I have cancer now is rather unnerving. I have a small cancerous area on the inside of my gums, next to my jaw. Nobody knows yet just how large or deep it may be. I plunged into fear—fear that I would lose the ability to eat at all, much less slowly and laboriously as it is now, that I would lose my lower jaw, that I would lose my face, or my life. When you learn something like this, your imagination runs as wild as a pet chimp let loose in a mall of horrors. What if this? What if that? What will they do to me? How much pain? Horror? Misery? Blood? The human mind is capable of both soaring sweetness and mindless, blundering fear.

However, there is a vast beaming City on a Hill (a hill of hope only, since Houston is so flat that the gutters don't flow) called MD Anderson. On going there last week, I met a team of brilliant doctors and speech pathologists and nurses and beaming staff, smiles and kindness at every turn. Capability everywhere brought to an acute point—you realize you are in the place where the best people are doing the most advanced and specialized things.

Instead of sadness and despair, people are undergoing treatment with hopeful eyes and confident faces. Treatments that are out there in the world look sci-fi: chemo, radical surgeries, skin and tissue grafts, skin radiated until it is literally glowing red. Out there we are great oddities, and people stare at us uncontrollably. (More on that later; I have thought about that a good deal over the last thirty years.) But inside MDA we are all just people being worked on, no big deal.

In a week I went from runaway terror to runaway giddiness after I finally got a dose of reality. A brilliant lady surgeon who made me feel a hundred times better within an hour and a chemo specialist whose intelligence and sense of humor were like a cool drink of water on a West Texas summer day when the grasshoppers are louder than the oil derricks. I am apparently to be surrounded by a team of doctors and researchers, all of whom would be considered the best in their fields in any hospital in the world. An oncological dentist whose mind, while examining me, begins to fly through vast expanses of possibilities and then quickly draw up tentative plans and ideas to make me better, almost whole, again. We ask her what she is going to do, and her answer is "I'm going to think!" And when she thinks, big stuff happens.

I like being in the care of women. It reassures me. There is nothing in the world more competent than a woman who has triumphed in a man's world, as this Western medical world surely has been for hundreds of years. As I observed to Kimmie afterward at late lunch at our favorite Houston bistro, Café Rabelais, you can bet that any girl who makes it this far would have been able to kick the classroom-ass of any guy in school, both because she is really, really sharp, and because she has had to work harder to prove it.

And, now, as the final, wild, impossible cherry on top of this sudden Gulf Coast Good News Sundae, the women (again) in speech pathology say I should be able to speak again. Uh-huh. I, in my sternest fashion, say that I come here with very little hope of that possibility. Jodi, the speech pathologist, is not fazed by my fatherly gravity. She sneaks up on me and jams a little white tube up my nose and down my throat and tells me to loosen up and quit whining. When she has it halfway to China, she tells me to breathe in and when I breathe out, say, "One, two, three." Okay. I breathe in, open my mouth, which I haven't used to speak a word in exactly thirty years, and out comes a gurgling, deep "One, two, three," and it is me, talking quite clearly. I look over and Kimmie has tears coming out of the corners of her eyes and down her sweet cheeks, and she says, "That is the first thing I ever heard him say." I laugh and say I sound like one of those movie swamp monsters. They ask me if I want to say anything else and instead of saying "I love you" to Kimmie, like I, played by Russell Crowe, will say when they make this movie, I just raise my hands in claws and gurgle, "AAAaaaaarrrrghhhhh," like a swamp monster. It gets a big laugh, but I notice that the other speech lady also has tears and she has to leave. My nose-tube taskmaster, Jodi, tells me about this patient she has who is in exactly the same shape I am in—no larynx, no tongue—but he is, like me, shaped correctly to be able to use this method to "speak" and has been now for six years. She will put me in touch with him so I can get it from the horse's mouth, via e-mail.

Yikes. As of today, I'm still walking around this one, kicking the tires and wondering if I can drive this baby or not. It is the Porsche Cayenne of my dreams, as Rodney (Crowell) said later. I am imagining the comic possibilities of this new toy, saying ridiculous things, cursing, singing in a monotone in a voice like Tom Waits. Let me at it. I can't wait to try this out. Surgery, schmurgery. Pain? Gimme morphine for my pain and red wine for my brain. The memory of pain is short. Me talking again? The crazed wonder of it is carrying me away on a river of impossible happiness.

So, that's what I been doing while school was out. Wish me luck and wait for the audio file of me singing "Picture in a Frame" to appear soon in this space.

Peace and Love,

Joe Gracey Jr.

March 30, 2009
It has been a hard week. I'm down to the last supper before my surgery at 5:00 a.m. Today the doctors laid out all the different things they are going to cut and splice and paste out, onto, and into me. I still feel eminently lucky to be here at this amazing hospital and am thankful for the dedication and ability of these people, but I am a little scared as I get closer to the reality of the thing.

I have learned a lot about dining out in Houston this week—Houston has become a much better food town in the past few years, and we have had some truly memorable meals here in preparation for a month of taking food in through a little plastic tube that will run into my nose and down to my stomach.

Today a nurse wrote on my skin "this side," so they would cut me on the correct side of my neck. I was reminded of thirty years ago when I had big red squares on each side of my jaw to aim the radiation machines at, and when Stevie Ray Vaughan and Bobby Earl Smith saw me, they went upstairs at the Rome Inn and got red markers and drew big red boxes on their faces in solidarity with me after some asshole at the bar made fun of me. I loved Stevie; he had a large, sweet heart.

And, as Paul Baumgartner would always say, "And so we go. . . ." See you on the other side!

Peace and Love,
Joe Gracey Jr.

April 10, 2009
It's Alive!
Dear Friends,
I'm out of the hospital recovering at a nearby hotel (the ZaZa, which Kimmie dubbed the "Zaspital"), thanks to their special "MD Anderson rate," and Monday I go back for a last series of tests and pokes and prods, after which I may get to go home. Some observations:

—Surgery is now much easier on the patient than it was thirty years ago. Last time I was in an operating theater for eight hours, the aftereffects of the anesthetic were almost as bad as from the surgery itself, and waking up in intensive care was miserable in every way. This time, the aftereffects were almost zero. Amazing.

No more cancer. Brilliant Lady Surgeon removed the cancer tissue, and this time a brilliant Zen master plastic surgeon took a hunk of unused muscle and tissue from my thigh and used it to fill in the gap. No cancer in the jawbone. None of my fears came true. No bone removal, bone grafts, mutilation, nada. If I can pass the swallowing test on Monday, I can get this plastic feeding tube out of my nose and make a beeline for my favorite Houston restaurants (Feast, Café Rabelais) and start inhaling soup in a serious fashion. And, as a nice present, the plastic surgeon miracle guy gave me a neck-lift!

As for the philosophical stuff, I must confess that one lingering effect of the anesthesia combined with the opiates (for pain) has been a rather dull mind this week, but a few random thoughts straggled to the surface after ten days of post-op recovery with a feeding tube and no food or drink by mouth allowed.

—Never, ever drink a glass of cold ice water again without stopping to enjoy it. I would scalp you and eat your eyeballs raw right now for a glass of ice water.

—Same goes for an ice-cold cerveza frosting the sides of a glass, foam dancing on top. I won't take this for granted again.

—This is much like my previous epiphany, only more basic; a cool glass of water, a spoonful of warm soup, the aroma of red wine as you tip the glass to your mouth. I'm being whipsawed by longing and gratitude in equal measure. Is it possible to regard such mundane things with tenderness? I am now. I bet I continue to, too.

—One of the larger ironies of this whole thing is that had I not had cancer again and come to this hospital for treatment, I might not have learned that I was a candidate for speech after thirty years of not speaking. Not pretty speech, or particularly easy to understand. But what the hell? Am I complaining? Do I look like such a putz?

—It is humbling and touching to be told "we are praying for you" or "we are sending good thoughts your way" or "our prayer group prayed for you today." While I remain a grumpy old skeptic, my heart is made tender by this constant inpouring of sweetness and faith directed into the ether on my behalf. Thank you all. I accept it gratefully.

—This has all happened so fast that it is almost impossible for (my) mind to process. From cancer diagnosis, with its plunging primitive fear, to "cured and healing" in a few weeks is as mind-blowing as any trip I've been on so far. I'm still way back there trying to deal with the past, and already the future is crowding it out.

—Nurses rule. Literally. They make the rules on the ground. We need more and the job finally pays good money, so think about it. Thanks to you all for your dedication, knowledge, and aid to the sick and helpless.

I shall return!

Joe Gracey Jr.

April 13, 2009

Flee! He's Coming Out!

Wow, sitting in the café at the hotel. Biopsies all clear, tubes out, stitches out, real clothes on, a Shiner Bock in front of me. Wow. What a lovely day!!

MMMmmmm, live it, boys and girls, live it while you got it. . . .

Thanks for all the prayers, thoughts, wishes, and dreams.

Peace and Love,

Joe Gracey

April 16, 2009

Home Again

Home is nice. . . . Stuff is where you expect it to be, the food is fabulous (Kimmie is making great soups for me now), and Miss Liliana the golden retriever and Mama Kitty are offering full support, no questions asked.

My emotions seem to be lined up in order, though—I should be dancing around the rooms in ecstasy, but instead I am apparently going to be forced to experience all of the old fear and sadness, and then after I do that, I get to feel all happy. Stupid lizard mind . . .

I still can't eat anything solid, or even semisolid, yet. So soup it is. I think we will make an asparagus soup tonight. It is asparagus season, after all. Easy as pie, too. Easier, actually.

— ASPARAGUS SOUP —

1 lb. white asparagus, or green, snapped in two,
blossom ends chopped into 1" pieces
1 yellow onion, roughly chopped
4 cups broth or cold water
1 cup heavy cream or whole milk
Good salt, freshly ground pepper
4 egg yolks
More heavy cream or milk

MAKES 4 SERVINGS.

Cut or break the tender ends of the asparagus stalks and reserve them. One good way to find the spot in the stalk where tenderness begins is to hold the ends of the stalk in each hand and bend it until it snaps. The root end will be too tough to eat pleasantly. Put the root ends and the onion into the broth and simmer for twenty minutes. Strain, reserving the broth, and put the blossom ends into the broth and cook until just tender, about ten minutes. Turn off the heat, add the cream or milk, salt, and pepper. Put the egg yolks into a measuring cup and add an equal amount of milk or cream to them and stir well. This is called a "liaison" and is a wonderful way to thicken a soup or sauce, but do not turn on high heat after you add, or it will turn into scrambled eggs. Add this liaison to the soup and stir. If necessary, turn on a very low heat until soup is just heated through, stirring, and serve.

April 20, 2009
I'm impatient. I want my full sense of taste back. I want the swelling to go down and go away so I can see what I am going to look like now. I want a new dental setup so I can chew real food again. I want my leg to stop feeling weird and numb and weak.

I feel slightly ashamed of this, because I should be grateful and gleeful. After all, a few short weeks ago I was climbing the walls of a deep, dark place in my mind, fearing terrible new ordeals and trials. Cancer had returned. I was facing more long, serious surgery and reconstruction. My thirty-year journey through the desert toward this new Promised Land was ending, with no idea what I would face when I reached my new destination.

And then, when the Promised Land did show up, it was beautiful. No serious aftereffects from the surgery. No involvement with the jawbone, and thus no awful complications. The plastic surgeon did amazing things with his part of the surgery, making my breathing much better, getting rid of some old scar tissue, making me look and feel better for the next thirty years, and making my eating and swallowing better with a tissue implant into the floor of my mouth. No involvement in the lymph nodes or surrounding tissue. All clean, all done, all healed. Nothing left but to rest, heal, and go back for follow-up stuff. Next stop, a way to perhaps speak again . . .

So why am I not happy and gay, to quote W. C. Fields? I am, but I am having to get used to the concept. After gearing up, girding myself, setting my muscles and my mind for a blow, the blow went past and nothing happened, and here I am sipping coffee in my sweet little office at my beautiful home, tapping out my thoughts like any old guy.

It is sort of like when they tell you a tornado is coming, and you do all the stuff you are supposed to do, the candles and foodstuffs and blankets and flashlights and battery radios and a good bottle of cognac and you run down into the wine cellar and the guy says, "Oops, already past, never mind." Okay. Well, then. Let's see, what were we going to make for supper?

Or in football where you see the middle linebacker coming at you to smash your brains out and you duck and weave just in time for him to miss you . . .

I think some people are wired to be positive and to go to the higher place every time. I seem to be wired to go to the place I am in and then whine about it. I am not proud of that; it is just an observation. It drives the positive types crazy. I have tried all my life to change this and get better about it, but it is a little bit like trying to stop being Woody Allen: good luck. I am one of the few human beings who could have his life, his face, his voice, and his sense of taste handed back to him after a close shave and then whine because I have a swollen place on my leg. And then whine about being such a whiner.

Another peculiarity about being this me is that almost nothing of what I say is really true. I seem to have several "me's," and the one I describe above is only one of them. I also have the tough-as-nails me who can do anything required and not give a damn, and just did. I have the completely happy me that is, in fact, out walking in the rain right now in the Texas Hill Country and so grateful and joyful that it would make a puppy sick. The whiner-me is just one facet of the total boy, but one that I must address as I rotate around to the next me in the circle. I have the happy, positive, laughing–me who is ready for the next stage of what has turned out to be a rather remarkable life, after worrying for years that I would be just average and not turn out well. I have the guy who goes out to a restaurant to celebrate with friends over a good bottle of Rasteau and is deeply grateful for every moment of life, of friendship, of happiness that comes his way.

Are we all built this way? Probably. I guess the trick lies in being able to choose the one who will lift you, take you up instead of down, do some good for somebody else along the way.

Although the thought just occurred to me that I may be experiencing the curse of the actor, who is equally adept at "feeling" all sorts of ways but sometimes doesn't know which one is real, or even if there ever is a real one. Am I an actor who is able to sort his personality into distinct types and then inhabit any one of them at will? This could explain a lot of things. Hmm . . .

May 4, 2009

Ripe Fruit

Peaches on the tree in the backyard. I'm still all stove up from surgery, but I am determined to pick as many of them as I can reach, standing precariously on a chair, fighting the yellow jackets for them. This tree rises from the middle of a giant rosemary bush, so as I plunge clumsy below trying to get to the ripe ones, the scent of rosemary swirls around me. A mockingbird sings the dove's song goofily. Ripe peaches have a scent, too, and these have none of the melony aspect that the supermarket varieties have, thank a loving God. I find myself doing something very human, cartoon-like, old as ancestors: I grab a branch and bring it down to me so I can reach the big ripe ones that hang against the sky above me. Some of them are already too ripe, too fed-upon by birds and hungry creatures, and they fall to the ground under the rosemary and I find myself thinking "the gods' share, of course," like a Greek pouring out the first tip of the wine to the gods, or a priest placing a bone wrapped in fat upon the altar so that the aroma might rise to meet Them/Him/Her/It and they be pleased. You cannot get every peach—the gods will have theirs, too! I expect a farmer learns this pretty fast. Peach ice cream soup tonight!

What better way to be reminded to love life, and love the earth, and love a ripe Texas peach? With sight, smells, sounds, tastes? To love my wife with a love like an ache, who, "like a fruitful vine," planted this tree long ago with a vision in her heart that is now real, here, now?

I'm very, very grateful.

JG

June 20, 2009

Some of my friends have asked for a medical update. Although I generally shy away from this type of blogging (I'd rather be writing about other things), I will give you the short answer: I just got back from MD Anderson. I am still cancer-free, as would be expected.

They tried to insert a TEP prosthesis, and for various reasons, it had to be removed. I am going back in late July to try again. Try Googling TEP and listen to the people using them; it is rather amazing. Not entirely new, but only about ten years old now and really good.

One of my doctors recommended that I not do the TEP, but I think he was wrong, and I am proceeding, based on the advice of the rest of my team there.

As for food, I am still on a liquid diet—i.e., soup, diet supplement drinks, and red wine. I am slightly dejected because it will be November or December before I can eat food again. Having built such a large part of my existence on cooking and eating and writing about food, you may imagine how miserable this makes me. However, soup is a good thing, and I am trying to accept what has been handed to me, and perhaps I will write a soup book or something. I started out in that direction when it hadn't really sunk in that it would last so long, so I am in the process of attitude adjustment now.

As I tell people, soup is just fine as long as it is not your only option three times a day, when it begins to pale. Going to a grocery store brings its own little agony every time I spot something and think, "Oh, I'll do that tonight!" and then remember I can't eat it, even if I do cook it. Some normal dishes actually do go into the food processor and become soup, even if it is mildly ridiculous, but any foxhole in a fight, right?

December 11, 2009

Well, here I have landed. After a thirty-year cancer recurrence last May, a bunch of surgeries and follow-ups and dental implants, new teeth, new speech prosthesis, some triumphs and some blasts of disappointment, I have landed here yet again.

Lots of dentists and doctors over the years said, "Nope, no dental implants for you, buddy—too much radiation, too risky, might bust the jawbone and ruin your life forever," so I gave up on that. One day the BLD (Brilliant Lady Doctor/Dentist at MD Anderson Cancer Center) said, "Oh, yeah, I can," and she proceeded to do so, and now I have implants and new, functioning teeth and a smile.

Lots of doctors over the years said, "I wouldn't operate on that neck flap area, too risky, might not heal. Sorry you look funny, but that's just life." One day the BCD (Brilliant Chinese Plastic Surgeon Doctor at MD Anderson) said, "Hey, let me do your new flap, and I will fix that old ugly stuff, too." and he did. He said I had plenty of good blood supply to the area, healing no problem. I'm fully healed, I look much more normal, and I can go to the grocery store without small children running screaming into their mother's arms pointing open-mouthed and speechless at the monster-man carrying the pigs' feet.

First thing the BLD surgeon said to me on my first day there was, "Hey, how long has it been? We should get you talking." Not "Sorry, this is going to be long and hard and may not work," or "Not sure what to do about this," or "Half your head and jaw are about to disappear," but "Hey, you should be talking." And now, I am. It took her three tries, the first two failures, third time the charm, and today I am talking. After thirty years of silence, writing pads, frustration, sadness, you name it—I am talking. Not pretty yet, kind of gurgly and burpy, but saying words and cussing my brother on the phone. He said I sounded just like "the old me—drunk." She didn't give up, shook off the advice from one doctor not to bother, kept on trying, and never stopped smiling with me.

I still can't eat solid food because I can't open my mouth wide enough to get any in there, or chew it once it is. But, the BL speech therapist is getting me a device to exercise my mouth and stretch the scar tissue in there, and one of these days I am going to inhale a bratwurst, a tamale, and an entire roast chicken, and then I am going to commence to eat some—by God—food like a real Texas man.

I am not saying bad things about those doctors who wouldn't or couldn't fix me. They were giving what was the best advice they had to give. I guess I am saying is that if you want to get something done and you have cancer, you should go where they are going to fix it, and usually can, and if they can't that day or that year, they probably will have invented a way to do it by the next.

JG

May 7, 2010

Mother's Day Altar

It being almost Mother's Day here in the US, I thought I would try to honor my own mother who passed away this year. I was reminded that Father Brian D'Arcy, our progressive Irish friend, once said to Kimmie, "Never forget to pray for the dead." That seems to me to be a very Catholic idea; growing up in the Disciples of Christ, a kind of liberal Protestant bunch, I don't think I ever heard anybody make that statement, and the only praying for the dead I ever heard was at a funeral where it seemed natural to do so on that day. However, we never lit candles or went out of our way to address the spirits of our ancestors, or worry about things like purgatory or hell or where our relatives had ended up. Nothing in our services ever addressed it as some sort of problem, or undertaking.

I think most Protestants miss the magic of some of the Catholic ritual, most without realizing it and be damned if they'd admit it. Humans apparently need ritual and magic and a sense of being able to address the gods somehow with some tool. We pay people to be our "ministers" or shamans, even the most steely-eyed Protestants of us. The story of Jesus as actually told in Protestant churches is impossibly filled with hoodoo and magic and spilt blood, allegory and horror, but all of that is merely alluded to. Only the Catholics come right out and say that it is really magic and that stuff really does happen in the ritual of the bread and wine, and that you really can help pray your relatives out of purgatory and into heaven, as I understand it anyway.

So it came to me that I would set up a little "altar" to my newly dead mother and my dead father and light a candle, like we see in all the big cathedrals we visit as tourists in Europe. I have no idea what I am doing, and barely why. I just feel a yearning to do something more concrete than mourn, or cry, or think about them. More concrete and yet totally allegorical and magical, in fact.

Mankind has been lighting stuff and waving it around and using the smoke to carry prayers for thousands of years, of course. Plants like sage in the Native American religions, remnants of slaughtered animals on the altars of the Jews, candles in cathedrals, those incense burners the priests wave in the mass. We hope the smoke, the aroma, will carry all the way to God and he will hear our pleas. We ritualistically roll a joint and pass it around the circle of friends as the fragrance of skunk-weed lifts to the sky. To me, the candle's flame is like an ongoing prayer for my parents' souls that carries my love and admiration and longing to them, I hope.

It is odd to me that I find myself doing this, or even thinking it. I am not religious. I have no concept of "God," do not particularly care if he exists or not, and do not find that worrying about my own afterlife is a profitable enterprise. I hope, but I do not worry. No religion has a hold on me, or power over me one way or another. I think one basically as silly as the next. So what on earth has possessed me to set up an altar now?

I think that trying to come to terms with my mother's death, in the midst of my own battle for life against cancer, has caused this. Mourning is difficult for me. Big boys don't cry, and Texas men are made of stronger stuff. My ancestors tell me to buck up and get on with it. Well, sometimes you just have to cave to the need for ritual, for healing balm, for something outside your own little tiny speck of self. I guess this would be it. God bless you and keep you, Mother and Dad. He'll be needing a good laugh, after all. . . .

JG

November 28, 2010

A Soft Landing in France

Somewhere in the Languedoc, southern France—Talk about a soft landing! After fourteen months of cancer surgery (gone), reconstruction surgeries (done), teeth implants (done), and one final operation to allow me to swallow again (plus a cut finger, but that's another silly story), I have landed in the most impossibly soft bed of French lavender.

Here in the Minervois in Languedoc ensconced in a village over a thousand years old, we wake up to the sounds of the birds and the breeze and the couple who walk their dogs; sometimes the dogs wear bells. This village was built as an outlying stumbling block on the way to Carcassonne. In the shape of a snail's shell, it winds around a central green, where the ancient church serves as the final refuge after every foot of the *circulade* has been defended. Under the Romanesque church, there is an altar from an even earlier chapel, which is easily as old as the first whispers of Christianity in Europe.

Now the village holds two hundred fifty people, mostly artisans, vignerons, ex-pats from various parts of Europe. We are only the second Americans to come here, and certainly the first Texans. I intend to put a Cathar flag and a Texas flag out front, soon as it warms up.

I had no idea when we first decided to buy a little home here that the area was teeming with history, both bloody and benign. This is the home of the troubadours and the Lenga d'oc, in which they couched their poems set to music: courtly love, knightly bravery, the beauty of existence. Later it became the center of the first Protestant movement, and the Pope in Rome used that as an excuse to join with the weak king in Paris to come here with a band of brigands and plunderers to dethrone the Count of Toulouse, who was as powerful as the king. Money, land, and power were, of course, the engines of this invasion, but Christianity was the cover story. Every single Protestant Cathar was slaughtered, starved, or maimed and marched away to death on a bonfire. The Catholic Church resumed its collection of tithes and lands, the counts were defanged, and the land became ostensibly Frankish, but in truth it never happened in the hearts of the people here. The accent still reflects the old Lenga d'oc, the sense of independence and grace still flourishes, and the food is very different.

It is almost December now, and cold by Texan standards—about 45° to 60° and going down. Last night it reached 34° or so. I finally learned how to wear enough layers and a wool scarf and heavy overcoat. Some locals are still going around in shorts or normal outfits, which beats hell out of me. Must be thicker blood.

This is wine and olive country and has been since the Greeks and Romans brought their cultivars here and planted them to foster trade. Grapes spring up here unplanted, like Johnson grass in Texas, and olive trees stand silvery in every little corner and wedge and otherwise unusable piece of land. Apricots, cherries, peaches are on sale everywhere during harvest.

The wine is in the tanks now, the harvest finished on about October 20. I will be tasting them this week and try to form a sensible opinion,

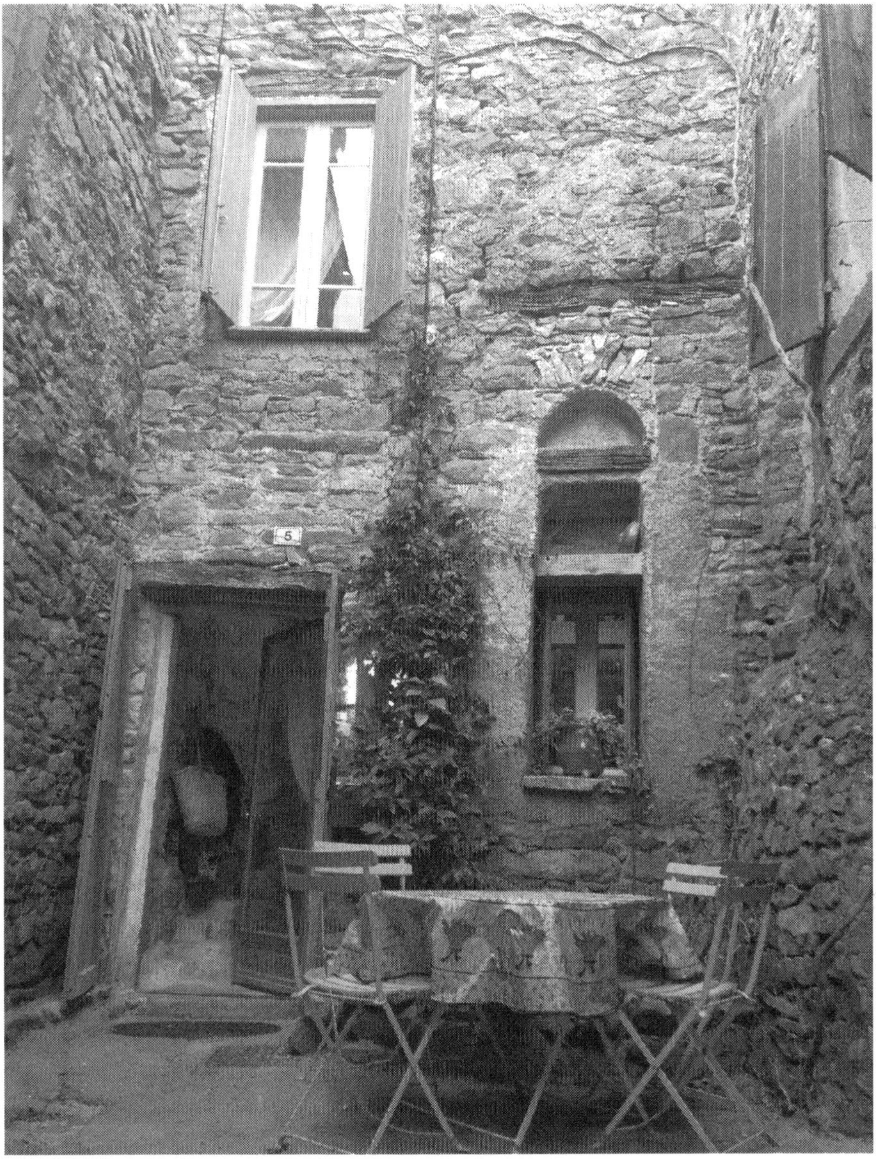

The renovated house, Languedoc, France.

though I don't really know what the hell I am talking about yet. That is my next mountain to climb—viticulture in this beautiful part of this ancient land!

August 20, 2011

Hello from Chemoland

Good morning from Houston,

I figure I should catch you up on where things stand in Graceyland Health World now that I have hit a landing place. I promise I will start blogging about interesting things very soon, now that I feel better, but therein lies this story . . .

I have been diagnosed with third/fourth-stage esophageal cancer since January. This pretty much "throwed me from my hoss," but as I have said before, you do what you must to survive. This has meant chemo every two weeks since then, with the strongest drugs I could ask for and withstand, since I figure the side effects (nails falling out, hair disappearing, weight loss, severe fatigue, neuropathy in limbs, stomach feeding tube—"Nil by Mouth" now joins me to Sir Roger Ebert—etc.) are nothing compared to an early death. It's like I told my oncologist, "Don't go easy on me, I don't need nice nails at my funeral."

However, one aspect of this bravado has been having to grind through the side effects in reality, not just in talk. So it has not been a very fun year thus far. I have gotten to go home some, see the family, cook a little bit (can't eat at the moment) just for the cook's pleasure, but most of my time has been spent in dealing with all of this and in going in and out of the hospital, as my white blood cell count dipped, and vicious little infections roared to life in me.

At last we came more or less to the end of the chemo and started radiation this week to try to kill or nearly kill some of the major cancerous spots that were beaten down by the chemo but not dead yet. Four more weeks of radiation and I'm catchin' the first thing smokin'—first to Paris, then to our newly renovated little home in the Languedoc for some actual Life Its Own Self and not just jabber about living longer. I'll come back to Austin for holidays and family and friends, but first I need my France fix, and it is almost harvest time there, and I can't wait to see the red grapes being hauled into town in the hopper trucks and taste the grape juice and eat some nice food at last.

So there you have it, minus all the little stuff that so interests the patient and so bores the friend.

I have more to say about the effects on my thinking, my life, and my newfound (again) love of this sweet existence, but that must wait for more energy to accrue in the batteries.

Thanks for your condolences, cards, and jokes, and I hope to repay you in the future!

Love

Joe Gracey Jr.

The following are excerpts from e-mails to Colman Andrews, Gracey's good friend and editor at Saveur *magazine.*

September 8, 2011

Subject: Progress is being made

Started radiation. It's coupled with a new fancy chemo drug that actually caused the test group to live twice as long, and the damned tumor is shrinking by the day. I can swallow fine now; all I need to do is pry my jaws open enough to eat.

Our daughter, Jole Goodnight, is coming (to France with us), and she wants a return trip to Cal Pep (she was there for the War and Pizza story), so we are planning a day in Barcelona and most likely a meal at the Empordà on the way home to Aigne as well. Perhaps this would be a swell place for you to jump in on October 26, 27, in there.

In any case I am greatly encouraged by my health and my direction of treatment. I have two weeks left here, then we board Air France for Paris and Dehillerin to pick up a few odds and ends before we head south on the TGV. We plan to be in Aigne from September 29 to November 3-ish.

Hope all is well there.

JG

September 11, 2011
Sorry you won't likely make it over—we'll be going back in the spring. Deal on my jaws is that old scar tissue from multiple surgeries is keeping my jaw muscles from opening. I have a machine that literally spreads my jaws open, stretching and dissipating the scar tissue just like you can massage it away. Three times a day for thirty minutes, and I should be able to eat small bites of softish things. Eventually I can get back to just about anything I want to eat after about six months of therapy. By the time I get to France I'll be eating soft foods, soup, soft insides of bread, etc.

The vocal valve had to go. I didn't like the sound it made, anyway. I still plan to investigate that Mac computer voice like Ebert got. I have lots of tapes of my radio stuff to use in reconstructing my real voice for the computer. Only eight more days of radiation; two weeks from today we'll be sitting in the new digs in France!

I may be going back for further chemo as it pops up in new places, but that beats dying. At one point I was convinced that I had until around Christmas, which was concentrating the mind, indeed, but I think now I'm looking at a few years and hopefully five or more, and maybe they will even pronounce me cured one day. It is rare, but it has happened. I just have to have very regular checkups. I ain't afraid of dying, but I will miss the oysters.

That sounds fantastic to have you guys here doing the music rounds. Hell, I might even get off my ass and go out on the town with you. Time to go take some morphine. This pain just won't quite go away.

JG

September 12, 2011
Four more days of radiation and then I'm Paris-bound. To Dehillerin for some pan lids and then the TGV to the south. We could have taken the plane, but by the time you get to the airport, the train is just as fast and a

hella lot more fun, and relaxing. Plus, I gotta stay away from that cabin air when possible. Apparently, the harvest is going on now, although I see we just got some rain there . . . and it's supposed to be a good one! What do you think of the chances for a coffee-table book, something like "A Vineyard Year in the Languedoc," with lots of big pics and me following the growers and vintners around for a full year?

We'll be home for Thanksgiving, Christmas, New Year's, etc. Probably go on tour in the spring and then end up at the house again for a month or two. Depends on my prognosis.

JG

September 22, 2017

Subject: Congrats

What a ride. That was an unexpected bit of news, frankly. I still have to come back here for tests and keep a sharp eye out for any new areas that are bound to pop up, but for now I am in remission and set free. Leaving for Paris Saturday and not looking back. The captain is already set to upgrade us to first class if there is any room up front.

JG

9

THE WHITE DOVE

KIMMIE RHODES AND JOE GRACEY

KIMMIE RHODES

WE KNEW THE WAR with cancer wasn't over, but we felt like we finally had at least a toehold on what had been a very slippery slope. Gracey was exhausted and needed to rest and think about something besides cancer for a change, so we booked a flight for France. After living at the Hotel Zaza in Houston for the better part of a year, we said our grateful goodbyes to the many friends we'd made on the hotel staff, and headed home to grab the things we needed before taking off for our vacation. We felt greatly relieved, hopeful, and alive.

Gracey had only been home once in three months, and then for only a few days before becoming anxious to return to Houston. He always felt like he would be so happy to be leaving MD Anderson, but in no time at all, he'd be ready to return. It's hard to describe the very strong sense of being safe from cancer that builds the closer you get to the hospital. The force from the collective consciousness of decades of souls striving with the hope of conquering cancer permeates the very air, creating a powerful aura. It's like the pull of a mega-magnet.

Our house had been sitting closed, locked, and quiet, except for my monthly trips back to pick up the mail and make sure everything was okay. The home where we had once watched the children run down the drive to catch the school bus and play in the water sprinkler on the summer lawn, celebrated holidays with friends and family, passed milestones, and lived the millions of moments that had etched our story into the half-acre grounds had become like the museum of the life we had lived before cancer had come to arrest us, leaving it empty and waiting for people, dogs, cats, goldfish, flowers, music, and food to reappear.

As we passed through the back door that day, our attention was immediately drawn to the only living thing in the house, a very large, pure-white dove! It was perched atop a container that had a cluster of three ceramic doves that formed the lid, which also seemed odd. We stood staring at it in disbelief, wondering how it had gotten into the house, and decided that it must have come in through the fireplace. It just sat there peacefully, with its head cocked to one side, looking at us. It felt eerie and ominous, like it was there for a reason, to tell us something. I walked over and picked it up in my hands. The bird was surprisingly weighty; it didn't struggle or flap around or try to fly. It just sat serenely in my cupped palms and looked me square in the eyes. I walked to the front door and held it up to the clear blue sky.

I was surprised by the sound of the muscular power of its wings as it stretched and spread them and achieved liftoff from my outstretched hands. I watched it soar straight into the heavens until it disappeared from sight. Amazed, I turned to Gracey, who shivered a bit and signed, "I'm not sure I like that." We decided to deem it a good omen and packed our bags to leave the next morning for Paris.

Some French friends pulled some strings and arranged for Gracey to get an upgrade on the flight. By the time we reached Paris, as the pulmonologist had said might be the case, the compression had caused Gracey some lung distress because of the damage caused by radiation. But even with that, he was feeling better by the time we got to Paris. We

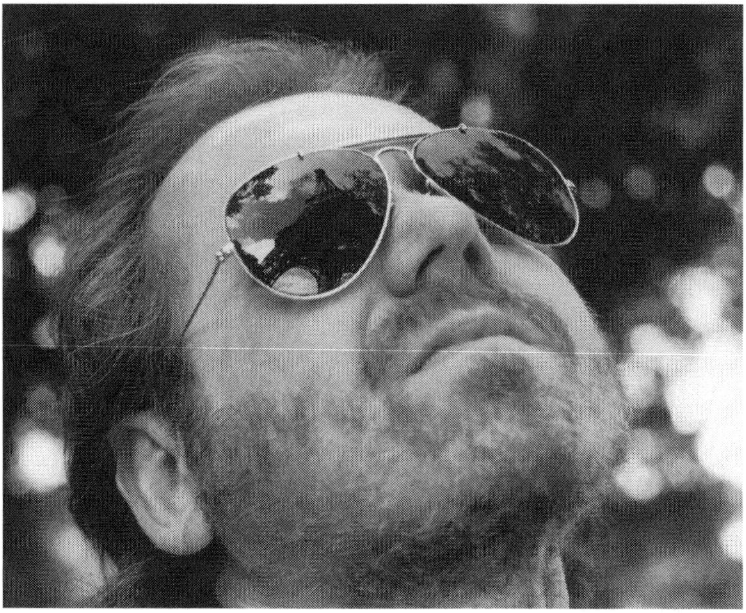

Gracey at the Eiffel Tower. Photo by Kimmie Rhodes.

had dinner with some friends, and he managed to eat a little bit and drink some wine. He even got strong enough to jump in a cab one day and run over to our favorite restaurant supply shop to buy a lid for one of his copper pans.

He wanted to take the train from Paris to Toulouse, so we packed a picnic lunch and jumped on the TGV. When we arrived we rented a car. Gracey even drove for the first time in months. It felt fantastic to be cruising down the road like "the good old days." We hung around the house and enjoyed the autumn weather. In the evenings he walked next door when the winemaker, Andrea, would arrive with a wagon-load of grapes from the day's harvest and dump them into the big hopper. Gracey watched with delight as the overflow of cherry-red juice literally flowed past our entrance and down through the streets of the village. He was really loving drinking the wine that Andrea offered him straight from the barrels.

One day I ran down to the hardware store in the neighboring village and surprised Gracey with a barbeque grill. I set it up in the courtyard, which had a table, chairs, and an umbrella. Then I strung up the

Christmas lights we'd bought the year before. Some friends traveled up from Catalonia to visit, and Gracey barbequed sausage for everybody.

A few days later our daughter, Jole, arrived, and we drove to Toulouse to pick her up at the airport. Gracey insisted on driving and was having so much fun being behind the wheel again that he even met with our French banker to get information on car insurance, with plans to buy a car. Brother Bill and his wife, Cathy, arrived later that week, and Gracey drove back to Toulouse to pick them up at the airport.

He was still improving, but the chronic coughing from the radiation damage was causing him a lot of soreness, so he had been taking codeine. He eventually ran out of it, and by the time we got in touch with a doctor in Paris to get a prescription and have it filled, he was already having some serious symptoms of withdrawal. At the time that Bill and Cathy left, he wasn't feeling much like getting out of bed. Jole and I came home early one evening and were alarmed to find him too weak to stand on his own, so we helped him into the car and drove him to the nearest emergency room in Béziers, about an hour away.

That is when the nightmare began. The small hospital wasn't equipped to accommodate much of anything really, especially someone with Gracey's complicated medical history, and they said as much when they admitted him. Our flight back to the States was booked for just a few days away. We were hoping to get some treatment for his withdrawal symptoms and have him feeling well enough to catch the plane back home. The doctor, a kind man, spoke English. The nurses, on the other hand, were like a coven of evil witches and, in fact, had treated us so poorly on the first night, that when the doctor came back the next morning and heard the report, he excused himself briefly and, with us watching, fired all five of them after giving them a good, loud dressing down—in French, of course.

Meanwhile, Gracey just kept going downhill, and it became clear that he wouldn't be able to fly home commercially. Jole and I were becoming increasingly exhausted because there was no place to sleep, and by then we were acting as substitute nurses in the hospital, although there was one really sweet nurse. Unfortunately, she was so incompetent that she nearly killed Gracey the one time I left the hospital for a couple of hours. After that incident, we knew we couldn't leave him, so we were living on the crackers and peanut butter that we'd grabbed on our way to the hospital on day two of the ordeal. I eventually became the only one experienced enough to keep Gracey breathing. I would break open these little plastic tubes of saline solution we'd arrived with, drip the liquid into his airway, and clear it with a suction device that had been brought to me and that I had figured out how to use. Luckily, Jole had learned French in school, and since by then I had learned the words for just about everything, between the two of us we communicated successfully and got what we needed. I finally just went into the hallway, where the medical supplies were kept, and stocked the room myself. I also found a mop and cleaned the filthy floor and bathroom.

I had finally managed to acquire pretty much every piece of medical equipment in the entire hospital, so I was able to monitor his oxygen level and blood pressure. Amazingly, all his vital signs had remained great throughout the ordeal except for his oxygen level. I called his doctor at MD Anderson. She was extremely helpful. She gave me her personal number so that we could keep in constant touch and I could text pictures of monitor readings, among other things. Once she became aware of the conditions at the hospital, she started insisting, "Please! Get him home so we can get his baseline back and restage his cancer and keep going!" The French doctor agreed that that was the best option, given that we were outside of our insurance coverage and running up a pretty good bill at the hospital. I started making arrangements for a "medical evacuation," or "repatriation," with an American company that has a fleet of small air ambulance jets. Without going into detail, I'd just like to say, "American Express . . . Don't leave home without it." It's amazing what they were able to help us accomplish that the French doctor could not.

Once the bottom line for the expensive trip home was tallied, the question came up: "What if it's the cancer and he is going to die whether you take him home or not?" My answer was that "even if it meant having to live by picking up cans for the rest of my days, I would happily do that before I would see his amazing life come to an end 'in this shithole.'" Luckily, though, we had what it would cost to cover the emergency flight plus the rather large tab we had run up at the hospital by then. Besides, I argued, we had very responsibly checked with all the doctors and received not only their blessing but even their encouragement that it was perfectly all right for Gracey to leave the country.

It had only been three weeks since we had all looked at a scan that had shown only two tiny microscopic spots in his lungs, so miniscule that nobody had even known for certain if they were cancer. That's when they had used the magic word: "restage." I had also promised Gracey's oncologist that after all he had been through in the past three-and-a-half years, he would most certainly not be dying from anything other than cancer on my watch!

We had finally managed to have him moved to the cancer hospital about an hour away, in Montpellier. After a couple of long phone interviews with the repatriation medical team, it was decided which equipment and staff would best suit Gracey's needs and accompany him on the flight back to MD Anderson. It was also determined that besides the pilot and copilot, an emergency medical first responder, a pulmonary specialist, and I should occupy the only three available seats. I was not invited along because I was the next of kin but because when the time came to clear his airway, only I knew all the unique physical quirks of his anatomy. I was a walking encyclopedia of his medical history as well, and, in case he said anything (which he did not), I could translate his sign language.

Jole left to go close up the house and fly home from Toulouse the next morning with all of our bags. It was heartbreaking to watch our tired, beautiful child summon up her courage, climb into the car, and take off driving for the first time in France, by herself and in the rain. I whispered a prayer for her and missed her terribly, as I waited by Gracey's bedside, promising him that it "wouldn't be long now" before we could take him home.

Because the emergency medical responders had been on a mission that involved traveling from Switzerland, it was the middle of the night and raining when the crew of big, strong men arrived at the hospital. It was such a relief to see them in the hallway outside Gracey's room, dressed in their crisp, classy jumpsuit uniforms with matching field bags and equipment. Like a scene from a *Star Trek* episode, it felt (and looked) like they had been beamed down by Scotty to rescue us. They had friendly, confident smiles, and there was a superhero air about them. In a thick southern accent one of them said, "Hello, ma'am. Don't worry. We've got you now. We take Americans home, and we pride ourselves in always delivering them to their destination in better shape than they were when we picked them up. We'll get him back home, and everything will be just fine."

They all liked me already because the rumor had spread that I'd told the big boss, who'd let me fall through the cracks for a couple of hours the day before, "I know you are busy, but I am going need you to focus." He'd found that amusing and told them I was a "live wire," so they'd all been having a laugh about that and were looking forward to meeting me.

It was all very exciting, and I kept taking pictures with my phone, thinking how fascinated Gracey, who loved airplanes, would be by the whole thing once he came to. An ambulance had been arranged to transport Gracey to the plane, and the rest of us took a taxi. Once we arrived at the runway, all of our passports were quickly handed over to an immigrations officer who was ready to meet us. It was all very well orchestrated except that we realized nobody had the correct currency to pay the cab fare. They only had a few Swiss francs, so I just apologetically handed over whatever change I had left in my purse to the extremely incensed driver and hurried onto the plane where Gracey had already been moved by stretcher and placed on a narrow bed that occupied one side of the tiny interior.

The crew instructed me that they would be monitoring my fluid intake to make sure I stayed hydrated during the seventeen-hour flight but that there would be one nine-hour stretch with no restroom. There was no space for baggage; my knees touched the seat in front of me, where the pulmonary specialist was sitting. The first responder was seated in front of him. I propped my feet up on the purse I was carrying. The entire fuselage was filled with oxygen tanks and medical monitoring devices. The plan was that we would first fly to the west coast of Ireland to refuel before flying on to Greenland, where we would be changing pilots. It was surreal to be humming through the sky in a Learjet in the company of these extraordinary beings who spent their lives in the air, "taking Americans home."

During the flight they offered me a job and really tried to convince me that I was "made of the stuff" that it would take to become part of their team. The first pilot extended his arm and escorted me into the tiny airport in Greenland, where he had to say goodbye and get some sleep. He asked me if the rumor that I'd told the boss to focus was true, and, somewhat embarrassed, I admitted that it was and tried to explain that I had been under a lot of stress. Then he also tried to persuade me to consider the gracious offer to come work with them. I was extremely flattered but told him that if fate ever allowed me to return to my normal life, I was really looking forward to just being a lowly songwriter again.

Gracey really never awakened during the flight, but a couple of times I was asked to step one foot in front of the other up the narrow aisle to assist the pulmonary specialist. The space was so limited that even Gracey's legs were strewn with wires, tubes, and small devices. Finally we landed in Houston, and, if there had been time, I would have kissed the ground when I disembarked. My saviors and I climbed into a taxi and followed the ambulance back to what felt like a homecoming, to the glorious heaven of the MD Anderson emergency room. I can't imagine ever accomplishing anything harder or greater in my life than that commando mission to get Gracey back there.

Inconceivably weary, I entered the hospital to find my faithful friend, Marilyn, who had helped make arrangements for the repatriation. I paused for a moment to lay my head on her shoulder and shed a tear from each eye, and then realized there wasn't time to release the flood that would follow. She handed me a sandwich and a cup of iced tea, which in my present state of mind (and hunger) struck me as a monumental act of human kindness. The crew had to hand Gracey over and head immediately on to their next mission, which was to bring someone home from Japan. I followed them back to the inner sanctum of the emergency room, where I found Gracey awake, cognizant, and relieved. I began trying to help relay an impossibly complicated chain of medical events to the perplexed doctor on call. As promised, the crew had, in fact, delivered Gracey home in better shape than he had been when he left France.

The crew members and I hugged each other, said goodbye, and wished each other luck; then they hurried out the door. I never saw them again, but sometimes I hear the sound of a jet and look up into the sky and think about how comforting it is to know that twenty-four hours a day, seven days a week, forever, they're up there accomplishing their mission, which is "taking Americans home." I guess I'll always wonder if I missed my true calling.

JOE GRACEY—E-MAIL TO COLMAN ANDREWS FROM FRANCE

October 20, 2011

France is great! Daughter is here, but I feel very funky due to tailing off radiation and chemo. I hope to recover fully before we have to leave. The little house is working perfectly with almost nothing left to buy or install or finish up. I still can't damn eat but I cook some anyway. Looking forward to being home now.

JG

KIMMIE RHODES

They moved Gracey to a room, and two physical therapists immediately got him, sitting him up on the side of the bed, and started massaging his legs and making plans to get him walking by morning. I slept beside him in a chairbed that night, and, knowing that he was in capable hands, I slept all through the night, surprised to wake to sunlight pouring through the window. The nurse explained that having heard our saga, she had attended to Gracey with a flashlight all night long, so she wouldn't wake me. Again, just one small tender act—kindness from a nurse—overwhelmed my heavy heart so much that one more tear per cheek escaped my eyes.

The day went well. I was spent and had nothing left to give. The crisis seemed over, so I met Marilyn at Hotel ZaZa, where the smell of the starched white sheets seemed uncanny, evoking a memory that seemed like it was from another lifetime, although it had just been a few weeks since I'd slept in the same bed, in the same room. I stood beside the king-sized bed, planning to undress and take a shower, but collapsed on the bed into a deep sleep. I awoke a little while later with my toes still touching the floor and my body splayed across the bed.

I jumped back up the next morning, skipping breakfast, and took the hotel shuttle to the hospital, like I'd done countless times before, and hurried to the room to find the gastroenterologist oncologist who had faithfully taken my texts and calls from the hell in France. She said, "Come here. I need you to see something." She walked me to a monitor at the nurse's station and put up the scan we had looked at just a few weeks before, when everyone had congratulated us and sent us off to France for what was supposed to have been rest. Then she said, "Here is the scan that came back this morning." We had been fighting one small tumor tooth and nail for nine months, and here before my eyes on the screen were innumerable tumors in every available space in Gracey's body. I asked her if she'd ever seen cancer spread that quickly before, and she replied, "No." She said, "We can't tackle this. The treatment would kill him immediately in the state he's in." I exhaled, "Then, let's move him to palliative care."

I was still so very glad I had gotten him home so he could have some last goodbyes with the family and friends who came to visit. When our friends Doug and Susan came to visit, I asked Gracey, "Do you love Susan?" He nodded yes. Then I asked, "Do you love Doug?" Gracey managed a laugh and shook his head no, but then he smiled and nodded yes. It was funny, and we all laughed at what would be his last worldly opportunity to be his favorite thing—a smart-ass.

It was his sixty-first birthday: November 14, 2011. Just when we'd gotten him settled in the room, some hospital volunteers burst through the door with a cake covered in candles, heartily singing, "Happy birthday to you!" I walked over and blew out the candles. When I looked up, I saw someone entering the room who asked if I would go to the next room and sign a medical power of attorney as a witness for a poor guy who was about to breathe his last breath. So I did that. I came back to the room and whispered, "I'm sorry, Babe. Thank you for trying so hard, but you're gonna have to let go now and go on. We'll be okay. I'll look after the kids." The last thing he ever signed to me was, "Okay . . . I love you."

I sat my laptop on his chest and started playing the music of every single person I could think of that he had ever loved and admired who had passed before him. I called it the "angel band" and said, "Just think! You'll be seeing Stevie, Jimmy, Jesse, Waylon, and Sir Doug. You'll be playing music with all your old friends soon!" The nurses came in, and, instead of thinking I was crazy (which I most certainly was), encouraged me by saying, "We wish everyone would do things like this." Those hospice nurses are very special people, like no others.

Finally, a male nurse whom I'd gotten to know and who was about to be off duty, plopped into a chair beside me, studied me hard with his lips pursed. He said, "Look, we see this all the time. You think you need to be here with him until he dies because you don't want to leave him. But what you don't see is that he's hanging on because he doesn't want to leave you here alone in this room." It made sense, and I knew he was right because I had already realized that I had been sensing the much younger healthy "essence" of Gracey moving about the room. They have a metaphysical name for the cord that attaches the spirit to the body. It's called the "silver cord," "sutratma," or "antahkarana," among other terms. He said, "Please, just at least go have dinner and see how you feel."

So I left to go have a meal with Marilyn at a really nice restaurant that we knew Gracey would have loved. On the way to the elevator, I was hit by a wave of separation anxiety and was about to run back to the room, when I realized that the wise nurse was right. I could walk straight back and be with him, but once Gracey had broken that silver cord, he couldn't return. I went on to dinner, and the more I felt anxiety pulling me back to Gracey, the more I felt like one of us had to let go, and I even began to feel a little bit selfish, like I was causing him to suffer because of his love for me. When I finally got back to the room, I kissed him on the forehead and told him, "I'm going to the ZaZa to get some sleep now, Baby. If you want to come with me, you can."

Once "the veil" lifts, unexpected things happen. I knew the very second Gracey died. I called the nurses' station and asked about him. The man who answered said that he'd just been in there but would be happy to go check on him. He came back and said that he had gone. I asked if there was anything I needed to do, and he said that I'd done all I could. Then I did something I'd have never dreamed I would do. I gave up the fight and let myself sink into a deep, deep sleep, where there were no dreams. Both grandchildren told me of visitations, where he had come to visit them that night. Louis woke with shivers and told his mother, "Pepe came and lied down beside me in my bed." Ruby said, "Pepe danced with me, and he spun me around in my polka-dot dress." She still has the picture Gracey had drawn of her one afternoon, the one of her wearing a polka-dot dress.

Many times in the coming years I would remember the whooshing sound of the powerful wings of the white dove that had flown from my hands and disappeared into the clear blue Texas sky.

JOE GRACEY—THEY DON'T LAST FOREVER

There is a debate, of course, on who is the best. I have worked with Tom Brumley (Buck Owens, Ricky Nelson), Buddy Emmons (Ernest Tubb, everybody), Leon McAuliffe (Bob Wills), Herb Remington (Bob Wills), and a lot of other players, including getting to watch Lloyd Green do a session with Gene Watson, and to my way of thinking, Jimmy Day had the ability to project more of his spirit into his playing than anybody. Obviously, all those guys could play their asses off, and most people probably give Emmons the nod as to technical proficiency, but for pure searing blue soul, it was Jimmy for me.

At Jimmy's funeral, his "Blue Darlin'" steel guitar and amp were set up and turned on next to the casket, ready to be played. This was pretty tough, but I was okay. But then they started to play some of his famous records—"Crazy Arms," Patsy Cline stuff, Willie, George Jones, and, finally, some of the stuff we did together for his last sessions with

Kimmie. The enormous depth of feeling in his playing hit me harder than ever before, and I couldn't help but cry like an idiot then. Man, steel is such an emotional instrument in the right hands. (Sometimes, when people would say something about how great his steel sounded, he'd hold up his long, beautiful hands and say, "These help," as a gentle, humorous reminder that it was the driver, not the hardware. He was not falsely modest, nor did he hold forth on himself. He just recognized that he was a single-purpose instrument and that he had accomplished what he was supposed to.

I am glad that Jimmy Day played on our most recent recordings. He played on every record that Kimmie and I have made. We recorded one of his songs, "Home John," on our *West Texas Heaven* album. I almost wish I could die right now just to hear Jimmy play steel with Bob Wills and Hank Williams. I am honored to have known him and loved him and recorded his otherworldly art. Sometimes, when I question my daily existence, I remember that I was the man who was lucky enough to be at the console to put his music on tape, and that is reason enough for me. Smoke 'em if you got 'em, boys and girls. They don't last forever.

Thanks, Jimmy.

JOE GRACEY—LETTER TO BOBBY EARL THE DAY DOUG SAHM DIED

I was very green when I first encountered Doug, and so I saw him as a kind of big-deal rock star, then gingerly got relaxed around him enough to actually get to know him. He was always extremely supportive and forgiving of my "kid-ness." He educated me on a lot of things from a perspective that anything was now possible. He was complex enough to be a really wonderful guy and a real asshole, too. I always remember how he went out of his way to take me and introduce me to Dylan, only because he knew how much it meant to me.

What I keep feeling is this huge place in the world that he occupied, now empty. You don't replace guys like Doug and Day; they just go

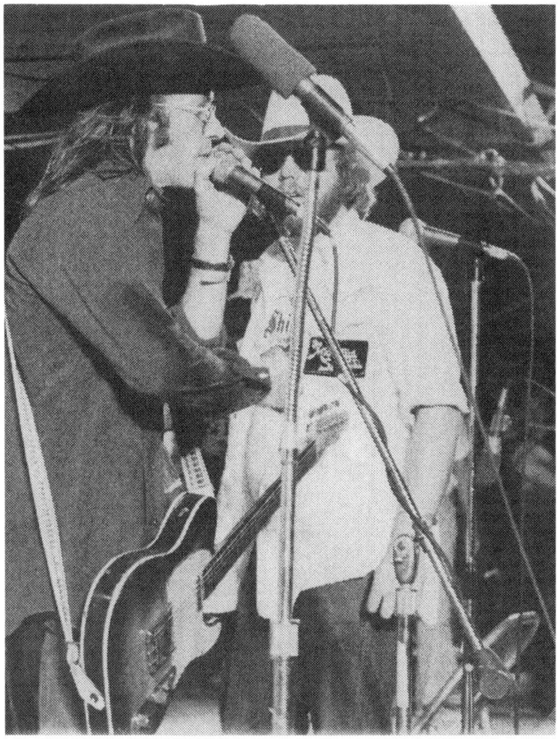

Gracey with Sir Doug Sahm.

away, and that's that. You know that gig we all did at the Spoke with Kimmie and him and Willie and Jimmy Day and Ely and Kristofferson is going to get more and more precious each time one of them sails away like this. I sure wish I could see him play just one more time.

KIMMIE RHODES

His absence filled the house and every waking moment, and then, at the end of every painful day came the nightmares of surgery waiting rooms, blue CT scans, rubber tubes, and the colored lights of beeping machines, as, night after night, my dreams began with a living, healthy mate, and, after struggling and pleading with nurses and surgeons in green masks, ended at a deathbed. Then another morning would start with the feeling of relief that night was over, mingled with the stark reality of another day of wading through memories that, whether good or bad, nonetheless burned.

Alone in our house I became this crazy person at dusk who called out to Gracey, "I need you. Where are you?" Sometimes I felt his spirit standing nearby, and sometimes he seemed to be off in the heavens, busy, but like me, also grieving. About every three days I locked myself in his office, the inner sanctum of his solitude, where framed pictures and pages of unfinished work loomed unfairly, still there to testify to a life that had once been lived in blissful ignorance of the fact that someday cancer would be returning to take him away. There I sought relief through the endorphins produced by crying, like returning to a drug. I sobbed into a pillow so the neighbors wouldn't hear me, and my faithful golden retriever, who had begun to understand the cycle, licked my tears and nuzzled her face into my lap.

One day I drank a glass of wine on an empty stomach before lunch and was amazed at how the edge of the emotional pain was instantly diminished a little bit. Proceeding with caution, I decided to begin drinking, only wine, as a means of survival and solace until the hands of time had more time to do their healing work. I sought a balance every day at sundown, which was the hardest part of the day, toggling between being out with friends and family until time for bed, being sure to be talking on the phone or otherwise distracted when I was at home alone, or getting completely smashed if none of the above had come about. This, coupled with the scheduled cries, seemed to work pretty well and helped with the nightmares because I began to sleep better.

I read some books on healing traumatic grief, where people who had lost children and loved ones and experienced death in ugly, tragic, and abrupt ways had shared their experiences. Since this seemed to be ultimately more comforting and productive than just getting drunk, I start preferring to stay sober in order to read myself to sleep and to awake reading works that inspired me, ranging from physics to spiritual practice and meditation, the biography of artists, the history of color, and so on. I began to write again, by practicing a Jungian process called "creative imagination," which I had discovered could be used to heal through analyzing images produced by the mind during sleep and/or meditation and taking notes.

So I began my "year of firsts," as the holiday season rolled around. Grace abounds at Christmastime, in stories, films, and songs about miracles and angels, and I was still drifting in a merciful grace that had descended to sand the sharp corners of all that was unbearable.

One morning I sat staring at the Christmas tree, which was decorated with memories from our travels, Daddy Pop's ornaments, the trinket from the flowers that had been delivered to my bedside on the day Jole was born, the cardboard star made by Lana that had been a prop atop the tree in my play *Small Town Girl*, the wooden trailer that represented the year that Jeremie had lived in Pecan Grove, Gabriel's terra-cotta saxophone, Gracey's University of Texas ornament. . . . As I squinted at the tree, I thought about how our life was like the ornaments and how if you looked at any one thing too closely, you might notice dents, scratches, worn places, tears, but if you took it all in as a whole, it was shimmering, luminous, and perfect. I felt Gracey beside me, just like he'd been every night when we would sit together on the couch, enjoy the beauty of our tree, and remember, laugh, and cherish all the wonderful times we had had traveling, eating, playing music, and just being with our family.

Those thoughts were interrupted by a knock on the door. My friend Jeff had arrived to do a walk-through of the house to make a plan to start putting things back in order and chase away the rats, which had moved in while we'd been away for years. At the top of the list was to finish building the fence, which in my mind had become the metaphor for when both the fence and our life had stopped moving forward that spring day in March when everything changed.

Jeff brought a guy named Joe Self with him to help with the work. Joe and I were sitting at the table while Jeff made notes. He looked at me and said, "You know, I died one time." And I answered, "Oh, I'm really interested in all that. Did you see a tunnel of light?" Then he started off into this whole story of how he'd been thrown from his motorcycle and how he'd felt the hands of a departed friend or "angel" holding him up, carrying him along as he followed his body in the ambulance down below on the way to the hospital. He told of how he'd hovered over a scene in the corner of a room and heard the doctors telling his family that they couldn't save him and that they should start making funeral arrangements. He said that at that moment, the spirit of his mother had appeared to him and said that, no, he was not going to die, but his life would have purpose like never before.

By now it was around 9:00 a.m., and I'm still on my first cup of coffee. I asked, "What did she look like?" He replied, "Like quicksilver." Then he said he had "flown back into his body," and they had rushed him into surgery and saved his life. He started to cry, looked me in the eyes, and said, "This house is heavy with the spirit of Joe Gracey." I said I knew that because he'd been hanging around all morning. Joe said, "Well he's here right now, and there are some things he'd like for me to tell you. He says that your life is your own now and he's not ever going to leave you, but he wants you to go on with your life and be happy." Then he paused and looked up toward his right, where I sensed Gracey was standing, and he continued, ". . . because he's happy . . . " He shuddered and rubbed his arms that were covered in chill bumps and then broke down sobbing and continued, ". . . because he doesn't have to suffer anymore." It was one of those Christmas miracles you hear about in movies and books. My paradigm shifted a little bit after that, and I began to realize that my life truly was my own, and I tried harder to choose happiness again.

I'd gone through life embracing the luxurious notion that memories were something that could never be taken away. One of the worst things about grieving for me had been the feeling that I'd never be able to have a treasured memory again without it hurting, so I had been banishing my memories from my thoughts. I devised a Christmas activity for myself that was a little bit like the twelve days of Christmas. I'd close my eyes and open a "gift box" in my mind's eye that contained a memory I loved, and when it started to hurt me, I would summon all the gratitude I still held in my heart for it. I discovered that the gratitude could overpower the pain. I reclaimed a lot of memories that Christmas season by giving them as "gifts to myself." One by one I placed them on a shelf in my mind until the shelf was overflowing.

I left Jeff and Joe to put the house back together and took off on the Blues Cruise with Delbert McClinton and sailed the high seas with dear old friends too numerous to mention. It felt really good to be traveling and singing again. Then I went directly from there to help celebrate my soul sister Emmylou Harris's twenty-fifth anniversary at the Grand Ole Opry. When I returned home, my children and grandchildren stayed with me a lot, so I rarely had to face being alone until I finally got to where I could be alone without being lonely.

WHEN YOU ARE IN THE TRENCHES, locked in a daily struggle, it's normal to be unaware of the wounds that are being inflicted on your psyche because the immediate focus is on survival. Once the challenging circumstances play out and time allows, the disregarded feelings creep into our thoughts, unexpectedly triggered by simple everyday things. I was surprised by a sudden flood of emotions while circling through a parking garage at a movie theater one night with a friend on the way to a movie. Curiously, this continued to happen every time I was in a parking garage. It finally dawned on me that Gracey and I had spent an unusually large amount of time circling through parking garages at the MD Anderson clinic on the way to appointments.

While it had nothing to do with parking, highly charged emotions of dread, fear, disappointment, relief, and hope, among other emotions, had become encoded and were associated with the daily activity of circling the stages of a parking garage. Understanding this helped, but I found that repetition was the only means to a change, since repetition is what had programmed the emotions initially. I was fortunate to have friends who encouraged me to share what had happened to us during the worst parts of the horrific experience, especially toward the end, when everything had careened out of control. Each time I told the story, I would reach certain parts where I would choke emotionally before being able to continue talking. The more I repeated the narrative, the less I had to pause during the telling. This, I later understood, was because traumatic events, whether they are immediately acknowledged, still program the brain for "fight or flight," and it takes the mind a while to realize that the struggle is over. I spoke with a therapist who explained how the primitive brain functions and that what I was experiencing was in fact post-traumatic stress. Without really knowing it, I had already been engaging in the therapy that was necessary to dissipate the emotional trauma by simply talking to friends. In fact, I remembered when I had been on the cruise and had run into my lovely friend Marcia Ball in an elevator. She sympathized, saying, "Kimmie, we can all see that you're hurting, but none of us knows what to do or say." I replied, "There isn't anything, really, but sometimes people listen and that seems to help."

Around this time, I remember sitting with John Gardner in his garden in Tennessee. John is my drummer friend who is like a brother to me. The two of us hatched a plan to gather some friends and make a record as a way to acknowledge our love and respect for Gracey. Instinctively, I knew I would write more ironic songs if I waited until I was able to see a little bit of light in the darkness and write from the point of view, or "line," that ran between that light and the darkness I felt. For years I'd dreamed of indulging myself by recording an entire album of other people's songs. I decided to select songs that would let others "speak for me," the way singers who aren't writers choose songs.

We assembled a band of family and friends and called it "Camp Kimmie," planning to spend days eating, partying, and playing music at our own Sunbird Studio in Austin. My friend Marilyn; John's wife, Jennifer; and Jole came to cook for everybody. John's whole family came with him. His son, Avery, manned the bass. His daughter, Deane, asked to "bless" the studio with a ritual using sage, oils, and orange water, and we all participated. Mike Thompson came from L.A. to play keyboards, and, of course, my main sidekick, trusted producer, guitarist, and above all, my son, Gabriel, was there to produce and play guitar.

I had worried about how my vocals would ever be recorded properly again without Gracey, who had known my voice so well, having recorded me for the three decades since the beginning of my career. Then, from the sky fell Bradley Hartman, celebrated engineer to many well-known stars. Even a new friend, Will McFarlane from the Muscle Shoals Band, showed up unexpectedly and offered to play guitar. With my loved ones gathered around me, I felt I might be able to safely open my heart again enough to sing a real vocal. Together we played, laughed, cried, and made music. I had always said in interviews that I feel so blessed to have my music, because without it I would be trapped inside myself with no way out, but as I sang each song in the solitude of my recording area, the pictures passing through my mind were not what I would have expected. I repeatedly saw myself sitting alone in the oncologists' waiting room, standing in line at the pharmacy, waiting

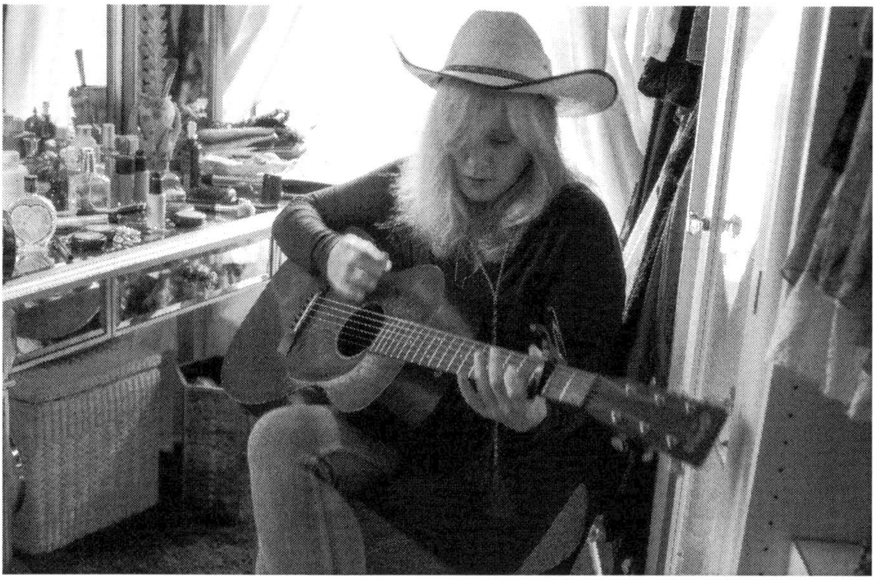

Kimmie at home in Texas. Photo by Alan Messer.

for Gracey at our table in the coffee shop at MD Anderson, but all the while I was singing the lyrics to the songs while the band played on, and once each song ended, I was almost surprised to find myself still in my studio.

Around that same time I had been asked to counsel Corky Hilliard, who was about to undergo a head and neck surgery (with the same MD Anderson plastic surgeon that Gracey had), because it was likely that she might lose her speech in the process. She survived the surgery without losing her voice, and we became fast friends, like sisters united not only by our experience with cancer and our gratitude for MD Anderson Cancer Center but also by our inherent belief that "if you can see it, you can have it." Corky, being a strategist and visionary, had reciprocated by counseling me on how to find my feet and move forward. It had been comforting to discover that there was actually a process that I could employ to dissipate the trauma and confront the memories in my mind where I was emotionally stuck.

With Corky as my companion, I decided to make a pilgrimage back to MD Anderson. I valeted the car with Bertha, whom I'd nicknamed "the parking angel" and walked past the struggling souls out front who were still in "the belly of the whale." Passing through the doors I was hit by the remembrance of the hope I had felt the first time I'd entered those same doors with Gracey by my side. (The visuals upon entering and the collective "vibes" of the place are really quite stunning.) In that moment I was finally able to truly realize how much better "now" was, compared to "then," at least for Gracey, despite our painful losses. I visited the oncologist and surgeon whose brilliance and cheerfulness had given us courage, and I saw past myself for the first time to realize that she had also grieved his loss. Her joy in seeing me made me understand that my being all that was left of him for others was not only a responsibility but also an honor. I passed through the pharmacy where I had stood in line with fellow caregivers so many times, walked the corridors, drank coffee in the coffee shop, and, finally, sat in the chair under a painting of a yellow clapboard house that looks like ours, where I had gone many times to sit for a while when I had been homesick.

Corky went with me to Hotel ZaZa, and as I walked through the front doors into the lobby, I finally felt the reality of the time that had passed and finally understood that "that was then" and that "this is now." I felt what was good about that thought as well as what was bad about that thought.

The plan worked, and I truly turned a corner after that visit to Houston and felt as though I was finally able to begin a new chapter of living. I had replaced the memories I had been "stuck in" with present-day realization, and the persistent lost hope that had survived beyond Gracey's death morphed into a new hope for whatever was next in my own life.

I learned something about hope from all of this. People can die because they are human, but hope, . . . it has no physical body; it lingers patiently and waits until you need it enough to find it again. It's always there. Hope doesn't find us; we find it, and while hope can change us, we must also sometimes change hope into what we need from it next. Like happiness, hope is a choice we make.

The one thing that rescued me was the love of my family and friends who stayed with me, kept me distracted and entertained, and above all just listened, knowing that there was no way to fix the situation but that just to be there was all that was required. I also knew that especially the married couples who had been together for years were looking to me for guidance, and I felt a sense of responsibility to get myself together and set a good example of how to find a way through those woods. All along there was an overriding grace that permeated my sadness, and by experiencing gratitude, a sort of alchemy transformed the bad things that had happened into a gold that I will never lose.

One time when I was just a little girl, I asked my babysitter, Bobby Carol, "Who is God?" She answered, "God is love." I then asked, "Then why does God let people go hungry?" She answered, "God doesn't let people go hungry, people do. God is love." I can look back on my life with humbling gratitude because no matter what else prevailed, there has always been love in abundance: the love of my parents, my children, my grandchildren, my friends and fans, and, by now, even a rather large herd of loyal pets have come and gone. I believe that maybe not everything we want but everything we will ever truly need is always somewhere around us or is on the way. If anyone ever tries to tell you people aren't good, don't believe them. And if you believe in magic, you have the universe at your command.

The following is the eulogy written for Joe Gracey by his dear friend and Jackalope Brother, Bobby Earl Smith.

"Well, friends," as Joe Gracey would say, we are gathered to celebrate Joe Gracey. To say "Thanks, Gracey" thirty-three years after the first "Thanks, Gracey" gathering held at the Armadillo World Headquarters, when he first began his brave, valiant fight with that old familiar "hellhound on his trail."

There's an old Scotsman prayer: "Lord, give us a good conceit of ourselves!" Gracey lived that prayer. He had the courage and "good conceit of himself" to reinvent himself, to redo, to remake, to do over, to award himself a mulligan, a second chance to perform, with each challenge and opportunity, no matter what hand fate dealt him. Joe, his own self, said, "I'm not afraid of dying, but I will miss the oysters." So today we celebrate the living of that life, that pearl of great price—the life of Joe Gracey.

His musical mentor and hero was Jack "Cowboy" Clement, whom Gracey credited for "teaching me that 'if you believe in magic, you have the universe at your command.'" When Gracey met Kimmie, the magic really began.

Joe's heart had ears. His soul vibrated with the music of the spheres. The music never got old and never stopped making everything else in life better. Still, Joe Gracey was so much more than that. Yes, his time in the magical, mystical Austin '70s was special, but he was so much more than that one moment in time.

My wife's mom, Yvonne, told him, "You do your talking with your eyes." Ol' Blue Eyes. . . . Years ago, I said, "Gracey, you can't call yourself Ol' Blue Eyes. That's what they call Frank Sinatra." Joe looked at me like I had just told him that the moon is made out of bean curd. "I am Ol' Blue Eyes," Gracey said. And, so he was.

His Magic Slate was, indeed, a thing of magic to behold, as Gracey held the red stylus, hovering over the surface until just the right thing to say, said in just the right way, came to him. When Joe wrote, I heard him in my head. Gracey talked to your heart. . . . "Let's have a heart-to-heart talk."

Joe and I were friends for thirty-eight-plus years. We were together the day we heard on the radio that Elvis had died. We were backstage at the Armadillo World Headquarters the night we heard that John Lennon got shot. We were in Dallas–Fort Worth in 1975, needing a dub of a master tape of ours. We drove out to Garland, Texas, to Autumn Sound Studios and arrived at the same time Bee Spears, Willie's bass player, walked out of the studio. Phil York, the studio engineer, asked us if we wanted to hear Willie's new album. Phil played the entire *Red Headed Stranger* album for us, the first time anyone other than Willie and the band heard it. Gracey, music director at KOKE-FM at the time, plugged that great and grand album when it was released, especially "Blue Eyes Crying in the Rain."

We were in Electric Graceyland in the basement of the KOKE building the day he met Kimmie, the true love of his life. Judy and I took our sons, Jon Marc and Eric, to the hospital when their daughter, Jole, the apple of Joe's eye, was born. What Gracey did, the things he did, are widely and well known. It is the "who" of the man that makes him so special and so loved. Family was all to Joe: the music, the writing and blogging, the joy of cooking and food writing, were outward manifestations of his creative nature, but family was the inner heart and soul of Gracey's life, the true expression of his love and passion in living. Family was all to Joe: daughter Jole is now "all growed up" and married to Jason Musick. Sons Jeremie Rhodes and Gabriel Rhodes were boys when he and Kimmie met and later married. Now Gabe has a family of his own, the grandchildren, Louis and Ruby Rhodes. Joe is their beloved "Pepe." Brother Bill Gracey and wife, Cathy, are here today, as are Joe's nieces Christy and Kate. Jamie Rhodes, Louis's mom, is very dear and special.

Gracey had the gift and joy of laughter. Joe said that he and Kimmie shared a sense of humor that bore them through good times and hard. W. C. Fields was his patron saint, and he, like Fields, perceived that which is absurd, hilarious, in the foibles and slight pretentions that abound in everyday modern living and life. Joe himself was a clever, yea, devious, rascal, with a nimble wit and devilish humor. One of Gracey's little terms of endearment for Kimmie was Kup, short for Kupcake, a moniker from back in our Kimmie Rhodes and the Jackalope Brothers days. In one of many messages from Houston, Joe said, "Kup is here now in all her glory; what a sweet girl she is. I'm a lucky man." Joe wrote, "I realized that I have had thirty years of a great life well beyond what I could have expected, and so I am grateful, regardless of if I go tomorrow or thirty more years from today. "Very few men have had the marriage, the love, the family, the experiences, and the friends that I have had! I've had a remarkable life indeed. Life is good." Another day, Gracey said, yet again, "By the way, I am not intending to say that I am afraid of dying."

"Onward, forward!" were Joe's watchwords. When we'd be out on the road years ago, if we got lost, he never wanted to turn around and retrace our steps. He would point toward the windshield and say, "Forward, onward!" Never look back. Always go right ahead. It was as if, as a small child, Gracey had heard the words "The man who puts his hand to the plow and then turns back is not worthy of the Kingdom of Heaven," and, boy, did he ever practice what he preached. Onward. Illness could not define him. He wouldn't let it. Though illness was the hellhound on his trail, he, like the blues singer, knew he "got to keep moving, got to keep moving . . ." and so he persevered on and on and on. "There is no one on earth like him."—Job 1:8. It is this that binds Joe

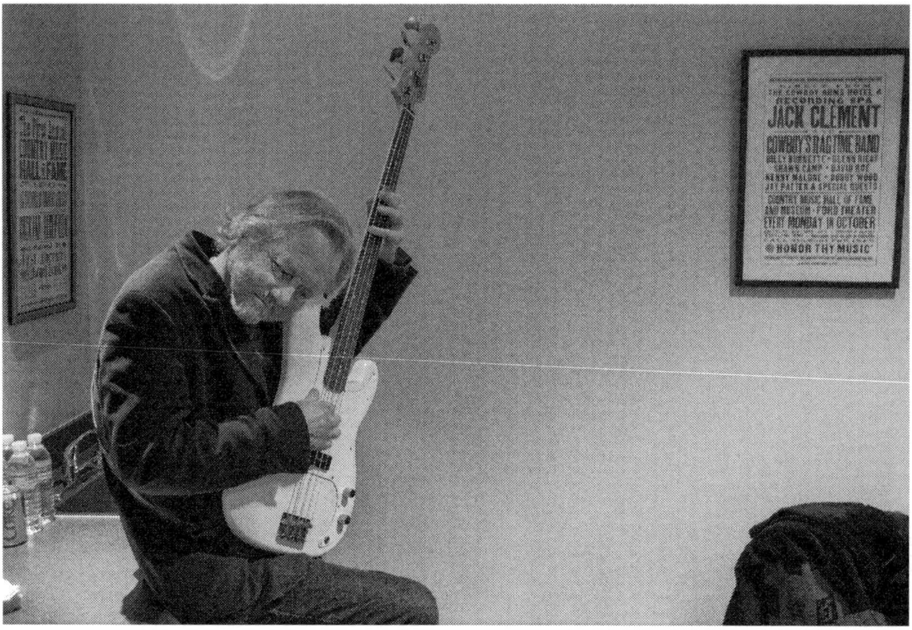

Gracey at the Country Music Hall of Fame, Nashville, Tennessee, 2009.
Photo by Alan Messer.

in our hearts. There is no one like him. While some may reject a chosen one or holy one, no one rejects Job. Joe, like Job, was simply a man. Not a saint but a comrade in arms and, more than that, a man who suffered. We identify with Joe, the man. A man who lived, and loved, and, yes, suffered, yet through it all clung to life with a courageous tenacity of spirit and spunk that defines Joe Gracey, this good, fine man.

Joe fought the good fight. A friend wrote, simply, "What a life. Playing in my head I heard this music on the radio. . . . Everywhere I turned, I tuned in to something you had to say. The angels play on their horns all day. . . . The whole earth in progressions seem to pass by, but does anyone hear the music they play?"

Joe Gracey heard that music. His life is that music that lives in our hearts today. "Someday when we meet up yonder / We'll stroll hand in hand again / In the land that knows no parting / Blue eyes crying in the rain."

Thanks, Gracey.

Adios, Amigo

The following is the obituary delivered by Joe Nick Patoski, November 28, 2011.

Friend Joe Gracey passed in mid-November, just after his sixty-first birthday, so his friends and family are throwing a big ol' bash for him on Sunday, December 4, at 2:00 p.m. at Austin City Limits Live in downtown Austin. Even if you never heard of Joe, if you dig Austin, Texas, music and all that is cool about this part of the world, you're invited to send off one of the tastemakers who made it so.

I am honored to have been asked by his family to write his obituary. God bless Kimmie, Jole, Gabe, Jeremie, Brother Bill, and all his friends and relatives.

After a well-spent life defined by a series of reinventions, each more outrageous and "way cooler than the previous one," Joe Gracey has left the building—this place we call Earth. Born near Fort Worth on November 14, 1950, Joe distinguished himself as a communicator at an early age. He built his own radio studio in the family attic in sixth grade, mowed lawns to get his first guitar, played in teen bands alongside fellow Fort Worthers Stephen Bruton and T-Bone Burnett, and projected gravitas and authority as a veteran newsman and familiarity and intimacy as a country music disc jockey for KXOL-AM and FM when the sixteen-year-old wasn't attending classes at Paschal High School. His mother drove him to work at the radio station.

Like many other young Texans of his generation, he gravitated to Austin to attend the University of Texas, where he graduated with a degree in American Studies while moonlighting on Austin's Top 40 radio station, KNOW-AM, and writing the first rock music column for the *Austin American-Statesman,* immediately overstepping his assigned category by writing about country and folk music, too, focusing on the unique country-rock musical hybrid that was incubating in Austin.

In 1974, he joined KOKE-FM in Austin, the first progressive country radio station in the world. Blessed with a warm, full-bodied voice with enough of a lingering drawl to leave no doubt where he came from, Gracey became an intimate friend to strangers who discovered they could learn a few things about music by listening to the radio; unlike his broadcasting peers, Gracey was fixated on what he said as much as how he said it.

Smart and a smart-ass both, he was a pillar of a burgeoning music community on the verge of being discovered nationally and internationally. He welcomed music fans to some of the most exciting and eclectic music being created as one of the voices who did radio commercials for the storied Armadillo World Headquarters. It was Ol' Blue Eyes, as he called himself, who coolly and casually opened his microphone so Willie Nelson and his friend Kris Kristofferson could perform an impromptu concert for listeners at home.

Gracey not only played Ernest Tubb and his Texas Troubadours; he took the time to explain ET's significance and line out Tubb's hip bona fides for a generation that had previously ignored their parents' and grandparents' music. He turned on music lovers to exotic sounds in their own backyard, such as Tex-Mex conjunto music—as articulated by his friends Doug Sahm, Ry Cooder, and Flaco Jimenez—and western swing, the almost-forgotten Made-in-Texas country-jazz hybrid popularized in the 1930s, kickstarting its revival by putting Asleep at the Wheel and Alvin Crow into heavy rotation. Gracey played a critical role defining "Super Roper Radio," as KOKE was known, demonstrating how the Rolling Stones and Gram Parsons were related to George Jones and Bob Wills and the Texas Playboys. In that respect, he was as influential as Willie Nelson, Austin's musical godfather, in bringing the hippies and the rednecks together through the common love of music.

With Gracey as program director, *Billboard* magazine crowned KOKE-FM as "Trendsetter of the Year."

Gracey's trendspotting abilities earned him the role as talent coordinator for the new *Austin City Limits*, now the longest-running music series on American television, when the series started in 1976. Through Gracey, the remaining Bob Wills's Texas Playboys, Flaco Jimenez y Su Conjunto, and Clifton Chenier and His Red Hot Louisiana Zydeco Band performed for national television audiences for the first time. His byline continued appearing in the *Austin Sun* and the literary country music journal *Picking Up the Tempo*.

In the summer of 1977, inspired by his mentor, Cowboy Jack Clement, he left KOKE-FM a few weeks before the station's format switched, and headed downstairs to the basement of the KOKE building, where he fashioned a four-track TEAC recorder and two windowless offices into the funky, duct-taped recording studio known as Electric Graceyland. The studio was the site of some of the first recordings of future blues legends Stevie Ray Vaughan and Miss Lou Ann Barton; The Skunks, Austin's first punk band; and Tex-Mex rockers Joe King Carrasco and the Crowns. Gracey also recorded the demo that scored the Fabulous Thunderbirds their first record contract and worked the dials for Lubbock songster Butch Hancock and his *Dixie's Bar & Bus Stop* cable television music series. He recorded Stevie Vaughan and Barton and the band Double Trouble at Clement's Nashville studio.

He used Electric Graceyland to collaborate musically with his partner in crime, Bobby Earl Smith, as the Jackalope Brothers. Gracey and Smith also did radio promotion for Alvin Crow and the Pleasant Valley Boys, while Gracey often opened shows for Crow with his brother, Bill, as the Amazing Graceys.

It was during this flurry of recording and promoting that Gracey was dealt the lousy hand of a cancer diagnosis that eventually robbed him of his gifted voice. Only twenty-seven, Gracey fought the hard fight medically while simultaneously adapting. A Magic Slate kids' erasable writing tablet tucked under his arm became a Gracey accessory so he could scribble a quick response to any questions and allow him to engage in conversations, followed by the soft, barely audible rip, as he cleared the pad to erase the message once his words were understood.

In 1979, his friend T. J. McFarland introduced him to the love of his life, Kimmie Rhodes, a singer-songwriter from Lubbock, as well as a playwright, painter, writer, and all-around creative force.

They married in 1984 and settled in Briarcliff, where he helped raise Kimmie's sons from a previous marriage, Gabe and Jeremie Rhodes, and their daughter, Jole Morgan Goodnight Gracey. A family band emerged, with Gracey playing bass, and Gabe, a talented producer in his own right, who absorbed all the nuances of the electronic recording art from Joe, playing guitar.

Kimmie and their neighbor Joe Sears started writing plays together, and Gracey joined the fun as an actor, playing the part of the skeleton barkeeper in the play *Windblown*, and the role of the clown in *Small Town Girl*, in addition to other performances.

He also worked the audio console at nearby Pedernales Studio for a

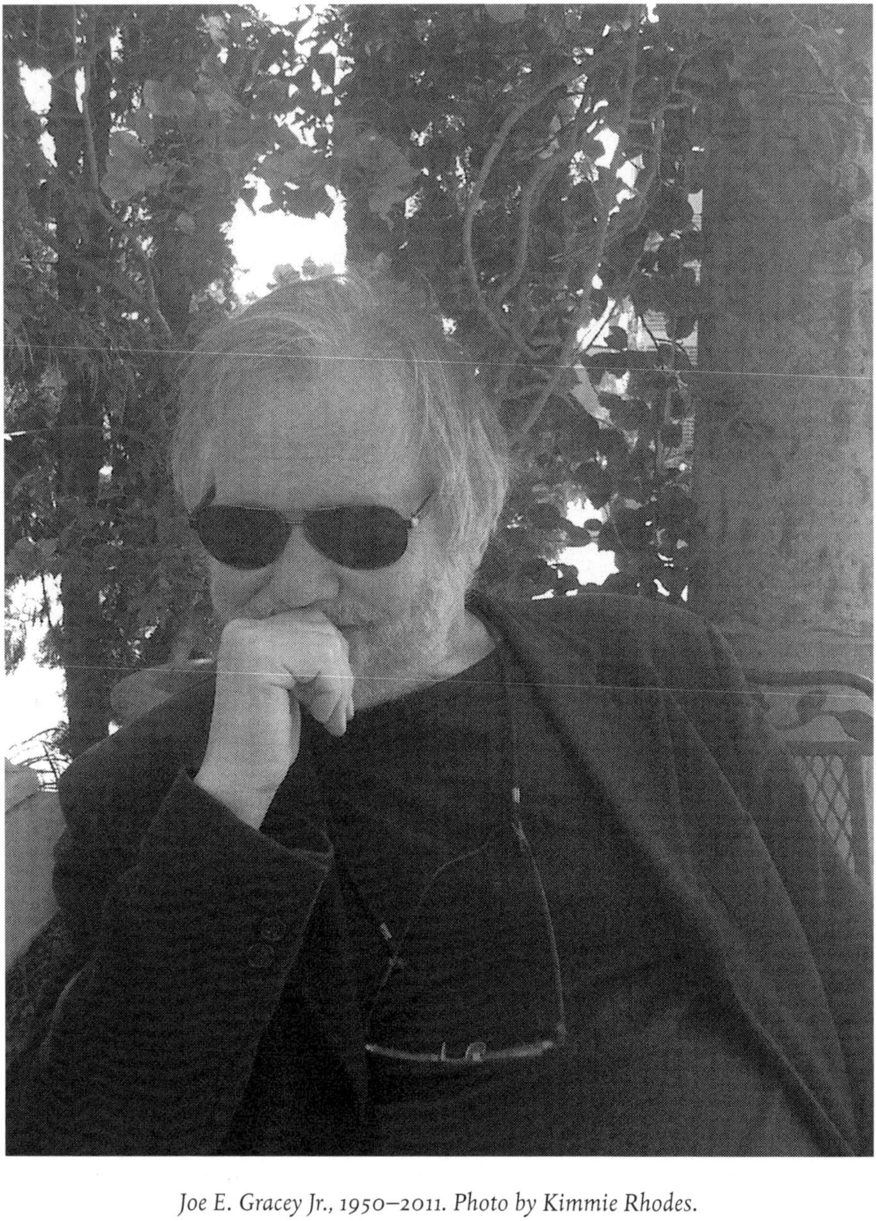

Joe E. Gracey Jr., 1950–2011. Photo by Kimmie Rhodes.

number of years, and in 1996 was at the controls for Nelson's groundbreaking album, *Spirit*, which inspired Nelson to redefine his live sound. Gracey and David Zettner built the small, simple recording studio in the back of Willie's Luck World Headquarters saloon, where Willie liked to hold court and make music at the spur of the moment, which yielded the albums *Picture in a Frame*, Willie's 2003 album of duets with Kimmie, and the Grammy-nominated collaboration between Willie and Ray Price, *Run That By Me One More Time*.

Rhodes and Gracey's shared love of food and fine wine (he learned how to keep boudin warm on his Cadillac's engine returning from a trip to visit Clifton Chenier in Lafayette, Louisiana), along with numerous European tours by Rhodes, launched another career for Gracey—food writer—as championed by their friend Colman Andrews, the editor of *Saveur* magazine, for whom Gracey did several pieces. Joe and Kimmie also taught cooking classes together. Their food adventures and Kimmie's continued popularity in Europe eventually led to the couple's renovation of a small thousand-year-old stable-farmhouse in the Languedoc province of France.

Gracey never stopped creating, and he started a blog, *Letters from Graceyland* (Graceyland.blogspot.com) to share his latest adventures with readers.

Cancer-free for thirty years, the beast reentered his life in 2009. The bad news was accompanied by good news, though. Doctors at MD Anderson hospital would embark on experimental surgery that led to a partial restoration of his voice. But the new cancer was joined by another cancer, leading to several months of treatments in Houston. Afterward, Joe and Kimmie were able to spend some weeks together in their French place again with friends and family before returning to Texas one last time.

Sickness never defined Joe's life. It was an irritant and obstacle to be overcome so he could pursue his many interests. He defined it; it didn't define him. And although so much of his professional career revolved around music, his life was much more than that, too, as his extensive network of family and friends that spanned the globe would attest to.

They all knew that Gracey's presence could never be ignored. He was not the kind of person to let that happen. Which is why despite his unplanned departure, he wanted his friends, family, and all the strangers he never met to hold close to their hearts the advice he dispensed whenever he signed off from another shift on the radio:

"Drink lots of water, stay off your feet, and come when you can."

"A red Bourgogne is the pinnacle of red wineness. . . . Give me Burgundy or give me death (or at least give me Burgundy as I die)!"

JOE GRACEY

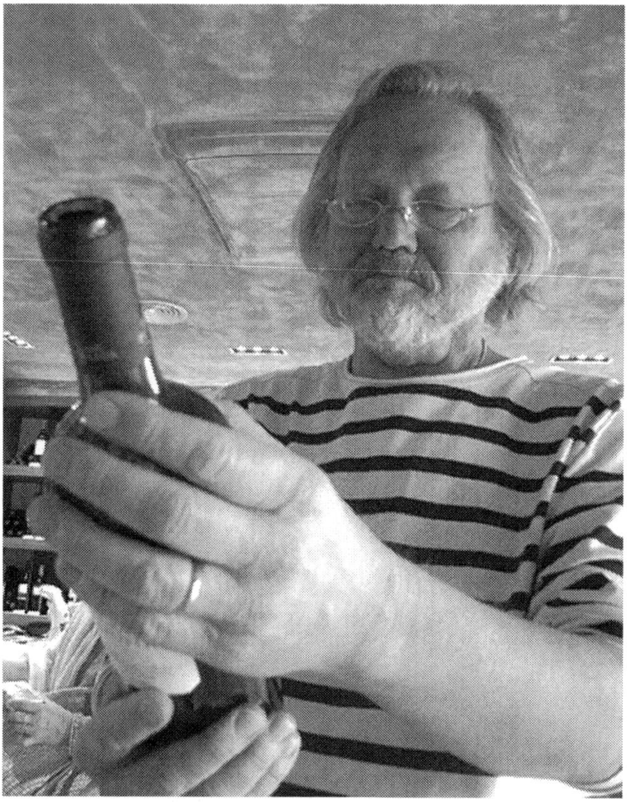

Gracey wine shopping in the Languedoc, France.

AFTERWORD

KIMMIE RHODES

LIFE WOULD BE unimaginable were it not going on before our very eyes. To wake to the vividness in just one ordinary room of a house is a miracle beyond comprehension. Simple objects speak the unspeakable, like when the sunlight hits a curtain turning it uncountable shades of white, the unseen green of the remembered grass and the blue sky outside, the chant of cicadas in a tree with blossoms, the silence filled with the whirring of a fan, a painting of the ocean, a hat woven in Mexico hanging from a mirror reflecting the opposites, a blank, dark television ready to transmit an infinite realm, framed multicolored butterflies in an insect collection that includes a giant stick bug, the crystals on a chandelier hosting a ray of dust motes floating in the rainbow prism of bent light, the scent of lavender flowers in an Irish porcelain vase, a coral shell covered in barnacles, a silk scarf from Venice, a silver chain, sunglasses, bottles of perfume, shoes, the pensive and quiet familiar presence of self, the observer and the space in the bed left forever empty by the loved one who disappeared, the magnificent grace locked inside grief, and the curious existence of gratitude . . . the key.

Outside the room from the windowsill onward, earth teems with unvisited jungles and mountains, colorful markets, skyscrapers, school yards, countries, people of every color and language, some aware of the miracle, and most distracted by the din and spin of a planet that is not even a speck in an infinite number of universes made of the same stuff beyond. What are the chances of this rare and beautiful existence? Everything that is so very here and with us now, when it is gone is so very stunningly gone that even the hard-earned raw emptiness becomes fascinating, extraordinary, and precious.

THANKS TO ALL of our family, friends, underwriters, supporters, and fans who helped bring these archives to light. Without their love and moral (as well as financial) support and patience, these unique and insightful communications written by Joe Gracey might have gone unspoken, waiting in notebooks that were buried in boxes or out floating unnoticed in the digital realms of the universe. We come into this world alone, we leave this world alone, but the beauty of life is that we are never alone because of the companionship of those who are lent to us to love and call our own.

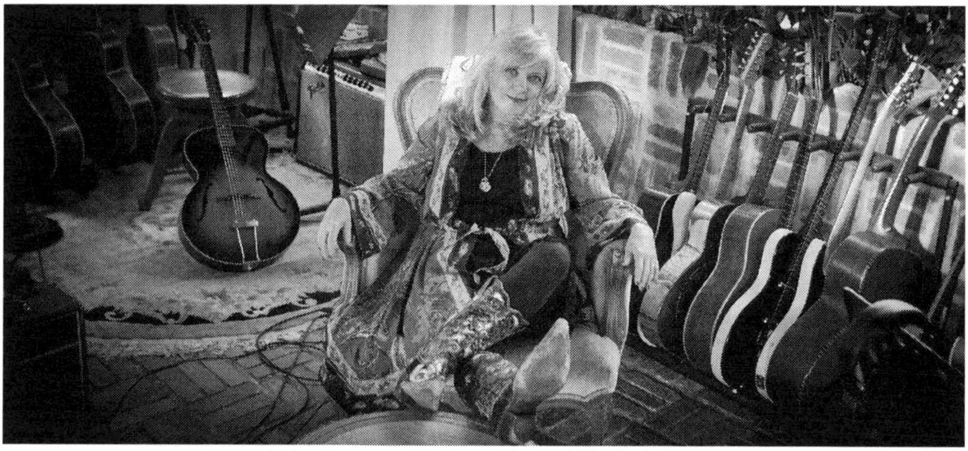

Kimmie at her Sunbird Studio. Photo by Gray Hawn.

ACKNOWLEDGMENTS

I AM PROFOUNDLY GRATEFUL to all our mentors, friends, fans, and family for your support. This labor of love could never have happened if not for you. Jole, how could I have ever braved this mountain of archives without you? Brothers Bill and Bobby Earl and sister Susan, you're angels. Thanks for helping me get it right.

Much love to the Myerscough-Harris clan for the shelter you have given me, to Trudie for looking after me, and to Bob and Miles for offering your experience and talents to produce the audio companion to this book so that the full story could be brought to light.

Special thanks to The Buddy Holly Educational Foundation for generosity and sponsorship and for the opportunity to serve as an ambassador in the mission to honor Buddy's legacy by keeping the magic and fun in writing songs and making music for future generations.

INDEX

Note: Numbers in italics refer to illustrations.

24026478R00204

Printed in Poland
by Amazon Fulfillment
Poland Sp. z o.o., Wrocław